KT-481-007

DISPOSED OF
BY LIBRARY
HOUSE OF LORDS

London's Mental Health

The Report for the King's Fund London Commission

Edited by

Sonia Johnson, Rosalind Ramsay, Graham Thornicroft, Liz Brooks, Paul Lelliott, Edward Peck, Helen Smith, Daniel Chisholm, Bernard Audini, Martin Knapp and David Goldberg

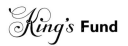

King's Fund

Published by
King's Fund Publishing
11–13 Cavendish Square
London W1M 0AN

© King's Fund 1997

First published 1997

All rights reserved. No part of this publication may be reproduced, stored in a
retrieval system or transmitted, in any form or by any means, electronic or
mechanical, photocopying, recording and/or otherwise without the prior written
permission of the publishers. This book may not be lent, resold, hired out or
otherwise disposed of by way of trade in any form, binding or cover other than that
in which it is published, without the prior consent of the publishers.

ISBN 1 85717 139 X

A CIP catalogue record for this book is available from the British Library

Distributed by Bournemouth English Book Centre (BEBC)
PO Box 1496
Poole
Dorset
BH12 3YD
Tel: 0800 262260
Fax: 0800 262266

Printed and bound in Great Britain by
Biddles Ltd, Guildford and King's Lynn

Cover photograph: Alison Forbes

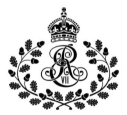

Contents

Contributors

Mr Bernard Audini
Research Worker, Research Unit, Royal College of Psychiatrists, London

Dr Sube Banerjee
Senior Lecturer, Section of Old Age Psychiatry, Institute of Psychiatry, London

Dr Veira Bailey
Consultant Child Psychiatrist, Hounslow & Spelthorne Community and Mental Health Services NHS Trust, London

Ms Ingrid Barker
Senior Consultant, Centre for Mental Health Services Development (CMHSD), King's College London

Dr Thomas Becker
Research Fellow and Honorary Senior Lecturer, PRiSM, Institute of Psychiatry, London

Dr Dinesh Bhugra
Senior Lecturer, Department of Psychiatry, Institute of Psychiatry, London

Dr Kamaldeep Bhui
Wellcome Training Fellow, Department of Psychiatry, Institute of Psychiatry, London

Ms Sara Bixby
Research Worker, PRiSM, Institute of Psychiatry, London

Ms Liz Brooks
Research Worker, PRiSM, Institute of Psychiatry, London

Dr Jose Catalan
Reader in Psychiatry, Academic Department of Psychiatry, Charing Cross & Westminster Medical School, London

Mr Daniel Chisholm
Lecturer, Centre for the Economics of Mental Health (CEMH), Institute of Psychiatry, London

Dr Mike Farrell
Senior Lecturer, Addiction Research Unit, Institute of Psychiatry;
Consultant Psychiatrist, Maudsley Hospital, London

Ms Vida Field
Reed Implementation Officer, Lambeth Southwark and Lewisham Health Authority, London

Dr Gyles Glover
Honorary Senior Lecturer, PRiSM, Institute of Psychiatry, London

Professor Sir David Goldberg
Commissioner, King's Fund London Commission
Professor of Psychiatry, Department of Psychiatry, Institute of Psychiatry, London

Dr Hilary Guite
Health Services Research Fellow/Consultant in Public Health Medicine, King's College
School of Medicine and Dentistry, London

Mr Gregor Henderson
Senior Consultant, Centre for Mental Health Services Development (CMHSD), King's
College London

Dr Sonia Johnson
Clinical Lecturer, PRiSM, Institute of Psychiatry, London

Dr Shaun Kerwick
Clinical Research Fellow, Department of General Practice, United Medical and Dental
Schools, Guys and St Thomas's Hospitals, London

Professor Martin Knapp
Director, Centre for the Economics of Mental Health (CEMH), Institute of Psychiatry,
London

Dr Paul Lelliott
Director, Research Unit, Royal College of Psychiatrists, London

Ms Ana Lowin
Research Worker, Centre for the Economics of Mental Health, Institute of Psychiatry,
London

Dr Jane Marshall
Senior Lecturer, Addiction Research Unit, Institute of Psychiatry;
Consultant Psychiatrist, Maudsley Hospital, London

Dr Edward Peck
Director, Centre for Mental Health Services Development (CMHSD), King's College
London

Dr Michael Philpot
Consultant in Old Age Psychiatry, Maudsley Hospital, London

Professor Amanda Ramirez
Professor of General Hospital Psychiatry, United Medical and Dental Schools, London

Dr Rosalind Ramsay
Honorary Lecturer, PRiSM, Institute of Psychiatry
Consultant Psychiatrist, West Lambeth NHS Trust, London

Dr Tom Sensky
Reader in Psychological Medicine, Charing Cross and Westminster Medical School,
London

Ms Helen Smith
Senior Consultant, Centre for Mental Health Services Development (CMHSD), King's
College London

Professor John Strang
Director, Addiction Research Unit, Institute of Psychiatry, London

Professor Graham Thornicroft
Director, PRiSM, Institute of Psychiatry, London

Dr André Tylee
Director, Royal College of General Practitioners Unit for Mental Health Education in
Primary Care, Institute of Psychiatry, London

Dr Simon Wessely
Reader in Psychological Medicine, King's College Hospital School of Medicine and
Dentistry, London

Dr Peter White
Senior Lecturer in Psychological Medicine, The Medical Colleges of St Bartholomew's
and Royal London Hospital, London

Foreword

In 1992 the King's Fund organised the first London Commission, which published its report **London Health 2010** on the changes that needed to be made to health services in the capital. Events moved much faster than anticipated, as this was followed by the Tomlinson Report, which led to far reaching changes in London's health services being introduced by the Government over a relatively short time scale.

The first London Commission did not consider mental health or services for older people, and these defects are to be remedied in the work of the second London Commission, which will report its work in the Spring of 1997. The Commission's objective is to suggest a comprehensive pattern of health services to serve London into the 21st century, and to indicate how such a pattern might be brought about by a carefully managed process of change. To do this the Commission has sought advice from experts both inside and outside the King's Fund, and has specially commissioned research work from independent contractors.

This research, reported in this book, is that upon which the London Commission will base its findings. It is the most detailed and wide-ranging picture so far assembled of London's mental health services. The aim is to gather together the best available information on what are the mental health services needs of Londoners and how far current services meet these needs. The report that follows represents the work of the four groups that were asked to address the state of London's mental health services: the PRiSM team at the Institute of Psychiatry, the Centre for the Economics of Mental Health, the Centre for Mental Health Services Development (at King's College London), and the Research Unit of the Royal College of Psychiatrists. These groups worked closely together, and their work was co-ordinated by a special steering committee. We acknowledge the unfailing support given to us by Dr Sean Boyle and Mr Huw Richards of the King's Fund, who have both played a major part in steering the work described in the pages that follow.

Because mental health services are complex and involve the participation of multiple agencies, and because good quality information about their functioning is rare, we have deliberately taken a multi-faceted approach. This allows us to explore where the results of different views of services coincide, and reinforces our confidence in our findings. We have reviewed previously available forms of information, including routinely collected official statistics from the Department of Health, quarterly returns from purchasers to the NHS Executive, the MINI (mental illness needs index), national unit costs data from the Personal Social Services Research Unit and elsewhere, data on sociodemographic characteristics which will affect the mental health morbidity of Londoners, as well as recent more focused papers produced by research and policy colleagues.

In addition we have conducted several new studies whose findings are presented for the first time in this report, including a survey of the numbers of in-patient and residential care places throughout London; a study of the views of purchaser and provider managers on the challenges they face, the obstacles they encounter and the services development needs they identify; a summary of the findings of the many recent inquiries, enquiries and reports into aspects of London's mental health services, a new study of the structure and functioning of the capital's mental health services, including for the first time a comprehensive assessment of the delays experienced in placing patients in suitable facilities; and a detailed consideration of the functions which a service should provide to fulfil the expectations and needs of service users and their carers. We also report here on fine grain studies of the range of service in three typical boroughs which represent inner, middle and suburban London, to throw light on the range and pattern of actual services in these areas; and finally, a health economic study has been carried out of current expenditure on mental health services in London, and the estimated costs of alternative systems of care which could be introduced.

We asked independent experts to prepare reports about specialist areas, and their names are shown on the chapter headings that follow. These areas include mental health services for the elderly, children & adolescent mental health services, services for substance misuse, services for HIV/AIDS, forensic mental health services, services for the homeless, liaison psychiatry services, services for minority ethnic groups and primary care mental health services. Wherever possible we checked our data against other sources of information, and by and large a consistent picture has emerged.

Where mental health services are concerned, London can be roughly divided into two parts: outer London, which seems to be broadly similar to other urban areas in Britain, and inner London, where problems seem to be worse than in any other part of the country. These problems are especially marked in the socially deprived areas of inner London, and in these areas problems are worse than in any other part of the country.

In the pages that follow we document these problems and provide suggestive evidence as to how the problems have come about. There are good reasons why the services are at present under severe strain, and we describe them fully. We also examine the perceptions of managers of the obstacles to change.

The picture is not all gloomy: we describe many admirable schemes, and show that the system is in a state of flux. Community mental health teams exist in most parts of the city, although no single area can be identified where there is a full range of services. Most in-patient units are available locally, rather than being provided from large mental hospitals at some distance from the patients' homes. It is our hope that by identifying the problems that now beset the mental health services in London, we will enable the second London Commission to produce firm recommendations which will lead to satisfactory and innovative services in all parts of the city.

David Goldberg
London Commissioner

Chapter 1

London's Mental Health: Executive Summary

David Goldberg

The findings outlined in this book describe a service in inner London that cannot be sustained because it is unable to meet the demands imposed upon it. Services in outer London are comparable with those in other English cities. The mental illness services are in a state of transition, and we describe admirable features in many parts of the capital. However, no single service appears to have a full range of desirable features. The crisis in inner London is not due to meanness among London's purchasers or to stick-in-the-mud attitudes among its providers. The formulae for allocating resources to deprived inner-city areas need to be revisited. London is shown to have greater needs even than the socially deprived areas of other cities, and the report explores some of the reasons why this is so.

What are London's main problems?

Mental health services in London are struggling to cope with extremely high levels of demand. As wards have been closed to raise finance for community mental health services, there is now a crisis in London's in-patient services, manifested by:

- Bed occupancy rates: these have been increasing steadily, at times reaching levels as high as 125%. Figures for London are worse than those for other inner cities in England (pp. 178–180; 182–183; 192). Rates for psychosis in inner London are double those for other inner cities in England (pp. 26–28).

- The numbers of assaults and cases of sexual harassment on in-patient wards are unacceptably high (pp. 178–180). Levels of violence among London in-patients are high in national terms and are above those seen among in-patients in other urban areas. A greater proportion of London patients are compulsorily detained than in other inner cities (pp. 175; 186).

- Equity of service provision in London compared with other parts of the country areas is in doubt, in that there are people with serious disorders who may benefit from admission but do not reach the very high threshold for admission in London, although they would be admitted in other areas of the country (pp. 177; 185–187; 189).

- In-patient facilities are being used inefficiently because inappropriately placed 'new long-term' patients remain there (pp. 178–180; 182–183; 186; 191–192). There is a more than threefold variation in the provision of these facilities across London (pp. 198–201).

- Only 8% of London hospitals surveyed had liaison services meeting minimum resource requirements laid down by the Royal College of Psychiatrists, and 14% had no liaison services whatever (pp. 82–91).

- Unacceptable delays are experienced by patients, their families and staff in provision of basic services. Median delay for admission to a secure unit is 24 hours; for allocation to a CPN or social worker 7 days; for a place in residential accommodation with 24-hour staffing 7 weeks; and for accommodation with a lower level of support 8 weeks (pp. 238–243).

- The concentration of resources on attempting to meet the needs of the most acutely ill has been associated with limited and patchy provision of other important elements in long-term care, such as day care, family interventions and employment schemes (pp. 243–248).

Services in the community are not sufficient to deal with the demand:

- A major contributing factor in this is a lack of residential places with 24-hour skilled staffing to which these patients can be discharged (pp. 39; 180; 192). There is a fivefold variation in the provision of these facilities across London (pp. 198–201).

- There is a tenfold variation in the provision of less intensively staffed residential care facilities across London (pp. 198–201).

- High intensity 24-hour community services, which may substitute for hospital admission when patients are in crisis, are almost entirely absent, and home treatment of moderate intensity, with daily visits on working days, is available in only few areas of London (p. 235).

- The voluntary sector is a major provider of day and residential care (pp. 281–284; 295–297). This is not a problem: but it is a new development, and must be taken into account in service planning.

- Local Authority Services are not taking the lead in providing general adult services in any of the three areas of London we studied intensively, although they play a larger part in services for the elderly. Indeed, the NHS has taken over some traditional social services functions, and it is a major provider of both acute and long-term day care. In one of the areas intensively studied, the NHS was providing work rehabilitation services (pp. 287–288; 288–292; 304).

Other aspects of London's mental health services:

- Services for ethnic minorities: Some specific services have developed for various of London's many and diverse ethnic minority communities, but the coverage they achieve in meeting a full range of needs within these communities is thus far very limited, and there is widespread concern that the generic services are not successful in meeting these needs (pp. 143–166; 230–234).

- Time trends: Over the country as a whole, as admissions become shorter readmissions become more frequent: the number of FCEs/100,000 at risk is increasing in all areas, but has reached an all-time high in inner London, with 911 FCEs/100,000 at risk for males aged 16–64 (p. 174).

- Staff recruitment. There are currently shortages of psychiatrists, clinical psychologists and community psychiatric nurses to run the mental illness services in London (pp. 40–41).

- Mentally disordered offenders (MDOs). Rates for social deprivation correlate highly (r = +0.75) with admission rates to medium and maximum security beds. Use of Special Hospital beds for Greater London is almost double that for the rest of the UK – with more than twice these high rates for Camden and LSL. Even when London is compared with other inner deprived cities, these differences remain (pp. 101–105; 183–184).

- Child and adolescent services. High rates of need are indicated by high rates of children in Local Authority Care and on 'at risk' registers (pp. 70–71).

- Managers do not feel able to manage the process of change, and are constantly striving to work with budgets which are not adequate to address the needs of the populations served. Most come from a practitioner background and have had no training in management, and there is considerable job instability (pp. 331–360).

Is London worse than other large cities?

Compared with other large English cities, London has:

- a proportionately greater number of patients needing services in inner London, especially marked in males aged 15–45 (pp. 172–174);

- more discharges going to NHS or LA residential services (pp. 175–176);

- more single, divorced or widowed patients (pp. 176–177);

- a higher proportion of patients with schizophrenia among those admitted to wards (pp. 177–178);

- 11 of the 26 recent national studies of homicides by mental patients have been in London (pp. 41–42);

- more children in care (102/10K inner London; 60/10K other cities; p. 70);

- more children on 'at risk' registers (58/10K inner London; 38/10K other cities; p. 71).

If **inner deprived areas of London** are compared with **inner deprived areas of other cities**, London has:

- 33% more FCEs (pp. 184);

- higher bed occupancy (pp. 182–183);

- four times as many patients in medium secure places (pp. 183–184);

- London's purchasers spend a 35% greater proportion of their total health budgets on mental health (pp. 185).

Are there reasons for London having high rates of illness?

Characteristics of inner London:

- London is at the extreme of the national spectrum for unemployment (pp. 24–25: inner London 16.5%, UK 9.2%).

- London has the six districts in England with the highest levels of social deprivation (pp. 16–19).

- Rates of mental illness near major rail termini are higher than those at some distance from them (pp. 26–28).

- The age structure of the inner London population is different from the rest of the country, with a greater proportion of the population in the age group 15–45 (36% compared with 29%), these being risk years for major mental disorders (pp. 19–20).

- More people in inner London live in single-person households (pp. 25–26: 54% compared with 27%).

Sociodemographic characteristics of Londoners (ideally, these require special forms of mental health services):

- London has the highest rates for ethnic minorities (London has 77% of the Black Africans and 58% of the Black Caribbeans, in the UK) – some of whom have very high rates of psychoses (pp. 20–22).

- More homeless people (pp. 118–130: 50% of the rough sleepers in the UK).

- The majority of refugees live in London (pp. 22–23; 148–149).

- Rates for substance abuse are higher in London than elsewhere: 75% of cocaine seizures in the UK are in London, and 35% of people starting treatment for drug problems are in London (pp. 75–81). The rise in rates for drug problems has not been matched by increases in service availability.

- London has almost 70% of the cases of AIDS notified nationally (p. 93).

Primary care services are significantly worse in London than in other deprived areas of inner cities:

- London services lag far behind those in other cities on such measures as percentage of practices reaching targets for cervical cytology, child immunizations and school age boosters. Far more London practices do not reach minimum standards, fewer have practice nurses, and more London GPs are single-handed. These disadvantages to London persist despite the LIZ initiative (pp. 131–142).

- Where mental health is concerned, recent figures confirm earlier figures, by showing that GPs in Manchester are better able to identify psychiatric cases than those in London (p. 135).

Are these problems due to London's purchasers?

London's purchasers:

- spend a greater proportion of their budgets on mental health (18.6% inner deprived London; 13.7% inner deprived other cities; 12.8% non-deprived London – p. 185);

- are more likely to have made comprehensive assessments of local mental health needs than purchasers in other cities (pp. 181–182). Since the system is in a state of crisis despite expenditure of large sums of money by purchasers, it is clear that the formulae used to allocate resources for mental health services for deprived urban areas are in need of urgent review by central government (pp. 362–363).

How completely has London introduced community mental health services?

London's services are indeed in transition, but measures that do not require initial expenditure have taken precedence over measures that are expensive.

Good features of London's mental health services include the following:

- Multi-disciplinary teams have been introduced in most areas (p. 225).

- Sectorisation has been introduced throughout the city. It is of interest that about 17% of Trusts have already moved to sectorisation by GP rather than by social services (pp. 222–224).

- User participation in service planning is reported widely (p. 230).

- There are many examples of innovative services (pp. 260–271), although no single Trust has all the components of a desirable service (p. 255). Detailed studies in three areas of London showed great heterogeneity of service models, with little guidance available about how best to organize services. A mixed economy of care has developed on all sites intensively studied, with the voluntary sector a major provider of daycare and residential care in each area. A range of private facilities are providing care, and the voluntary sector has become important (pp. 272–304).

Poorly provided facilities include:

- Providing proper premises for mental health teams in the community (pp. 225–226: over 60% of Trusts either have none or only have them in part of their area).

- Providing services in the community on a 24-hour basis. Thus, most community services are confined to office hours, and A&E departments are central to emergency provision out of hours: A&E departments are the most frequently used facility for emergency assessment, inside or outside office hours (pp. 228–229; 235–236).

- Intensive home-based treatment is not routinely available in most areas (p. 235: 48% never available; 44% sometimes or some of catchment area).

- Acute day hospitals are frequently unable to respond quickly enough to pre-empt admissions (p. 244).

- There is a severe shortage of CPNs available to carry out the Care Programme Approach: a 'good supply' [= available for >90% of those needing the service] of nurses is reported only by 42% of the best parts of higher UPA score Trusts, to 21% of the worst served parts of lower UPA score Trusts (p. 237).

- Sheltered work is only available in good supply to about 22% of Trusts, and schemes providing support in open market employment are universally poor (pp. 245–247).

- Few areas can actually provide the recommended 'spectrum of care': mental health professionals attached to primary care were not available or in severely short supply in 58%; Court Diversion schemes in 43%; and schemes for the homeless in 60%; support for carers in 56% (p. 248).

These shortages result in unacceptable delays in providing care:

- Significant delays were reported in the time taken to allocate a CPN or a social worker to someone needing the service (pp. 237–239).

- Delays for someone needing residential care were even worse, with delays of over 2 months being widely reported (pp. 242–243).

- Where beds were concerned, delays of between 2 and 3 days are reported by some Trusts to obtain an intensive care unit bed (p. 241).

Are resources distributed according to need?

- The London Boroughs vary greatly in their levels of service provision, service availability, degree of community-orientation and adequacy of functioning, with substantial variations even within catchment areas. Sociodemographic variables explain these variations to a degree, although considerable unexplained differences still persist between areas characterised by similar degrees of social deprivation (pp. 193–249).

- The Mental Illness Needs Index (MINI) was used to compare actual provision with likely need, using statistical indicators derived from census data to take account of variations in social deprivation. The original assumptions on which the MINI was based are shown not to be appropriate for inner London: it assumes that needs are normally distributed (and they are not), and gives estimates for requirements for services which do not fit with any of the evidence outlined in this book (pp. 206–207). A revised version of MINI produces a model which better fits with the service as we found it (pp. 207–208). The figures show what would have to be provided in each London borough to produce a service with 85% bed occupancy, using no ECRs, and with no patients unnecessarily detained in hospital because there were no facilities in the community. Extra hospital beds and extra community facilities are needed in most areas of London (pp. 217–218).

What are the cost implications of our work?

- Costs in London are higher than those elsewhere, and reasons for this have been examined (pp. 306–308).

- A set of 'actual costs' was computed by multiplying the number of services provided by unit costs, and these were compared with the 'predicted costs', using values derived from the various versions of the MINI (pp. 315–325).

- There are large variations in expenditure per 100K population at risk (pp. 316–318). Greatest expenditure on residential accommodation is on acute wards, with hostel wards and 24-hour staffed accommodation also being expensive items (p. 320).

- Where London Health Authorities are concerned, costs of residential accommodation range from £2.5–3M per 100K at risk for areas like Bromley, Hillingdon and Croydon, to £6.5–7.0M for KCW, LSL and E. London & City (pp. 321–322).

- Ten outer London boroughs, and four inner London boroughs, would appear to be functioning at about the predicted level of expenditure, or somewhat in excess of it (p. 323).

- Nine authorities are substantially underspent to the tune of between 3 and 4 million. (p. 324).

- These cost differentials have been analysed by type of facility (p. 325), indicating substantial underspends on acute beds and 24-hour staffed accommodation in both inner and outer London: only hostel wards in outer boroughs appear to have more spent on them than predicted by our models. Health authority cost differentials have also been explored, indicating that 'actual costs' are less than predicted needs by over 8 million in 5 health authorities (p. 324).

Possible Ways Forward

The evidence assembled from a variety of sources in this report demonstrates clearly that mental health services in London are working in a way that is not sustainable. The perspectives of service users and of carers need to be fully represented in future assessments of needs for services in London. Similar levels of home support should be available in all parts of the capital – currently the very wide variations between areas mean that services are far from equitable.

Resources for recurrent expenditure (NHS)

- The present national formula for allocating resources to purchasing authorities still fails to meet the needs of deprived inner cities. The York formula for taking the mental health needs of inner cities into account has only been partly introduced, as the Department of Health treats 24% of health expenditure as 'unweighted', and this was not the intention of the economists who produced the formula originally. If the York formula was introduced as it was intended, it would go a long way towards remedying the inequalities that we have drawn attention to. An urgent review of the allocation formula is required (p. 363).

- Many London purchasers are seriously overspent, and are likely to balance their budgets by reducing their mental health spend still further in 1997/1998. This will exacerbate a situation that is already dangerous. Central planners need to reconsider the problems posed by an increased demand for mental illness services in our inner cities.

New facilities (capital expenditure)

- Acute beds are one component of a system of care and should not be considered in isolation from other elements whose availability is likely to have substantial effects on acute bed occupancy. In some parts of London, some further acute beds may be needed in the short term to alleviate pressures on staff and patients (p. 364).

- More high support residential placements (including facilities with 24-hour waking nursing staff) need to be available, for placement of the most disabled patients who currently remain for long periods on acute wards (p. 364).

- Where teams are based at sites distant from the sectors they serve, more local community premises need to be provided (p. 365).

Extension of desirable practices

- For those who do not require 24-hour care, the supported tenancies being developed in some areas of London promise to be a very useful model (p. 364). Permanent tenancies with varying levels of support according to current need allow flexibility, and may be more acceptable to younger people who have not experienced long-term institutionalization and have higher expectations regarding privacy and autonomy than the generation discharged from the asylum.

- Agreed minimum standards should be established and implemented for acceptable maximum waits for appropriate residential care. We suggest that an acceptable level of service is that all patients should normally be placed in appropriate accommodation within one month (pp. 364–365).

- Minimum standards should be set for community teams' speed of response and the intensity of support they can provide, and ways should be found of implementing these throughout the city. We propose that a reasonable minimum is that it should be possible for acutely ill or relapsing patients to be visited at least once every working day when required, for initial contact to be available within 24 hours, and for longer-term allocation to a CPN and/or social worker caseload to take place within two weeks. These standards could not possibly be met with existing levels of resource in many parts of London (p. 365).

- Family interventions for people with psychotic illnesses and their relatives should be readily available in all areas of London. Services should actively seek to give families the opportunity to be directly involved in the care of their mentally ill relatives and fully informed about their care (pp. 367–368).

• Specific services supporting carers of people with severe mental illness should be available throughout the city (pp. 367–368).

• Procedures for maximizing the safety of staff dealing with those severely ill patients who may become violent should be developed as soon as possible (pp. 371–372).

Inter-agency collaboration

• Co-ordinated procedures should be established within each local area for monitoring services across health service, local authority and voluntary sector (pp. 361–362).

• A single multi-agency group should collate and disseminate all relevant local information within an area, avoiding any wasteful parallel procedures and ensuring maximum interpretability and availability of data (pp. 361–362).

• Reporting systems should be set up to allow the collation of data relevant to service provision and service comparison across London (this would be best organized by commissioning authorities; pp. 361–362).

• A multi-agency review of levels and types of long-term day care and of employment schemes should be carried out, with particular attention to the needs and preferences of younger people and of members of ethnic minorities (pp. 365–366).

The need for better information systems

• A regularly updated system of collection and collation of data across London as a whole should be instituted, allowing more accurate future assessment of how far services across the capital meet needs (pp. 361–362).

• Collation of information should take place at a Health Authority or Borough level, but should take into account the wide variations in service availability found between areas within the same catchment area. The services available to the population of each part of the catchment area must be considered (pp. 361–362).

• Standardized formats should be developed for recording service provision by all agencies, with clearly defined service and client group categories (p. 287).

• Future assessments of local services should not only examine numbers of places in use, but also service availability, including delays experienced and needs for service provision which cannot be met (p. 287).

• There should be an expansion of shared care registers between primary care and community mental health services (pp. 141–142).

• Detailed recommendations about special groups are to be found on pp. 46–166; 368–371.

The need for new knowledge

- A major review should be carried out of the causes of difficulty in recruiting and retaining staff, and of ways of improving working conditions and attracting adequate numbers of appropriately qualified staff to work in the capital (pp. 371–372).

- Research needs to be commissioned into the causes of the apparently rising demand for in-patient services for young men. Reasons for this are not well understood, but may include unemployment, increasing substance abuse among people with psychosis, or the alienation from community services of young men from ethnic minority backgrounds (p. 363).

- Research needs to be commissioned evaluating the effectiveness in preventing admission or reducing the length of in-patient stays of intensive 24-hour community services. It remains uncertain how far care of this type can be substituted for in-patient provision, as those currently admitted to London wards are usually very severely disturbed (p. 364).

- Improved bed management strategies and a centralised emergency bed service may have some role in prevention of large numbers of ECRs – this needs evaluation (p. 364).

- Research should be commissioned into the effectiveness of initiatives developed in partnership with ethnic minority communities, which may include training in cultural sensitivity for all mental health professionals, changes in the environments provided in mental health facilities and public information campaigns targeting ethnic minority communities (pp. 162–166; 366).

- Research should be commissioned into the nature and effectiveness of advocacy services currently provided, and whether users find them helpful. Where there is evidence that advocacy services are found helpful by users and carers, their funding should be placed on a more secure long-term footing (p. 368).

Chapter 2

Introduction to the Report

Rosalind Ramsay and Sonia Johnson

Summary

This chapter describes how we collected information about Londoners' mental health needs and about how far the services meet these needs. The report will identify gaps between need and current provision, and ways of improving services to bridge these gaps.

Because of the complexity of the questions addressed and the deficiencies in much of the data obtainable on routine service provision, the report makes use of multiple approaches and information sources.

The report includes discussion of:

- epidemiological evidence about population needs
- the national and local policy context
- the current state of sub-speciality services
- previous reports and research on London's services in the 1990s
- levels of in-patient and residential service provision
- the extent to which a full spectrum of community, day and residential services is available throughout London
- equity in service provision – are needs met to an equal extent in all areas and for all groups within the city's population?
- costs attached to current services and the cost implications of change
- innovative service models being developed in some areas
- recommendations for improving London's services

The report has been produced by four London research groups: PRiSM, CMHSD, CRU and CEMH, with PRiSM taking an overall co-ordinating role. The timescale has been very short, which has resulted in some limitations in the quality of the data.

2.1. Aims

This report describes current knowledge about needs for mental health services in Greater London, and about the degree to which services are currently succeeding in meeting these needs. It draws both on previous research and reports in the 1990s and on a large new body of data collected for the report.

The major questions which we set out to answer are:

- Are the mental health needs of Londoners different in extent or degree from those of the rest of the UK's population?
- Does the functioning of London's mental health services differ from services in the rest of the country?
- How far has a community-based model of care been implemented in the city?
- What is the current evidence on the state of acute wards in London and on the availability of alternatives to admission?
- To what extent is a comprehensive range of facilities readily available for the city's mentally ill, including accommodation with a variety of levels of support, day care and leisure facilities, home support, advocacy services and employment schemes?
- Is there equity in London's provision, with the populations of different parts of the city and members of the many different ethnic minority communities all having their needs met to an equal extent?
- What costs are associated with current provision and what would be the resource implications for different areas of London of adopting innovative models of care?
- How might purchasers and providers move towards the planning of comprehensive long term strategies for each area, taking into account the full range of needs of the local population?
- What obstacles currently exist to planning such co-ordinated and comprehensive services?
- How might the capital's mental health services be improved so that they meet the mental health needs of Londoners more fully?

2.2 Approaches and methods

No single set of information or single perspective is currently available which can fully answer these questions. This report therefore draws on of a variety of approaches and information sources. Levels of analysis used vary from identifications of trends in Greater London as a whole, through descriptions of services and service use at Health Authority, Trust and Borough catchment area levels, to evidence about the characteristics of individual patients in London.

2.3 Teams involved

The following four London research teams have collaborated in preparing the report: Section of Community Psychiatry (PRiSM), Institute of Psychiatry; the Centre for the Economics of Mental Health (CEMH), Institute of Psychiatry; the Centre for Mental Health Services Development (CMHSD), King's College London; and the Royal College of Psychiatrists Research Unit (CRU). Overall co-ordination of the work and final editing of the report was carried out at PRiSM by Rosalind Ramsay, Sonia Johnson and Graham Thornicroft.

2.4 Limitations and timescale of the project

The time available for each of the four teams to complete data collection and report writing was short. The co-ordination of the project started in January 1996 with the first draft prepared by 31 August 1996 and the final version of this first edition submitted for publication in November 1996. CRU and CMHSD were required to submit their reports by April 1996. This short timescale led to some difficulties in completing data collection, particularly as it proved very difficult to obtain responses from purchasers and providers during the final three months of the financial year (January to March). Time was also too short for it to be feasible to carry out full and independent checks on the reliability and validity of the data supplied by purchasers and providers, and our impression, discussed in more detail in Chapters 7, 8 and 10, is that there may be some inconsistencies and inaccuracies. Uncertainties about the accuracy and interpretability of routinely collected data have been a further reason why we have presented data from a variety of different sources rather than relying on a single study for information. In this way we have sought to identify patterns where evidence from multiple sources may reinforce our confidence in our findings.

2.5 Main components of the report

The report has three main sections: Chapters 3 and 4 set out the policy and epidemiological background for the report, Chapters 5 to 10 discuss in detail the evidence on London's current service provision and the degree to which this meets needs, and Chapters 11 to 13 discuss the gaps in services, the opportunities for improvement, and the obstacles which exist to change.

2.6 Overview of the chapters

Considering each of these sections in more detail, Chapter 3 outlines the epidemiological evidence on London's mental health needs. Characteristics of London's population which influence needs for services are discussed and studies which enumerate and describe London's mentally ill population are summarised. Chapter 4 provides a background from the point of view of public policy and of previous reports: it outlines the national policy context and also the previous reports and initiatives which have specifically addressed difficulties in London's services. It also discusses a series of public inquiries into homicides perpetrated by mentally ill people in London, some of which have had a considerable impact on the views of the public and on national policy.

Chapters 5 to 10 describe and evaluate London's current service provision from a variety of points of view. Chapter 5 focuses on major sub-groups of the mentally ill population with particular needs: older people, children and adolescents, substance misusers, people with HIV infection or AIDS, mentally disordered offenders and homeless people. It also provides an account of service provision in primary care and in general hospitals, and of the specific service needs of people from ethnic minority backgrounds. Chapter 6 summarises the information on London's mental health services in the 1990s which is available from routinely collected statistics and from previous research. Chapter 7 is based on a large data set collected at PRiSM in early 1996, which quantifies levels of in-patient and residential service provision in all London Boroughs. Variations between Boroughs and their associations with epidemiological characteristics are discussed, and actual provision is compared with a model which predicts expected levels of service provision on the basis of epidemiological characteristics. Chapter 8 uses a further PRiSM London-wide survey carried out early in 1996, which addresses two major questions: how far has a community-based model of care been adopted across London, and to what extent is a comprehensive range of in-patient, residential, day and community services available in all London catchment areas? In Chapter 9, a framework for developing comprehensive, needs-based services in London's catchment areas is set out by the Centre for Mental Health Services Development, and innovative London services which promise to be more appropriate ways of meeting local needs are identified. Finally in Chapter 10, the focus is shifted to a detailed view of the diverse ways in which services are delivered in three London Trust catchment areas.

In the final section, Chapters 11 to 13, questions about the feasibility and desirability of change are addressed more directly. Chapter 11, from the Centre for the Economics of Mental Health, discusses costs attached to current resources and the economic implications of the adoption of innovative service models. In Chapter 12, barriers to change experienced by managers in purchasing authorities and in providers are described on the basis of a study carried out by the Centre for Mental Health Service Development in summer 1996. Finally, Chapter 13 draws together evidence on the current state of London's mental health services and on the degree to which Londoners' mental health needs are being met, and proposes solutions to the difficulties faced.

Chapter 3

Londoners' mental health needs: the sociodemographic context

Sonia Johnson, Rosalind Ramsay and Graham Thornicroft

Summary

- London is at an extreme on the national spectrum for unemployment, homelessness and overall social deprivation, all of which are strongly associated with high rates of psychiatric disorders, including psychosis.
- A high proportion of Londoners come from ethnic minorities, and in many parts of the city, a large variety of different communities are represented within a small area. Some ethnic groups have increased rates of illness, while members of all minority communities have specific needs for services to be made appropriate for them. Currently, these needs are frequently unmet.
- Most of the UK's refugees live in London. Their mental health needs are not yet well understood, but are likely to be considerable.
- Young people are disproportionately represented in the population, and this is associated with increased needs for services for psychosis.
- Londoners are more likely than people elsewhere in the country to live alone: this is both associated with higher rates of illness and likely to lead to greater requirements for support from services for those who become ill.
- Inner London is an extreme outlier on the national spectrum for most of these demographic characteristics, whilst many outer London areas are intermediate between inner London and the national average.
- Epidemiological studies indicate that inner London has rates of psychosis around double those found in suburban or rural areas.
- Mentally ill individuals in inner London are more likely than those living elsewhere to belong to an ethnic minority, to have a history of homelessness, to have been compulsorily detained in hospital, to have a history of violence and to have been imprisoned. They are less likely to live with family or relatives.
- Several of London's sociodemographic characteristics are not only associated with higher rates of mental illness, but also lead to requirements for specific forms of service – examples are homelessness, unemployment, and the high rates of refugees and ethnic minority groups.

3.1 Introduction

> **'Mental health needs in London are undeniably much greater than in most other parts of the country and services require more attention to keep pace with growing need.'**
> **(NHS Executive, 1996b).**

This opening sentence from a recent NHS Executive briefing paper restates the premise behind many of the reports discussed in Chapter 4: that London has needs for mental illness services different in scale and kind from those experienced in other parts of the country. In this chapter, we examine the reasons for holding such a view.

The evidence supporting this view comes from two major sources. First, several socio-demographic indicators have been found to have marked influences on the prevalence of psychiatric disorders and on mental health service utilisation. These include rates of unemployment and homelessness, ethnic composition of the population, age structure, and overall social deprivation. This chapter will begin by describing those socio-demographic characteristics of London which are likely to have a significant impact on its population's needs for mental health services. Second, the prevalence of various psychiatric disorders in London has been directly measured in some recent studies, and this epidemiological work also provides valuable evidence on the likely extent of Londoners' mental health needs. The latter part of the chapter will summarise this work.

Throughout this book, the term 'London' describes the 32 Boroughs which correspond to the area of the former Greater London Council (1936-86). The G.L.C. covered an area defined by 1938 legislation on the metropolitan green belt – this was based on the extent of contiguous urban development at that time (Bardsley & Hamm, 1995). Sixteen purchasing authorities now cover an area almost co-terminous with that occupied by these London Boroughs. Within this area, acute mental health services are delivered by 27 NHS Trusts (see maps 1 and 2).

Recent OPCS mid-year estimates (Office of Population Censuses and Surveys, 1993) indicate that London has a population of almost 7 million people, representing approximately 14% of the population of England and Wales. The Boroughs (excluding City of London) range in size from 138,000 in Kingston upon Thames to 323,000 in Croydon, and the purchasing health authorities range from 240,000 (Hillingdon) to 729,000 (Lambeth, Southwark and Lewisham).

3.2 London's socio-demographic characteristics and their implications for needs for mental health services

3.2.1 Social deprivation
The relationship between psychiatric disorder and various measures of poverty, low social class or social deprivation became a major focus for psychiatric epidemiology in the first half of the twentieth century. Many positive findings have been reported since the original observation in the 1930s in Chicago that there was a higher rate of admission for psychosis in poorer central areas than in more prosperous outer areas (Faris and Dunham, 1939). A series of subsequent studies have confirmed this tendency

Map 1 London mental health trust catchment areas

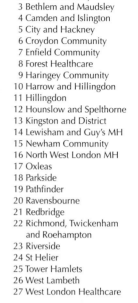
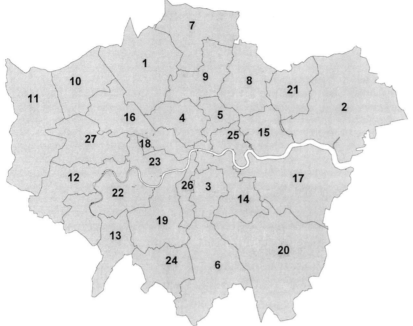

Legend
1 Barnet
2 BHB Community
3 Bethlem and Maudsley
4 Camden and Islington
5 City and Hackney
6 Croydon Community
7 Enfield Community
8 Forest Healthcare
9 Haringey Community
10 Harrow and Hillingdon
11 Hillingdon
12 Hounslow and Spelthorne
13 Kingston and District
14 Lewisham and Guy's MH
15 Newham Community
16 North West London MH
17 Oxleas
18 Parkside
19 Pathfinder
20 Ravensbourne
21 Redbridge
22 Richmond, Twickenham
   and Roehampton
23 Riverside
24 St Helier
25 Tower Hamlets
26 West Lambeth
27 West London Healthcare

Map 2 Local authority boroughs of London

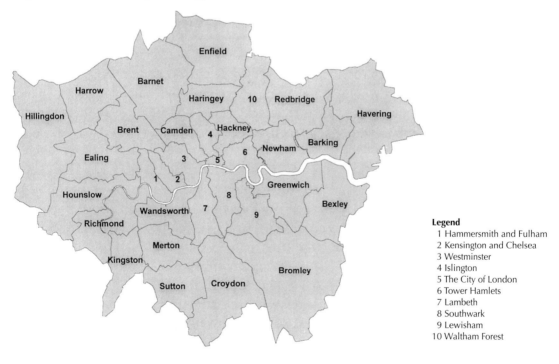

Legend
1 Hammersmith and Fulham
2 Kensington and Chelsea
3 Westminster
4 Islington
5 The City of London
6 Tower Hamlets
7 Lambeth
8 Southwark
9 Lewisham
10 Waltham Forest

for people with psychotic disorders to be concentrated in inner cities (Eaton, 1985; Giggs and Cooper, 1987). These effect are particularly clear for schizophrenia, and there has been a debate over whether people born in the inner city are at high risk of psychotic illness ('social causation hypothesis'), or whether this finding is the result of mentally ill people tending to migrate to inner cities even if they are born elsewhere ('social drift hypothesis'). Recent research has tended to support the former view, that there is a true increased incidence of schizophrenia in individuals born or brought up in an urban environment (Castle et al, 1993; Dauncey et al, 1993). However, it is likely that 'social drift' operates as well, with numbers of individuals with schizophrenia in the inner city inflated by migrants from more prosperous areas (Buszewicz and Phelan, 1994).

More recently, exploration of the characteristics of areas which predict high rates of mental disorder has been aided by the development of specific indicators of social deprivation. In studying links between deprivation and psychiatric disorder at an area level, the most widely used composite indicator in recent UK research has been the Jarman index, or Under-Privileged Area score (UPA score: Jarman, 1983; Jarman, 1984). This has been shown to be highly correlated with psychiatric admission rates for Health Districts in the North West and South East Thames Regions (Hirsch, 1988; Thornicroft, 1991), and across the whole of England (Jarman et al, 1992; Jarman and Hirsch, 1992). Harrison et al (1995) have carried out similar analyses studying admissions by diagnostic group, and find that this relationship between admission rates and deprivation principally applies to schizophrenia and other psychotic disorders, for which they found the correlation between admission rate and UPA score to be 0.77. They suggested that for affective illnesses and other non-psychotic disorders, admission rates may be influenced more strongly by service availability. Finally, Harvey et al (1996) have used Jarman scores to model differences in prevalence of schizophrenia between individual electoral wards in an inner London area, and find they perform well, predicting 36% of the variation in prevalence between wards.

Studies carried out at an individual rather than an area level have indicated that low social class increases the risk of schizophrenia by a factor of two or three (Eaton, 1974). Importantly, social class not only influences illness prevalence, but is also likely to have a significant impact on needs for mental health services because of its effect on the course of illness. It is associated with longer duration of episode, greater risk of relapse, poorer treatment response and clinical outcome, disproportionate use of psychiatric services and differing perceptions of mental illness (Thornicroft, 1991).

In community surveys, neurotic disorders such as anxiety and depression also show a clear relationship with indicators related to social deprivation. The finding of a higher prevalence of such disorders in more deprived areas has been replicated a number of times (Lewis and Booth, 1992; Platt et al 1990). At an individual level, the UK National Morbidity Survey, a large community survey, has recently indicated that the highest overall rates of neurotic disorders and of drug and alcohol dependence are in Social Classes IV and V (Meltzer et al, 1995). For child psychiatric disorders (Richman, 1985; Wolkind and Rutter, 1985), rates again appear to be higher in the inner city, probably because of the clustering in such areas of known specific risk factors such as poor parental mental health and housing, family conflict and poor schooling.

Thus even this very brief overview indicates that the evidence for an association between social deprivation and psychiatric morbidity in various forms is strong. Considering the implications for London, parts of the metropolis are at an extreme in relation to the rest of the country. According to the Jarman index, the most deprived districts in England are six London boroughs: Hackney, Islington, Lambeth, Southwark and Tower Hamlets in inner London and Newham in outer London (Bardsley and Hamm, 1995). Even within the more affluent boroughs, pockets of severe deprivation occur, with, for example, 9.6% of the population of Barnet living in wards whose Jarman UPA scores are within the most deprived 10% for the country.

The extent of deprivation in inner London may be increasing. Between the Censuses of 1981 and 1991, proxy indicators for poverty and wealth from the Census (unemployment, economic inactivity, socio-economic group, car ownership and educational attainment), show evidence of relative increases in the degree, extent and intensity of poverty in inner London (Green, 1994).

Thus population-level composite indicators of deprivation already suggest that Londoners' mental health needs may be particularly great. A number of individual demographic characteristics are also good predictors of mental health needs and service use, in some cases appearing to predict variations in service use more powerfully than composite deprivation scores (Kammerling and O'Connor, 1983). London's position on the indicators most relevant to mental illness will now be considered.

3.2.2 Age structure

London deviates markedly from the rest of the country in its age structure, in that the city in general and the inner city in particular have proportionately more young people than England and Wales as a whole. OPCS mid-year estimates for the year 1993 showed that in inner London, 36.3% of the population was aged between 15 and 45 compared with 29.4% in England and Wales (Office of Population Censuses and Surveys, 1993). London has a lower proportion of elderly people than England and Wales as a whole, and again this is particularly marked for Inner London, where 12.6% were over 65 in 1993, compared with 15.9% nationally. There is often a pattern of young people from other parts of the country initially moving into central London, but later, as they get older, moving to outer London suburbs and beyond (Bardsley & Hamm, 1995).

This difference in age structure has significance for population needs for mental health services. Most people with psychotic illnesses present to services for the first time below the age of 45, and research on the course of psychotic illness suggests that for the majority, needs for admission and social care will be greatest during the earlier years of the illness. Eating disorders, drug abuse and personality disorders are other forms of psychiatric disorder for which epidemiological evidence suggests that young adults are likely to have the greatest needs for services.

The age of the patient population is also likely to influence the type of service required. Many existing community facilities were developed for the generations who were the first to be discharged from the large asylums and who are now approaching old age. Surveys of day centre and residential facilities have indicated that many 'general adult' facilities are occupied by a population largely aged over 45 (Shepherd et al, 1995; Orrell and Johnson, 1992). The younger generation who predominate in London have generally grown up without the experience of long-term institutionalisation and with different expectations. The facilities and activities provided for a previous generation may interest them little, and they may be unwilling to accept the same conditions, for example where bedrooms are shared in residential accommodation (Morris, 1991). Further, it has been suggested that there is a particular sub-group among the younger generation of urban users of mental health services who present particular management problems – this group has been described in the extensive US literature about them as 'young adult chronic' patients (Bachrach, 1982). Whilst institutionalisation and negative symptoms may be less common than among the previous generation who had often been long term in-patients for many years, some younger individuals with psychosis appear to have a particularly disrupted clinical course, marked by frequent crises, failure to engage consistently with services, impulsive behaviour, high rates of substance abuse and disrupted social histories. As further discussed in Chapter 9, they may need particularly intensive and highly staffed services to engage them.

3.2.3 Ethnic minorities

Ethnic composition is another aspect of London in which it differs markedly from the remainder of the UK, even the other metropolitan areas. In view of the great importance of the topic and for completeness, we briefly describe London's ethnic characteristics and their implications for service provision here: section 5.9 provides a much fuller discussion of the needs of ethnic minority communities and refugees, with full references.

Map 3 shows the proportions of the population of each London mental health Trust who are from an ethnic minority background. At the 1991 Census, 45% of Britain's ethnic minority population was resident in London, and 20.3% of London's population was from an ethnic minority. Ethnic groups vary in the degree to which they are concentrated in London: communities predominantly living in London rather than

Map 3 Minority ethnic groups in London

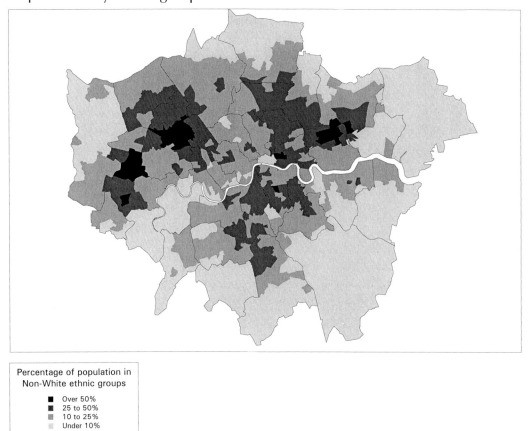

Percentage of population in
Non-White ethnic groups

■ Over 50%
■ 25 to 50%
▪ 10 to 25%
░ Under 10%

elsewhere in the country include Black Africans, with 77% of UK Black Africans resident in London, as well as 58% of the nation's population of Black Caribbeans and 52% of Bangladeshis. Almost all other major British minority communities apart from the Pakistani community are substantially over-represented in London (Travers and Minors, 1995). Generally the proportion of people classified as non-white is highest in inner London, apart from the Indian and Pakistani populations, who are concentrated in outer London. Distributions across the city vary considerably. Some communities live predominantly in one areas, such as the Bangladeshi community in the area of Tower Hamlets adjacent to the City, while communities such as the Chinese and Vietnamese are more widely dispersed (Travers and Minors, 1995; Bardsley and Hamm, 1995).

This ethnic diversity has a number of very important consequences for London's mental health services, which we summarise here. Further discussion of these is found in Section 5.9, which is specifically devoted to ethnic minorities, and this theme recurs throughout the book, indicating its centrality to consideration of Londoners' mental health needs.

First, a number of studies have suggested that different communities have different patterns of prevalence of mental illness. The commonest focus in such work has been on Black Caribbean people, with several studies indicating that they are at higher risk than their White neighbours of being admitted to psychiatric hospital (Moodley & Thornicroft, 1988) or diagnosed as suffering from schizophrenia (Harrison et al, 1988; King et al, 1994). The reasons are uncertain, and it is possible that the finding results more from the very high levels of social disadvantage experienced by this group than from any true ethnic difference. Evidence about the prevalence of psychosis among other minority groups remains incomplete and inconsistent: some studies in the South Asian community show rates similar to the white population (Thomas et al, 1993), whilst others have suggested that rates of psychosis are high in a variety of different immigrant communities (King et al, 1994). For more minor psychiatric disorders, there are again inconsistencies in prevalences estimated for various groups, but reports in early studies of low rates of neurotic disorders among Black Caribbeans now seem likely to be attributable to low rates of detection (Burke, 1984; Jacob et al, 1996), while among South Asians there is evidence that prevalence is high, especially among women (Ahmed, 1995). A particularly worrying finding is a markedly elevated suicide rate among young Asian women (Soni-Raleigh and Balarajan, 1992). The inconsistencies between prevalence studies may be at least partly attributable to the fact that analyses by broad ethnic group miss major differences between the histories, present circumstances and composition of minority communities living in different areas within the UK.

Secondly, there is considerable evidence that mentally ill members of some minority ethnic communities have different patterns of service contact and report different experiences of the mental health services from the White community. This is particularly striking for Black Caribbeans with psychotic illness, who appear less likely to have voluntary contact with the services and much more likely to be subject to various forms of coercive control, such as detention under the Mental Health Act (Davies et al, 1996). Among at least some sections of this community and its leaders, there appears to be a strong feeling of alienation from the statutory services and of suspicion of these services (Christie, 1995; Fernando, 1995). This resonates with the conclusion of a series of reports and inquiries (see Chapter 4) that services appear to have limited success in engaging this population in voluntary treatment.

This tendency not to reach psychiatric care via voluntary channels has also been observed for Black Caribbeans with milder mental health problems (Burke, 1984). South Asians have been found to have lower rates of referral to secondary psychiatric services despite identical rates of primary care consultation, with again a greater tendency for psychological disorders to go unrecognised (Brewin, 1980, Jacob et al, 1996). Chinese and Vietnamese people are the largest minority group after South Asians and African and Afro-Caribbeans, but are widely dispersed rather than concentrated in particular areas, which has probably militated against the provision of specific services for them. Wang and Xiang (1995) report a survey of the Chinese population in Oxford which indicates very limited use or knowledge of local health services.

A third implication of the presence of a large variety of ethnic minority communities is that members of these groups have important specific service needs. Failure to meet these needs may account for some of the differences in service use. Section 5.9 of this report and Bhui et al (1995a) have described some of the general needs of ethnic minority populations, including those for interpreters and bilingual staff, appropriate public information campaigns, access to a full range of services including psychological interventions, sensitivity to prevailing religious and cultural imperatives, ethnic monitoring of services, training in cross-cultural working for all staff and black-led action research on appropriate services.

Thus the remarkable ethnic diversity of Londoners is likely to lead to an increased requirement for resources and training to make services appropriate, and may also lead to a higher prevalence of psychiatric disorder. London is particularly distinctive in that, whilst other parts of the country have high concentrations of one or two ethnic groups, many areas of London are home to substantial numbers of members of a wide variety of different communities. Thus setting up parallel services for one or two ethnic groups will not usually meet local need comprehensively, and the ethnic sensitivity of generic services becomes a central issue.

3.2.4 Refugees

Refugees constitute a sub-group among migrants to London who need specific service provision, and the size of its refugee population is another characteristic in which London differs markedly from the rest of the country. A recent study in East London gave an estimate of 116,000 refugees living in the capital (Gammell et al, 1993), while the Refugee Council (personal communication) believes 90-95% of the estimated 200,000 refugees in the UK are in London.

Refugees have experienced multiple losses of family, friends, home and culture, many have experienced torture, persecution and imprisonment, and their future in London may be very uncertain. Thus one might predict a significant prevalence of mental health problems among them, although obviously they are a heterogeneous group, with diverse experiences. Information is limited, but several District Health Authorities have recently commissioned local surveys. For example, a study in Newham has examined demographic data on refugees in the area, their health needs and use of services

(Gammell et al, 1993). Considerable deprivation was found, with high rates of unemployment, overcrowding, and living in rented accommodation. Only half the refugees had been in the UK for more than two years, and many had spent their first year unable to communicate in English. This inability to communicate was associated with poor self-assessed health and depression.

Overall, one-third of the refugees reported depression (44% women, 25% men), with the highest rates in Iranians, Palestinians and Zairians. Rates of depression increased with the age of respondents, but decreased with the time they had spent in the UK. Refugees who had left children behind rather than other family members were also more likely to report depression, as were those whose main activity was housework or childcare. Uptake of counselling and psychiatric services was low (7% of the total sample), but most of those reporting depression wished to see a professional counsellor who spoke their own language. In a smaller more recent questionnaire survey of refugees in Lambeth, 49% reported depression, but again a large proportion had sought no support or help (Grant and Deane, 1995).

Thus there may be significant unmet needs for mental health care among London's growing refugee population, and again specific attention is needed to making services accessible to them and appropriate for their needs. Like other black and ethnic minority people refugees may have current fears of racist abuse and attack, but they are also likely to have feelings of fear related to past persecution. They may be wary of statutory services because of experiences of dealing with government organisations in their country of origin and while applying for asylum, and may also be suspicious of mental health workers as authority figures and may fear that disclosing their mental health problems could affect their status or application for asylum. Although these groups are all entitled to receive health and social services, the Asylum and Immigration (Appeals) Act (1993) has limited asylum seekers' access to public housing even if they fit the criteria for being in priority need and many face homelessness or bed and breakfast accommodation (Jacobs, 1995).

3.2.5 Homelessness

The specific needs of London' homeless population are discussed in greater detail in Chapter 5.7 and are referred to at several other points in the report – only a brief summary will therefore be provided here of the evidence on London. Although there are difficulties in ascertaining precise numbers of homeless people, the evidence suggests that homelessness is another demographic indicator on which London scores high compared with the rest of the country.

Regarding rough sleepers, the 1991 Census (OPCS, 1991) counted 2,703 people sleeping rough in England and Wales, of whom 1,275 were in London, although the methods used mean that substantial numbers are likely to have been missed. Much larger numbers are placed in temporary accommodation, and an estimate of the total homeless population in London in November 1995 was 85,414 people, of whom 1,275 were street homeless, 3,273 living in hostels and 72,570 in temporary accommodation (Health Action for Homeless People, 1996). Non-statutory homelessness and the number of people sleeping rough appear to be higher in inner London than outer London, while statutory homelessness is high in both inner and outer London boroughs

(Peace and Quilgar, 1996). Over the last decade there has been an increase in the number of homeless people in London, largely attributable to increases in homelessness among younger people, women and ethnic minorities.

The implications for population mental health needs of London's substantial homeless population are again considerable. Recent research in the UK suggests that the homeless in hostels and night shelters and on the street probably have a rate of mental illness of between 30 and 50%, and that psychoses predominate (Scott, 1993; Timms and Fry, 1989; Marshall, 1989). These homeless mentally ill individuals are often younger adults with psychotic disorders, and not, as often presumed, former long-stay in-patients (Dayson, 1993). As discussed further in section 5.7, the homeless population includes a variety of sub-groups with different patterns of psychiatric illness, including young families, women, refugees and elderly people.

Conventional psychiatric services often fail to contact or engage the homeless mentally ill, so that specific services are needed. For example, clinics may be provided in places where the homeless tend to congregate or assertive outreach work carried out on the streets. The needs of the homeless are particularly likely to be multiple, with many requiring interventions for physical health, psychological and social problems, so that there is a particularly important need for services which can provide a range of types of intervention and for good inter-agency co-ordination for this group.

3.2.6 Unemployment

For unemployment rates, inner London is again an outlier on the national spectrum, and is markedly different from outer London. London Research Centre data indicate that in February 1995 the unemployment rate for London as a whole was 11.9% of potentially economically active individuals, three points above the national average of 8.9% (Travers and Minor, 1995). However, Outer London was close to the national average at 9.2%, whilst the rate in Inner London was almost double, at 16.5%. This represented 407,000 individuals in London as a whole. Map 4 shows variations across London in rates of unemployment.

London's unemployment problem appears to have become more marked than that of the rest of the country during the 1990s. In 1984, London's unemployed accounted for 12.2% of the national total, and this figure scarcely changed during the 1980s, yet by 1995 they accounted for 17%. The recession had a particularly marked effect on London, with a rise in unemployment in the capital of 67% between 1989 and 1995, compared with 23% for Great Britain as a whole. The severity of Inner London's unemployment is indicated by the fact that in 1995 the 7 local authorities with the highest unemployment rates were all London Boroughs. Hackney, Tower Hamlets, Newham, Southwark, Haringey, Lambeth and Islington had unemployment rates ranging between 18.2% and 23.3.% (Travers and Minor, 1995).

With regard to the likely impact on needs for services in London, both in the Depression of the 1930s and in the recent period of high unemployment of the 1980s and 1990s, a series of studies has demonstrated that unemployment appears to have a considerable negative effect on mental health, with associations including depression, poor self esteem, anxiety, substance abuse and negative effects on relationships (Jahoda, 1979; Frese and Mohr, 1987; Crawford et al, 1987; Warr et al, 1988; Bhugra, 1993).

Map 4 Unemployment in London

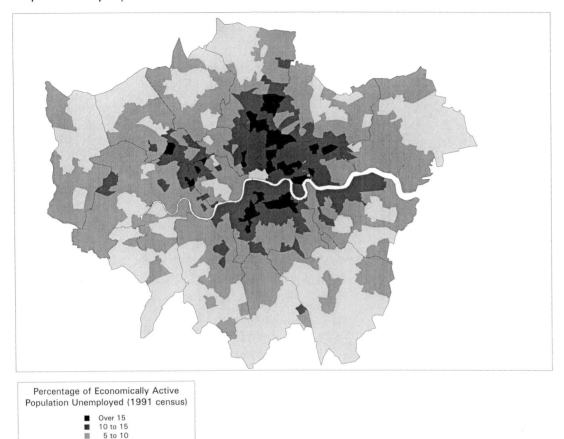

Percentage of Economically Active
Population Unemployed (1991 census)

■ Over 15
■ 10 to 15
▓ 5 to 10
▒ Under 5

Kammerling and O'Connor (1995) have found unemployment to be the best predictor of admission rate, reporting a 0.94 correlation between these two variables. A study in north east London found that local rates of unemployment accounted for 81% of the variance in the rates of accumulation of new long stay patients in different health districts in the area (Thornicroft et al 1992). High levels of unemployment and suicide rates have been found to be correlated in several Western countries (Pritchard, 1992, Platt et al, 1992). Thus this demographic characteristic again suggests that the needs for mental health services in the London population are likely to be at the extreme end of the national spectrum.

High unemployment rates may also have an impact on the types of services needed by the long term mentally ill. Whilst they may be able to find jobs in times of full employment, they are a group who are likely to be especially vulnerable to losing or not being able to find work when the country is in recession. Needs for help with employment and with activity in general are thus likely to be currently at a high level among London's long term mentally ill.

3.2.7 Household composition

Inner London has a much higher proportion of households consisting of only one person than the rest of the country – 54% compared with 27% nationally (NHS Executive, 1996b). Several studies have indicated high correlations between the proportion of people in an area who are living alone and rates of psychiatric disorder

(Shapiro et al, 1985). Similarly, the OPCS household survey of psychiatric morbidity indicated that lone parents and people living alone are the people at greatest risk of neurotic disorder or substance abuse (Meltzer et al, 1995).

The high rate of people living alone is also likely to have implications for the type of support required by people who become mentally ill. A smaller proportion of patients than elsewhere are likely to be living with informal carers or to have very good social support, so that a more intense service input is likely to be required for services to succeed in supporting severely ill people at home.

3.2.8 Residential mobility

Census data indicate that, as well as being more likely to become homeless, Londoners move more frequently than people elsewhere in the country. For example, whereas 4% of the population of England and Wales had lived at a different address a year before the 1981 Census, the figures for the Borough of Camden were 17% in the northern part and 18% in the southern (Harvey et al, 1996). This high level of mobility again has implications for primary and secondary care and social services provision: continuity of care will be more difficult to sustain when people move frequently, and people who need help are also less likely to know how to get access to services in their local area.

3.3 Londoners' mental health needs: direct epidemiological evidence

The second source of epidemiological evidence on Londoners' mental health needs is more direct, although not as comprehensive or as plentiful. A number of recent studies carried out in the city have measured the prevalence of illness in London or studied the social and clinical characteristics of mentally ill Londoners. Some of this evidence will now be briefly reviewed.

3.3.1 Studies of the prevalence of mental illness in London

The following studies provide information on the prevalence of psychosis in London:

(i) In the Camden Schizophrenia Surveys (Harvey, 1996; Harvey et al, 1996), a key informant method was used to identify all people with a possible psychotic illness who had any contact with local health services, GPs, social services, voluntary sector services for the mentally ill, hostels for the homeless and probation services serving the Borough of Camden. Standard research criteria were then applied to identify subjects with schizophrenia. This yielded a point prevalence for broadly defined schizophrenia of 5.3 per 1,000 resident population, representing 698 individuals. This has been compared by the authors with the Nithsdale study (McCreadie, 1982), a survey carried out using closely similar methodology in a largely rural area of Scotland, which gave a point prevalence of individuals meeting broad criteria for schizophrenia of 2.4 per 1,000 resident population. In both studies, the stricter Feighner criteria for schizophrenia were also applied, giving a rate of 3.1 per 1,000 in Camden and 1.7 in Nithsdale.

(ii) The PRiSM study at the Institute of Psychiatry in London has also used a key informant method to identify all individuals with psychosis within two South London sector catchment areas. This yielded 566 cases with evidence of psychosis in a population of 83,000, giving a one year prevalence of 6.84 per 1,000 resident population. Data from an outer London sector (in Croydon) using the same methodology are also available – here 141 cases were detected in a population of 38,000, giving a one year prevalence of 3.74 per 1,000 population, about half that found 8 miles further north.

The OPCRIT package (McGuffin et al, 1991) was used to assign research diagnoses by standardised criteria from the evidence of casenotes and informants. Prevalence rates of schizophrenia (defined by ICD10 standard criteria) in the inner London sample have been compared with rates in one of the Nithsdale surveys, which used the same methodology (McCreadie et al, in press). This again showed a higher overall prevalence rate in the urban areas than in the rural area. However, unlike the Camden surveys, the substantial differences are almost entirely attributable to an elevated rate of schizophrenia among the non-White population of South London. The White population in South London had a rate of schizophrenia close to that of the almost entirely White population in Nithsdale, whereas for the South London non-White subjects, the risk of meeting research criteria for schizophrenia appears to be between two and three times as high as for the White population in South London or Scotland. The authors speculate on possible reasons why there is no urban-rural difference among the White population, and suggest as a possible reason the fact that, unlike Camden, the areas of South London studied do not have major rail termini and may be less subject to 'drift' into the city.

(iii) The Kensington, Chelsea and Westminster Mental Health Census (Gath and Higginson, 1995)

This study again used a key informant method, but was based on slightly different inclusion criteria, aiming to ascertain the number of adults aged 16 to 64 who had severe long term mental health problems and resided in the catchment area of the Kensington, Chelsea and Westminster Health Commissioning Agency. The study used clear criteria to identify individuals with a substantial disability and/or risk to self or others, and with either at least an eighteen month history of mental health problems or a total of six months spent as an in-patient in the past year. Within the total catchment area population of 320,000, 2,369 residents of the Boroughs who met these criteria were identified. This represents a point prevalence of severe long term mental health problems of 1.2% of the population aged between 16 and 64. Of these, 61% had a clinical diagnosis of psychosis, 33% affective illness and 14% severe personality disorder.

The point prevalence for a clinical diagnosis of schizophrenia or other non-affective psychoses found in this survey is 7.08 per 1,000 population between 18 and 64. The authors compare their results with various other recent studies of the prevalence of psychosis, and conclude that prevalence is higher than in all other areas studied except Camden. The PRiSM data from South London allows calculation of the prevalence of clinical diagnosis for schizophrenia and other non-affective psychoses per 1,000 population between 15 and 64, and gives a figure of 6.14. The proportion of identified cases who are Black Caribbean, Black African or Black Other in the Kensington, Chelsea and Westminster sample was 15%, compared with 31% in South London, but despite this, the Kensington prevalence figure is slightly higher. Thus overall this evidence suggests that elevated illness among the Black African and Caribbean population may be used to explain high rates of psychosis in the South London sectors, but that other factors, perhaps related to a more transient population and greater homelessness, need to be invoked to explain the very high figures both in Camden and in Kensington, Chelsea and Westminster.

With regard to the prevalence of milder mental disorders, Bebbington et al (1981) surveyed a representative sample of the population of Camberwell, which led them to estimate that over the previous month 10.9% of the population of Camberwell had had symptomatic psychiatric disorder of some form, in most cases anxiety or depression. There was a marked sex difference, with 14.9% of women reporting disorders. compared with 6.1% of men. However, this survey was carried out in 1978, and subsequent social changes, including increasing unemployment and homelessness and changes in the ethnic composition of the population may well have affected morbidity.

Results available so far from the recent OPCS household surveys of psychiatric morbidity (Meltzer et al 1995) unfortunately do not give specific London results – data have been published for differences between urban and rural areas and for different NHS Regions, but not for individual cities. The general urban-rural differences found in this survey are quite marked: the prevalence of generalised anxiety disorders, depressive episodes, phobias, psychosis, and alcohol and drug disorders was overall twice as high in urban than in rural areas. The analyses by region are difficult to interpret as they group areas of London together with very prosperous parts of the South East of England.

3.3.2 Characteristics of people with psychiatric disorders in London

The second area where epidemiological studies carried out in London yield important information is regarding the characteristics of people with mental illness. This section summarises information from major epidemiological studies, emphasising studies where some comparison has been made with areas outside London.

(i) Ethnicity

Table 1 shows the ethnic origins of individuals identified as mentally ill in the population-based samples discussed above.

Table 1 Ethnic characteristics of people with psychosis in London and Nithsdale

Ethnic group	Camberwell (clinical diagnosis of psychosis) n = 548	Croydon (severe and enduring mental health problems) n = 141	Kensington/Chelsea/ Westminster (clinical diagnosis of psychosis) n = 2,591	Nithsdale (OPCRIT diagnosis of schizophrenia) n = 161
White	64.8%	72.9%	75% (White UK – 56.5%)	100%
Black Caribbean	25.2%	10.0%	9.7%	0
Black African	5.7%	3.6%	3.7%	0
Black Other	0.2%	0.7%	2.8%	0
South Asian	1.5%	6.5%	2.6%	0
Chinese	0.4%	0.7%	0.6%	0
Other	2.3%	5.7%	6.6%	0

As would be predicted from the high prevalence of mental health problems found among certain minority groups, the diversity of patient populations is still greater than that found among the general population, so that providing ethnically sensitive services is obviously one of the most significant additional requirements for services in London, compared with a rural area such as Nithsdale. It is worth noting that the outer London area, Croydon, is as ethnically diverse as the KCW catchment area, demonstrating that ethnic sensitivity is an issue for services throughout London, not only in the central area. The complexity of needs for services for minorities is also evident from these figures. In Camberwell, the large Black Caribbean group is a clear focus for development of specific services, but otherwise patients are dispersed among a variety of different groups, with large 'Other' categories in both Croydon and KCW. The KCW survey distinguishes White UK from other White individuals, revealing the diversity existing even within the White population – almost 20% of KCW's patient population (almost 500 individuals) are Irish or 'White Other', and the specific needs of such individuals have not generally been examined.

The KCW study also provides information on patients' first languages, of which 56 were identified. The commonest apart from English were Arabic, Spanish, German, Polish, Farsi, Portuguese, Italian, French and Amharic/Ethiopian. Again this is an indicator of demands on London's services unlikely to be encountered on a similar scale elsewhere.

(ii) Living situation

Table 2 shows the current accommodation of people with a clinical diagnosis of psychosis identified in three of the London surveys discussed above.

Table 2 Housing of people with psychosis in Camberwell, Camden and Croydon

Type of housing	Camberwell (psychosis – clinical diagnosis)	Camden (schizophrenia – broad criteria)	Croydon (psychosis – clinical diagnosis)
Mainstream housing	81.5%	67%	95%
Homeless/ temporary accommodation/squatting	2.5%	7%	1.4%
Supported housing	15.2%	22%	3.6%
In-patient	0.8%	excluded from calculation	0%

Thus in the inner London areas, there is a tendency for people to be in supported rather than mainstream housing (this reaches statistical significance for the differences between Camberwell and Croydon and between Camden and Croydon).[1] Camden has much the highest figure for homelessness, and the KCW survey gives a still higher figure of 19% (n = 54) for homelessness or residence in temporary accommodation – these data thus support the idea that homelessness may contribute to the high rates of psychosis found in these two areas.

---

[1] Statistical tests reported in this section were carried out on SPSS PC using chi-squared tests to examine whether the different samples were likely to be differently distributed across categories. Results are reported here as 'statistically significant' if they reached the conventional $p = 0.05$ level.

The Camberwell, Croydon and Camden surveys also all include information about household composition (Table 3).

Table 3 Household composition of people with psychosis

Lives with	Camberwell (psychosis – clinical diagnosis)	Camden (schizophrenia - broad criteria)	Croydon (psychosis – clinical diagnosis)
Alone	41%	30%	39%
With partner ('spouse' specified for Camden)	23%	14%	31%
With other family members	21%	21% (13% – with at least one parent)	26%
With people who are not family members	16%	35%	5%

Thus people in the Croydon survey were most likely to live with family or partner, and those in Camden were least likely to do so. Conversely, numbers living with people who are not relatives or spouse were highest in Camden. All these differences reach statistical significance, but it should be noted that some of those living 'with people who are not family members' in the Camden survey may have been living with partners, but unmarried. Harvey (1996) compares the Camden results with one of the Nithsdale surveys and with a number of community surveys from elsewhere, and concludes that fewer people in Camden are living with relatives than in samples resident in other areas, including some studies carried out in other cities.

The Camden survey was carried out almost a decade before the others, and it is possible that the situation has changed in this period. In both the recent surveys, more than a third of patients were living alone, indicating that the support required from services to maintain them at home in a crisis or if they are severely ill is likely to be considerable.

(iii) Symptoms

Harvey compares the Camden data on symptoms with data from Nithsdale. Positive psychotic symptoms (such as hallucinations and delusions) were common in the Camden sample, whilst negative symptoms (such as inactivity, lack of motivation and emotional flatness) were uncommon. The reverse was true in the rural sample.

(iv) Compulsory admission

The following shows rates of ever having experienced compulsory admission in the various samples:

Table 4 History of compulsory admission

Sample (& inclusion criteria)	% who have experienced at least one compulsory admission
Urban: Camden (broad diagnosis of schizophrenia)	57%
Urban: Camberwell (clinical diagnosis of schizophrenia)	67%
Suburban: Croydon (clinical diagnosis of schizophrenia)	47%
Rural: Nithsdale (clinical diagnosis of schizophrenia)	49%

The difference between Camberwell and each of the others reaches statistical significance, and Camden also has a significantly higher rate of history of compulsory admission than either the suburban or the rural area.

(v) Violence and contact with criminal justice system

Comparable data is available from Croydon, Camberwell and Nithsdale on lifetime history of violence, imprisonment, and, for Croydon and Camberwell, criminal convictions (Table 5).

Table 5 Lifetime history of violence/contact with the criminal justice system

Area (all samples – individuals with a clinical diagnosis of schizophrenia)	History of violence	Ever been to prison	Ever had a criminal conviction
Camberwell	51%	23%	30%
Croydon	34%	4%	15%
Nithsdale	41%	8%	no data

Differences between Croydon and Nithsdale do not reach statistical significance on any of these variables, whereas Camberwell's rates of violence and history of imprisonment are significantly greater than either of the other areas, and its rate of convictions is significantly higher than that for Croydon. Another noteworthy aspect of these data is that the disparity between Camberwell and the other areas is considerably greater for history of imprisonment than for history of violence: one may speculate that responses to violent or deviant behaviour may be different in inner city areas from elsewhere.

(vi) Employment

Among people under 65 with a clinical diagnosis of schizophrenia in Camberwell, 81% were not in any form of employment, 12% were employed in the open market (full-time or part time), 1% doing voluntary work and 6% in sheltered employment. In Croydon, among subjects of all ages with a diagnosis of schizophrenia, 20% were in some form of open market employment, 3% doing sheltered work, 7% retired, 1% full time students, and 68% unemployed. In the Camden sample, which was collected before the worst of London's recession, 19% of people with schizophrenia of all ages were employed and 2% in sheltered work. Thus most people with schizophrenia in London do not work, and the contribution made by sheltered work is notably small.

(vii) Substance abuse

A possible unmet need for services for people with a dual diagnosis of substance abuse and psychotic illness is discussed in Chapters 5 and 9, and debate about why the demand for acute beds may be increasing in London has sometimes referred to the possibility that increasing substance misuse among people with psychosis may contribute. This is a problem which has received considerable recent attention and is believed to be increasing in the US, but has only recently entered British discussions about needs for psychiatric services (Cantwell and Harrison, 1996). A survey among patients with in contact with the secondary mental health services has been carried out in Camberwell (Menezes et al, 1996), and has indicated a one year prevalence of evidence of a substance abuse problem of 36%, with an association between such 'dual diagnosis' and a longer hospital stay. Comparable data from other areas is not as yet available. This suggests that substance misuse may have a significant impact on severely mentally ill Londoners' needs for services, a possibility requiring further exploration.

3.4 London as an Extreme Metropolitan Area

The chapter gives multiple forms of evidence that, as a large urban area, London can expect to have a population with mental health needs at the upper end of the national range. How far are these needs extreme compared with other parts of England? We have shown that London has the single largest concentration of factors associated with psychiatric morbidity in the country, and that Londoners with mental illness are at risk of having multiple forms of clinical and social disadvantage. The sheer scale of the inner metropolitan area also means that inner city residents find access to work, social, and other facilities and services more difficult than if they lived in a socially deprived district within a smaller city. Overall, the demographic and epidemiological evidence points strongly to a substantially raised need for mental health services in the capital. We shall quantify the extent of this increase in Chapters 6, 7 and 8.

Acknowledgement
We are grateful to Richard Hamblyn of the King's Fund for preparing the maps for this chapter.

Chapter 4

London in the context of mental health policy

Paul Lelliott, Bernard Audini, Sonia Johnson and Hilary Guite

Summary

- London, together with the rest of England, is now in its fifth decade of moving towards a community-orientated mental health service.

- An accelerating series of statutory requirements and guidance documents has appeared over the last decade setting, a framework for mental health service provision and clinical practice.

- London's services have attracted unprecedented levels of public attention during this decade. A series of widely publicised reports have emphasised a group of common themes:

  - severe pressures on acute psychiatric beds
  - a requirement for further development of community based services
  - inadequate inter-agency collaboration
  - poorly developed services for minority ethnic groups
  - poor arrangements for care following discharge from hospital
  - incomplete assessments of risk
  - inadequacies in the numbers of residential care places.

- Several reports have highlighted particular difficulties experienced by patients who move address between different catchment areas, producing discontinuity in service contact.

- A crisis in recruitment and retention of mental health professionals appears to have developed in London and threatens to be one of the most serious problems faced by London's mental health services over the next ten years.

4.1 Introduction

'Mental health services are of interest not only because of the large burden they impose, but also because they have been subject to more change than virtually any other type of health service over the past four decades' (Raftery, 1992).

Because of radical changes in public health policy and in professionals' views of what constitutes a good service, mental health services in London have been in a state of transition for the past four decades, and remain so. In considering the service system in London it is thus essential to remember that it is not a system which has as yet achieved any period of equilibrium or stability – in the 1990s, professionals, managers and users in many parts of London have had to adjust to extensive changes in their local services and in national mental health policy almost on a yearly basis. In this section, we shall describe some of the forces driving these rapid changes and some of the previous commentaries on their effects on London. Section 4.2 begins by describing the national policy context in which London's services have developed. Policy initiatives particularly targeting London and reports on the state of the city's services will then be outlined in section 4.3. Finally, London's psychiatric services have been prominent in public awareness at various times in the 1990s because of a series of tragic incidents involving mentally ill people. In particular, homicides perpetrated by people with severe mental illness have been reported extensively in the media and may have had widespread negative effects on public attitudes to the mentally ill and to community care. The conclusions of the public inquiries which have followed these incidents in London will be discussed in section 4.4.

4.2 The national policy context: four decades of change

Mental health services in the UK are moving into the third stage of a progressive shift in the locus of patient care. The first stage was the decision, arising in the 1950s from reforms in the hospitals themselves, to reduce NHS bed numbers and close large psychiatric hospitals. The second, which reached its peak in the 1970s and 1980s, was the development of small local psychiatric units, often on district general hospital sites, with a limited range of community services to meet the needs of those who no longer required hospital accommodation.

The third stage, heralded by the white paper 'Caring for People: Community Care in the Next Decade and Beyond' (Department of Health, 1989a), is intended to divert people from community based residential services into their own homes.

The factors which precipitated these radical changes can be summarised as:

1   The focus of psychiatric care in large institutions, which often had restrictive regimes, did not accord with the social climate of the 1960s and 1970s which emphasised personal freedoms and rights. The anti-psychiatry movement reflected the mood of the time as it questioned not just the appropriateness of regarding psychiatry as a medical speciality but also the existence of mental illness itself.

2   A number of well-publicised scandals in the 1950s and 1960s which awakened public interest and concern at poor conditions and standards of care in some of these large institutions.

3   The demonstration, by pioneering social psychiatrists, of the feasibility of caring for people with severe mental illness in settings outside the large institutions. Later, understanding of the impact of family and social factors on relapse in severe mental illness, and the development of psychosocial interventions lessened the influence of those who advocated the primacy of physical treatments in medical settings.

4   The introduction of neuroleptic drugs, effective in reducing positive psychotic symptoms, which meant that some existing patients could be freed from the hallucinations and delusions hindering rehabilitation and resettlement, and that new episodes of illness could be shortened.

5   The (mistaken) political assumption that community care would be cheaper.

4.2.1 Key mental health policy and guidance, 1959-1996

The key changes in mental health policy and guidance accompanying the extensive changes in services over the past forty years will be summarised in this section. Section 6.2 supplements this with an account of changes in provision, service use and staffing over this period.

1959   **The Mental Health Act** (House of Commons, 1959) emphasises the hospital's role as a place for treatment and not merely custody. The Act places a duty on local authorities to provide residential and other services for the mentally ill.

1961   **Enoch Powell's 'water tower' speech** (Powell, 1961) states the government's intention to dismantle the asylums.

1962   **The Ministry of Health's 'Hospital Plan for England and Wales'** (Ministry of Health, 1962) predicts that by the early 1970s the requirement for psychiatric beds would have fallen by about 50% (to 180 per 100,000).

1970   **The Local Authority Social Services Bill** (House of Commons, 1970) makes the new local authority social services departments responsible for providing personal social services for the mentally ill. This creates a split between health and social functions which previously have been interactive.

1972   **A departmental circular (Circular 35/72)** gives planning guidelines for 12,000 residential places for the mentally ill in the community.

1975   **The white paper 'Better Services for the Mentally Ill'** (Department of Health and Social Security, 1975) sets out the government's four broad policy objectives for mental health services: i. an expansion of local authority personal social services; ii. the relocation of specialist services to local settings; iii. the establishment of good organisational links between settings and agencies; iv. a significant improvement in staffing to enable multi-professional assessment of needs and earlier intervention and prevention.

1983 **The revised Mental Health Act (Department of Health and Welsh Office, 1983)** brings the legislation relating to detention of mentally ill people more into line with the principles of community care and reinforces the rights of mentally ill people.

1985 **The Social Services Committee (Department of Health and Social Security, 1985)** restates the elements that make up the comprehensive district service. It also refers indirectly to aspects of the development of community care that were progressing slowly: these include poor provision for new long-stay patients, failure to provide new facilities before old ones are closed and the difficulty in releasing money from hospital closures.

1989/90 **The White Paper 'Caring for People: Community Care in the Next Decade and Beyond' and the NHS and Community Care Act – implemented in 1993** (Department of Health, 1989a; House of Commons, 1990) makes local authorities the lead community care agency from April 1993. Two key objectives are to promote services to support people living in their own homes wherever feasible and to encourage 'the development of a flourishing independent sector alongside good quality public provision'. Local authorities have a duty to assess the needs of individuals and, through the development of a care plan, the services to meet these.

1990 NHS guidance on the **Care Programme Approach** is intended 'to provide a network of care in the community' which will minimise the risk that people with severe mental illness lose contact with services (Department of Health, 1990). The introduction of the CPA reinforces the message that before patients are discharged from psychiatric hospital services should ensure that 'proper arrangements are made for their return home and for any continuing care'.

1991 The **'Reed Report'** emphasises that mentally disordered offenders should, if appropriate, receive care and treatment from health and social services rather than in custodial care (Department of Health and Home Office, 1991).

1992 Mental illness is one of the five Key Areas in the white paper '**The Health of the Nation: a Strategy for Health in England**' (Department of Health, 1992a), whose stated objective is to 'reduce ill health and death from mental illness'. Three main targets are set: i. to improve significantly the health and social functioning of mentally ill people;

ii. to reduce the overall suicide rate by at least 15% by the year 2000; and iii. to reduce the suicide rate of severely mentally ill people by at least 33% by the year 2000.

1993   As the final phase of the implementation of the NHS and Community Care Act, **money is transferred from the Department of Social Security to local authorities social services departments**. From April 1993, local authorities become responsible for assessing needs of new applicants and for funding the residential placements of those who cannot afford fees. They are expected to become 'enabling authorities' with a purchasing and contracting role, rather than acting solely as direct providers. It is hoped that a 'mixed economy of care' will result, making use of voluntary and private providers. This will be catalysed by the requirement that local authorities spend 85% of the DSS transfer element of their community care grant in the independent sector. There is an expectation that a considerable proportion of the DSS transfer will be spent on the development of day and domiciliary services as an alternative to residential care.

1993   The secretary of state announces a '**10-point plan**' for developing successful and safe community care of discharged psychiatric patients' (Department of Health Press Release H93/908)

1994   The introduction of **supervision registers for mentally ill people** from April 1st 1994 is announced (NHS Executive, 1994a), requiring all health authorities to ensure that provider units identify, and give priority to, patients at significant risk of suicide, of doing serious harm to others, or of serious self-neglect.

1994   Following the publication of the **Ritchie Report** into the care of Christopher Clunis (Ritchie, Dick and Lingham, 1994), the Department of Health issues further guidance on the discharge of mentally disordered people, emphasising that 'no patient should be discharged from hospital unless those taking the decisions are satisfied that he or she can live safely in the community, and that proper supervision and care are available' (NHS Executive, 1994b).

1996   The **Mental Health Act (Patients in the Community)** is passed.

1996   In 1996, the **Mental Health Patients' Charter** is published.

1996   The NHS issues guidance that health authorities should commission more **24-hour nursed beds** for mentally ill people (NHS Executive, HSG (96)6).

4.3 London's mental health services: reports and initiatives

Accompanying the national policy developments outlined above, a series of reports, inquiries and policy initiatives has focused specifically on London, some dealing with health services in general, some with mental health in particular. This reflects a persisting concern that London has a particular set of problems, different in kind and degree from elsewhere because of the current state of its services and the extremity of need encountered particularly in the inner areas (discussed in Chapter 3).

Public concern with the increasing numbers of people sleeping rough in parts of Central London was reflected in the government's announcement of the Homeless Mentally Ill Initiative in June 1990. This was a £20 million initiative, including up to 150 specialist hostel places. Kingdon and Jenkins (1996) report that developments under this initiative have been the opening of five hostels, plans for several further hostels, and the development of five multidisciplinary community psychiatric teams which provide outreach, support to hostels and in resettlement.

In 1992, both the Tomlinson report (Department of Health 1992b) and the Kings Fund Commission (1992) reported on London's health services in general. Both emphasised a need to strengthen London's primary and community care structure, and both suggested that in general the outer ring of the capital has been under-resourced compared with the centre. Of considerable relevance to planning of mental health care was the Tomlinson report's finding that standards in primary care in the capital seemed dangerously inadequate, with 46% of general practices reported to be 'below minimum standards'. Commenting specifically on mental health, Tomlinson emphasised the need to develop fully resourced community teams responsible for both acute and continuing care, backed by a range of sheltered accommodation and day care close to patients' homes.

The Tomlinson report was followed at the beginning of 1993 by the setting up of LIG (London Implementation Group), as an initiative to promote radical changes in London's health service, with a large-scale shift of resources towards primary and community care. As described in 'Making London Better' (Department of Health, 1993c), £170 million expenditure was planned within the London Implementation Zone (LIZ), including £75 million for pump-priming voluntary sector developments. LIG included a mental health reference group, which aimed to encourage a range of primary and secondary care community developments, and to promote strategic purchasing. LIG continues to be a source of specific funding for mental health developments in London – information collated by the King's Fund indicates that in 1995/6 LIG moneys funded 81 projects concerned with mental health, making up a total mental health expenditure of just under £10 million. This has supported a variety of community projects, with home-based care, mental health workers within primary care and day care prominent on the 1995/6 list. A fuller discussion of LIG funding and its effects on London's mental health services is found in section 5.8 of this report.

Two of the most highly publicised incidents involving people with mental illnesses occurred around this time. In December 1992, Christopher Clunis, an individual with paranoid schizophrenia, stabbed to death Jonathan Zito, a complete stranger, on Finsbury Park tube station platform. This led to a highly publicised public inquiry (Ritchie et al, 1994, see next section), and the setting up of a Trust by Jonathan Zito's widow Jayne Zito, which has campaigned vigorously for various improvements and changes in London's psychiatric services. At the beginning of 1993, Ben Silcock, also diagnosed as having schizophrenia, climbed into the lions' den at London Zoo and was mauled.

The Ritchie inquiry described Clunis's care as 'a catalogue of failure'. The report's many recommendations included needs for improvement in care planning and in inter-agency working, for all keyworkers to be trained staff, for highly intensive care to be available for the most difficult to manage individuals, for advocacy services, for a greater range of residential care, for better and more clearly recorded assessments of risk, and for greater attention to making services appropriate for ethnic minorities.

Following this, extra expenditure of £10 million was announced for London services, with funding for 170 more medium secure beds in the Thames regions before 1995. In February 1994, the Mental Health Task Force was commissioned by ministers to report on London's mental health services (Department of Health, 1994a; Moore, 1996). Their report encompassed the 12 purchasing authorities within LIZ and drew on visits and collection of a variety of data about service activities. Major recommendations from their report included:

- Pressures on acute beds needed to be addressed, with a reduction in the out of district placements which were draining resources from local facilities. Solutions to this problem would involve commissioning more beds in some health authorities, but would also be likely to require bed management strategies and alternatives to admission, including accommodation with 24-hour skilled staffing. A better understanding was required of the causes of pressures on beds.
- Further development of community based support was required, including housing, social support, day time opportunities and outreach.
- Inter-agency collaboration between health service, social services and other key agencies needed to be improved.
- Services needed to become more responsive to the needs of members of ethnic minorities.
- Plans for closure of long stay hospitals and reprovision should be reviewed to ensure that timetables were manageable: 'Before agreeing to further closures of psychiatric beds, DHAs must satisfy themselves that demonstrably effective alternative services have been established.'
- Some innovative services did seem to be highly successful in meeting local needs – examples identified included the TULIP team providing intensive community outreach and support in Haringey, St Mary's early intervention service, the Feathers Project (a work scheme in Greenwich), the Star Centre drop-in in Hounslow and the Forward Project which provides residential care and psychotherapy services targeting black service users in Hammersmith. MISG (the ring-fenced Mental Illness Specific Grant, available to all local authorities nationally for mental health service development since 1991) funding seemed to be a successful way of promoting some such initiatives.
- Spending on mental health services varied very widely between authorities, in ways that could not always be readily explained in terms of variations in levels of need.

The Task Force agreed specific six month action plans with each purchaser, and then worked with them on the implementation of these. A follow up report after six months (Department of Health 1995b) reviewed progress on these plans. It concluded that in general some progress had been made, with reports of better collaboration between health services and local authorities, prioritisation of severe mental illness, increased availability of community support in some areas, some improvements in the availability of ethnically sensitive services and some increases in bed numbers.

In 1995, a Ministerial review was carried out of current and planned Health Authority purchasing throughout the UK. Ten out of sixteen London authorities were judged to have comprehensive plans for development of local services – a figure slightly better than the national average. Following this, a further allocation of additional mental health funding was announced early in 1996 – the Challenge Fund is intended to speed up service development in those health authorities which were above resource allocation targets or had furthest to go in implementing comprehensive local services. This makes available approximately three and a half million pounds for London (NHS Executive, 1996b), to fund a variety of hostels, community and crisis services, and one employment scheme. This central funding is to be matched by the health authorities pound for pound. Seven of the London purchasing authorities have been awarded funding from this initiatives – the amounts vary widely from around £100,000 in Merton Sutton & Wandsworth to nearly a million and a half in Lambeth, Southwark and Lewisham, the largest purchasing authority.

In early 1996, the NHS Trust Federation's Mental Health and Learning Disability Committee produced a report addressing inner city mental health in general, but focusing particularly on London. Major recommendations emerging from this report include:

- That pressures on acute psychiatric beds in London must be relieved: an emergency bed service is proposed as a means of helping resolve this, by providing immediate London-wide information on bed availability.
- That clear targets should be set and implemented in every area for acceptable bed occupancy and acceptable access to acute, intensive care and medium secure beds.
- That the development of alternatives to hospital services should be encouraged.
- That out of hours crisis services require improvements.
- That agreements should be reached on appropriate caseloads for keyworkers for the CPA and supervision register.

In August 1996, the NHS Executive published a briefing paper on London's mental health services (NHS Executive 1996b). This summarises previous developments in London's services and the major issues which have been raised, including pressure on acute beds, high rates of mentally ill offenders and homelessness, and the need to strengthen primary care involvement. It also gives a number of case studies of innovative services which are apparently providing community-based services effectively in London.

Many of the concerns discussed in these two recently published reports are ones which have been raised in previous reports. However, both highlight one important issue which is not prominent in previous work – both draw attention to very serious difficulties now arising in London in recruiting and retaining mental health professionals of all disciplines. Many services are reported to have levels of agency and other non-permanent staff over 20% of total complement, with shortages of psychiatric nurses, psychologists, occupational therapists and psychiatrists of all grades. A similar concern with 'burnout' among mental health staff is beginning to appear in the research literature – Audini et al (1994) suggested that staff demoralisation was one of the major reasons why an innovative community service in inner London failed to sustain its initial good outcomes, and Prosser et al (1996) have recently found high levels of 'burnout' and poor psychological health among community mental health staff in three South London sector teams. Reasons for difficulties in recruitment and for high staff turnover are not as yet well understood, and research on the causes of this crisis is needed as a matter of urgency. Making jobs in London more attractive and improving staff support so as to prevent 'burnout' is likely to be one of the major future challenges for mental health service providers in London. It is also remarkable that this crisis has developed against a background of high levels of unemployment, so consideration should be given to the potential role of local training initiatives in staffing London's mental health services.

4.4 Key recommendations from recent London enquiries, inquiries and reports

In the decade from 1978 to 1988 there was only one independent inquiry into a homicide in the UK by someone with a mental illness. Sheppard's (1996) compilation for the Zito Trust of inquiry reports includes 26 reports on homicides published in the UK between 1988 and 1996, of which 11 related principally to London services. Since 1994 Health Authorities have been advised to carry out an independent inquiry in all cases of homicide where the offender has been in contact with specialist psychiatric services. Table 1 lists major London inquiry reports published since 1988.

Reports from such inquiries provide valuable information in the form of detailed accounts of how systems of care can work or fail in practice. Many of the recommendations have been reiterated in successive inquiries, and, as shown in section 5.6 (mentally disordered offenders), there are close resemblances between the results of the first of these inquiries, the inquiry into the care of Sharon Campbell and the inquiry into the care of Christopher Clunis published several years later. During this period, a series of reports on the state of the nation's health services has also appeared and made sometime similar recommendations. Major reports of the 1990s have been:

- Better off in the Community: the Care of People who are Seriously Mentally Ill (House of Commons Health Select Committee, 1994a)
- Priorities for Action (Department of Health, 1994a)
- Finding a Place: a Review of Mental Health Services for Adults (Audit Commission, 1994a)
- One in Ten: Report into Suicide and Unnatural Deaths (National Schizophrenia Fellowship, 1995)
- Report of the Confidential Inquiry into Homicides and Suicides by Mentally Ill People (Royal College of Psychiatrists 1996)

Table 1 Published homicide inquiries in London 1985–1996

Year	Principal author	Title	Authorities	Victim
1988	Spokes	Report of the Inquiry into the care and aftercare of Sharon Campbell	Bexley HA	social worker
1992	Collins	The Independent Inquiry into Kevin Rooney	North East Thames HA	former patient known to Rooney killed at her home
1992	Langley	Findings of the Independent Review on the management of the case of Erieyune Inweh	Kingston & Richmond	voluntary worker at hostel
1994	Ritchie	Report of the Inquiry into the care and aftercare of Christopher Clunis	South East & North East Thames HA	stranger
1994	Higginbotham	Report of the Inquiry examining the care of Michael Buchanan	North West Brent	stranger
1994	Gabbott	Inquiry into the deaths of Jason and Natalia Harry	Haringey Child Protection Committee	her two children
1994	Woodley	The Woodley team report	East London & City HA, Newham Council	stranger (another patient at a day centre)
1995	Hughes	The Independent panel of inquiry into the circumstances surrounding the death of Ellen and Alan Boland	North West London HA	mother
1995	Mishcon	The Independent Inquiry into the care and treatment of Kenneth Grey	East London and City HA	mother
1995	Mishcon	The Hampshire Report	Redbridge & Waltham Forest HA	wife
1996	Main	Report of the Independent Inquiry team into the care and treatment of NG	Ealing, Hammersmith & Hounslow HA London Borough of Hounslow	stranger

The following list is a synthesis of the most frequently recurring major themes emerging from the general reports on mental health services and from five of the enquiries on homicides (those led by Collins, Higginbotham, Ritchie, Woodley and Hughes). The numbers in brackets below indicate the number of separate reports in which they figure (maximum = 10).

Theme 1: **Poor communication between agencies (7)**; particularly between health and social services (5), between mental health services and housing departments (3) and between specialist mental health services and GPs (3). A related theme to this is that of poor joint working (4) which is at all levels from commissioning and strategy (2) to multi-disciplinary care delivery (3).

Theme 2: **Problems with discharge from hospital (5).** This particularly relates to failure to follow Section 117 procedures, assess need, develop an aftercare plan and communicate this adequately to other agencies.

Theme 3: **Poor assessment of risk of violence (6).** This emphasises particularly the need for better and more training in risk assessment (4) and the importance of disclosure of risk factors to those with a need to know.

Theme 4: **Liaison with police and probation services (5).** This relates both to the involvement of police in receiving or providing information about people receiving care from mental health services (2) and the need for greater involvement of mental health care workers in diversion from custody services (3).

Theme 5: **Confidentiality and professional ethics (4).** These are reported as barriers particularly between health and social services (2) and between mental health services and the police (2).

Theme 6: **Adequacy and allocation of resources (9).** The inadequacy of, or the need to protect, numbers of residential care places in London (including hospital beds) is a common theme (8). Specific mention is made of short-stay admission beds (4), medium secure provision (4), and the importance of maintaining a wide range of community-based residential services (4) with DoH guidance on levels of provision. Comment is also made on the inadequacy of numbers of community workers (2) and of provision of day care services (2). Allocation of resources is commented on both between competing groups e.g. children, elderly etc. (1), between health and social care (1), between areas of high and low need (2) and for the targeting of the most severely ill (3); as is the need for bridging money or ring-fencing of money as services move from a hospital to a community focus (2).

4.2.5 Conclusion

London's mental health services, like those in the rest of the country, have been in a state of transition for the past forty years. A series of recent reports, initiatives and inquiries focusing specifically on London reflect a widespread concern that successful implementation of national policy and attainment of the standards of mental health care now viewed as acceptable have been especially difficult in the city. Many of the reports have commented on the extreme demographic characteristics of London and their effect in making it more difficult to meet demands and needs. Several recurrent themes are identifiable in the reports and enquiries: the importance of effective inter-agency working, the need to develop fully a range of community services, the pressure on acute beds and lack of alternatives to admission; the difficulties services have in engaging and meeting the needs of members of ethnic minorities; weaknesses in primary care provision and in links between primary and secondary care; and finally, the apparently high level of effectiveness achieved by a small number of innovative community services scattered around the city. A further difficulty coming to prominence in recent reports is in attracting and retaining mental health professionals of all disciplines in this hard-pressed inner city environment. A striking feature of this series of documents has been the tendency for the same difficulties to be reported and the same recommendations to be repeated year after year through the 1990s, suggesting that the effectiveness of initiatives following the earlier reports may have been limited.

Chapter 5

Special areas of need for mental health services

Introduction

Whilst most other sections of this report focus either on mental health service delivery in London in general or on services for younger adults (18 to 65 years), this chapter seeks to redress the balance by discussing some groups with specific needs for mental health services. Some of these groups, such as children and the elderly, are served by specific psychiatric sub-specialties, whilst others, such as members of ethnic minority groups, are the concern of professionals across all the specialties within psychiatry.

Nine experts or groups of experts on different areas of need were asked to write reports on service provision in their field. The groups of service users represented were the elderly, children and adolescents, substance misusers, people with HIV infections and AIDS, mentally disordered offenders, members of ethnic minority communities, the homeless, general hospital patients in need of consultation-liaison psychiatric services, and people who receive services at a primary care level. Each expert provides an overview of the area, including both general historical development and policy initiatives; and recent developments, including recent changes in service provision, the current state of services and any particular difficulties being encountered.

Chapter 5.1

Mental health services for older people in London

Michael Philpot and Sube Banerjee

Summary

- There is evidence of considerable progress over the past two decades in developing old age psychiatry as a profession and appropriate services for older people with mental illnesses in London.
- However, considerable variation remains across the city. There are examples of innovative services which maximise autonomy and provide high levels of home support, enabling patients to remain in their own homes as long as possible without excessive strain for informal carers. However, this quality and intensity of care cannot be matched in all parts of London.
- There is a relative dearth of community residential accommodation in London, with private sector provision in particular having grown less quickly in London than elsewhere. This appears to be leading to the 'export' of elderly people to Outer London boroughs and beyond, cutting them off from familiar surroundings and social networks.
- For the 65 to 74 age group, admission rates are higher in Inner London than in Outer London, other large cities or the rest of the country, but rates over 75 are lower than in other large cities or the rest of the country. Admission rates specifically for organic disorders are also relatively low. Possible reasons for these lower rates in the oldest groups and among people with dementia include competition for resources from younger age groups, lack of intensive social care elsewhere in the country, and the 'export' of the frail elderly from London.

Possible strategies which may increase the effectiveness of services for older mentally ill people include:

- Developing the role of 'trained carers' (employed by the NHS), who can assist in the practical day-to-day support of mentally ill elderly people in London.
- Expanding the use of care management (as exemplified by the Lewisham care management scheme described in this section), possibly by diverting part of the budget identified for residential and nursing home placements.
- Developing the use of full multi-disciplinary teams.
- Commissioning evaluative research into old age psychiatry provision, so that service development is led by evidence rather than by dogma.

5.1.1. Historical development

(i) United Kingdom

Specialist services for the elderly mentally ill developed in London as in the rest of the country from services provided in the county or borough asylums. Until the late 1960s, the elderly mentally ill were cared for largely as in-patients in these hospitals, or in out-patient clinics based in general hospitals. Care for elderly people with mental illness was not differentiated from that of other patients with mental illness, and general psychiatrists managed both groups. Patients suffering from chronic or progressive disorders who could not be discharged were transferred to the long-stay or back wards.

The pioneers of psychogeriatrics were motivated by a number of factors: the increasing need for psychiatric care for the elderly as a result of the increase in life expectancy, growing knowledge about late onset mental disorders, and the success of geriatric medicine (Wattis, 1994). The separation of mental health care for the elderly from that for other adults seems to have had its roots in a need to overcome institutional age-related prejudice and the identification of dementia with old age rather than in any biological imperative (Murphy & Banerjee, 1993). In addition, Jolley (1995) has pointed out that the speciality developed without the use of randomised controlled trials of treatment methods or service structures. In reality it grew from a pragmatic approach based on a passionate advocacy for the patient group and a struggle to identify funding and facilities. As a result many services in the UK and abroad have been based on a blueprint that seemed to work rather than adopting a scientifically evaluated service model.

During the early 1970s a London-based group of psychogeriatricians, now known as the 'Coffee House' group, started to meet regularly to discuss service developments and research. This formed the basis of the old age group of the Royal College of Psychiatrists (founded in 1973) and the specialist section of the College (founded in 1978). Ultimately, this group worked to the formal recognition of old age psychiatry as a speciality within the NHS (1989). During the late 1970s it had become health service policy to provide at least one psychogeriatric consultant in each district. The number of psychogeriatricians in the UK has steadily grown from 20 in 1973 to just over 370 in 1992 (Banerjee et al., 1993). Tom Arie was the first psychogeriatrician awarded a chair when he became a professor of health care of the elderly at Nottingham in 1979.

(ii) London

Aubrey Lewis first identified the need for special facilities for elderly patients with mental illness and in 1949 set up Gresham ward at the Bethlem Royal Hospital for the care of 40 patients with functional psychiatric illness over the age of 60. This was possibly the first such unit in the UK. Felix Post was appointed as the consultant responsible for these patients. He studied the characteristics and course of mental illness in the elderly and was a major influence on the training of future generations of psychogeriatricians.

A survey of three mental hospitals in London covering the late 1940s and 1950s (Norris, 1959) makes grim reading. The author found that there was a very high death rate in patients with dementia, and survival and discharge from hospital were more likely in patients with depression or mania. Overall, mortality rates were higher in men but women tended to become long-stay patients. There was a lack of precision in diagnosing dementia and cases of acute confusion, and affective disorders were often misdiagnosed leading to therapeutic nihilism.

The first comprehensive psychogeriatric service was probably that at Goodmayes Hospital, set up in 1969. This was certainly the first to have clearly identified aims and principles and it introduced an important community component. The principles were easy accessibility and flexibility, home-based assessment by a senior doctor, good communication with GPs and other specialists, and an emphasis on improving and maintaining staff morale (Arie, 1970). During the year following the introduction of the service (which catered for an enormous population of 42,000 elderly people) there was a 20% increase in admissions, a 70% increase in discharges and a 25% reduction in deaths. The resources which made this possible led to the development of 'norms' for bed numbers and personnel which are described in more detail below.

Service developments continued during the 1970s although there is a dearth of descriptive or statistical literature. Examining returns made to the Mental Health Enquiry, only 14 out of 55 hospitals in London with mental health units reported having old age psychiatry wards, accounting for 269 (1%) of the total 27,299 beds available (DHSS, 1985). While these figures may be subject to significant reporting bias, they do indicate the relatively undeveloped nature of specialist old age psychiatry services at the time. A small survey carried out in 1983 in London found that at least seven districts (out of 20 who replied to the survey [total =31]) had no consultant specialist and only six had specific beds for the elderly mentally ill. The author's conclusion was that 'London districts virtually all appear to have poor services for their psychogeriatric patients' (Cunningham, 1983). Reanalysing data collected in a national survey of old age psychiatrists, Banerjee et al. (1993) reported that by 1992 there were 51 consultants in London working full or part-time in old age psychiatry.

Academic developments paralleled those in the clinical field with Elaine Murphy being appointed the first professor of psychogeriatrics in the UK at Guy's Hospital, and shortly after Raymond Levy and Brice Pitt were appointed to similar posts at the Institute of Psychiatry and St Mary's Hospital respectively.

(iii) Routinely collected data on psychiatric services for the over 65s

The use of routinely collected data to examine old age psychiatry provision and activity in London is problematic. First, the methods of data collection and presentation have changed frequently over the last 20 years making longitudinal comparisons difficult. Second, the present system of hospital episode statistics (HES) cannot separate geriatric, general psychiatric and old age psychiatric episodes (Department of Health, personal communication). Also, the data generated for 1987/8 and 1988/9 are of such poor quality that they are unusable and subsequent publications have concentrated on 'finished consultant episodes' rather than admissions and discharges. Third, there is generally no separation of older people on general/long stay/rehabilitation units from those in specialist old age psychiatry services so that data can only be presented by age group rather than by service used. Fourth, the Mental Health Enquiry (MHE), which functioned up to 1986, and subsequent government publications have separated variables such as admissions, residence and discharge by region rather than by district. London data are therefore embedded in a combination of the four Thames regions.

Given the marked differences between London and the rest of south east England, a presentation of combined Thames data is no more likely to give an accurate representation of the situation in London than data for the whole of England.

In spite of these difficulties, routinely collected data can aid understanding of the importance of psychiatric service provision for those aged over 65 years. As there is unlikely to be an age-related statistical bias in data collection, useful comparative data can be generated. We therefore present data on first admissions and readmissions to psychiatric units, by age, for England as a whole.

(iv) First admission to mental illness hospitals and units

Table 1 presents the numbers of first admissions to mental illness hospitals and units in England by age group from 1956 to 1986.

Table 1 Mental illness hospitals and units in England, first admissions (thousands) by age group 1956–1986

	1956	1960	1964	1968	1972	1976	1980	1984	1986
0–64	33.4	40.8	56.9	67.9	45.3	41.5	36.2	34.8	32.5
65+	11.0	14.1	19.3	20.7	14.8	15.6	16.8	19.0	19.1
65–74	6.0	7.0	9.1	9.8	6.8	6.8	6.9	6.6	6.6
75–	5.0	7.1	10.2	10.9	8.0	8.8	9.9	12.2	12.6
Total	44.5	54.9	76.2	88.6	60.1	57.1	53.0	53.8	51.7
% 65+	25%	26%	25%	23%	25%	27%	32%	35%	37%

Sources

1956: The Registrar General's Statistical Review of England and Wales for the three years 1954, 1955 and 1956. Supplement on Mental Health. London, HMSO, 1960.

1960: The Registrar General's Statistical Review of England and Wales, 1960. Supplement on Mental Health. London, HMSO, 1964.

1964: Ministry of Health. Inpatient Statistics for the Mental Health Enquiry for the years 1964, 1965 and 1966. Psychiatric Hospitals and Units in England and Wales. Statistical Report Series No. 4. London, HMSO, 1968.

1968: Ministry of Health. Inpatient Statistics for the Mental Health Enquiry for the year 1970. London, HMSO, 1972.

1972-80: Department of Health and Social Security. Inpatient statistics from the Mental Health Enquiry for England, 1982. London, HMSO, 1985.

1984-86: Department of Health and Social Security. Mental health statistics for England, booklet 12: mental illness hospitals and units, diagnostic data. London, HMSO, 1988.

In absolute terms more new admissions during the time period were in the 75 to 84 age group than in any other age group, accounting for around a fifth of all new admissions. The over 65s made up just over a third of all new admissions by 1986 compared with a quarter in 1956.

The age-specific rate of first admission per 100,000 population was also strikingly age-related with an increase from between 102 and 111 per 100,000 for age groups between 20 and 64 to 151 for the 65 to 74 group, 341 for the 75 to 84 group and 504 for those aged 85 or more. These age specific rates were stable from 1972 to 1982.

(v) Readmissions to mental illness hospitals and units
Table 2 presents data for readmissions to mental illness hospitals and units in England by age group from 1956 to 1986.

Table 2 Mental illness hospitals and units in England, re-admissions (thousands) by age group 1956-1986

	1956	1960	1964	1968	1972	1976	1980	1984	1986
0–64	25.7	44.1	70.4	71.7	94.8	98.0	94.2	96.7	97.6
65+	8.7	8.3	12.2	13.5	20.3	23.7	33.0	41.8	47.9
65–74	4.7	6.1	8.4	8.9	12.7	14.0	17.1	18.7	20.9
75–	4.0	2.2	3.8	4.6	7.6	9.7	15.9	23.1	41.7
Total	34.4	52.4	82.7	85.1	115.0	121.5	127.2	138.4	145.6
% 65+	25%	16%	15%	16%	18%	20%	26%	30%	33%

Sources: as in Table 1

Again it is clear that there has been a steady increase in the over 65s, both in terms of absolute numbers and in the proportion of all admissions (except for 1956 when the total number of readmissions is low). Between 1960 and 1972 the proportion of over 65s stayed fairly constant but in the years between 1972 and 1986 the proportion of readmissions aged 65 or over almost doubled from 18 to 33%.

As with first admissions, the age specific rate of readmission per 100,000 population is powerfully age-related with a steady increase from 337 per 100,000 for the 25 to 35 age group up to 378 per 100,000 for the 55 to 64 age group. After this there is a sharp rise to 428 for the 65 to 74 group, 684 for the 75 to 84 group and 810 for those aged 85 or more. Over the 10 year period from 1972 to 1982 the age specific rates for the over 65 age group increased each year in comparison with younger age groups which remained relatively stable.

A further insight into the impact of the elderly is provided by a consideration of the data on all admissions to mental illness hospitals and units for 1982. Again the same pattern is observed with rates (per 100,000 population) between 458 and 499 for those aged 25 to 64 and then a rise to 579 for the 65 to 74 group, 1,024 for the 75 to 84 group and 1,314 for the over 85 group.

(vi) Trends in service use

These data help to clarify the relative importance of mental health problems in the elderly compared with younger people. Those over 65 years account for a substantial proportion of all new admissions and all readmissions. Up to 1986 these proportions were increasing. In terms of resident patients in mental illness hospitals and units in 1982, 38,745 out of a total of 70,881 were aged 65 or over, 55% of the whole hospital population. Age-specific rates also increased with age. Subsequent comparison is hampered by difficulties with central data collection and analysis (but see section 5.1.4). However the importance of the elderly as consumers of psychiatric resources is clear.

5.1.2. Policy initiatives

(i) General developments

The 1962 Hospital Plan provided the impetus to reduce the numbers of beds for mental illness and this undoubtedly stimulated the development of alternative forms of residential provision for elderly patients with chronic or progressive mental disorders. The recommendations of the Seebohm committee (1968), the formation of the Hospital (later Health) Advisory Service (1969), the reorganisation of the NHS in 1974 and 1982, and the Mental Health Act (1983) all had important effects on psychiatric and social services which were not exclusive to the elderly.

During the past 10 years a number of government initiatives have been more specifically relevant to old age psychiatry. 'Caring for People' (Secretaries of State, 1989) emphasised the need for health purchasers to give priority to the development of day care and day respite services, practical support for carers, proper assessments of need and case management.

The introduction of the Care Programme Approach (Department of Health, 1990) is of particular relevance to the elderly as the criteria include a history of self-neglect which is very often a feature of patients with moderate to severe dementia and those with severe functional illnesses. To date, there have been no published accounts of the application of CPA registers in elderly mentally ill populations although local experience suggests variability in the numbers of patients included on registers, even within relatively small districts (Maudsley Hospital, 1996).

Lastly, 'NHS Responsibilities for Meeting Continuing Health Care Needs' (Department of Health, 1995c) sets out the requirement that by 1/4/96 local and health authorities should have consulted and drawn up eligibility criteria determining which patients are entitled to continuing care funded by or provided in NHS facilities. The criteria are to have been negotiated locally suggesting that there could be considerable geographical variation. Decisions on individual patients are intended to be made on a multidisciplinary, multi-agency basis. A local appeals procedure should have been set up to enable patients or their representatives to challenge the decision-making process (i.e. whether the correct procedure was followed in arriving at the decision to discharge a patient rather than keep them in hospital). It is too soon to know what practical effects this new requirement will have but it could well lead to greater delays in discharging elderly patients from acute hospital beds, and more time for professionals spent in attending meetings, writing reports and defending their decisions.

(ii) Defining the patient group

'Services for Mental Illness Related to Old Age' (Department of Health and Social Security, 1972) identified three groups among the elderly mentally ill: patients who had entered mental hospitals before modern methods of treatment were available and had grown old in them, elderly patients with functional mental illness, and elderly patients with dementia. The first group were largely cared for by general psychiatrists until the 1960s and 1970s when the first consultant psychogeriatricians were appointed. Many patients (particularly those who had developed dementia during their long stay in hospital) were then transferred to psychogeriatric care but a substantial proportion of these 'graduates' remained under the care of general psychiatrists. This has an impact on our ability to determine the resources available to the elderly mentally ill between the 1950s and the 1970s as bed numbers were identified by the specialism of the consultant responsible while patients (i.e. their admissions, discharges and deaths) were classified by age and diagnosis.

(iii) Levels of service provision

'Hospital Services for the Mentally Ill' (DHSS, 1971) included the first guidance on the level of service provision, in terms of beds and day-places, for elderly patients with a functional mental illness and this was expanded on in a subsequent report 'Services for Mental Illness Related to Old Age' (DHSS, 1972). These figures are shown in Table 3.

Table 3 Recommendations for service provision

	DHSS[1]	Royal College of Psychiatrists[2]
Consultants		1 WTE/22,000

Acute assessment beds:
   Functional illness
   Dementia
   Total
	0.5/1000	0.5/1000
		1.0/1000
		1.5/1000

Continuing Care beds:
   Functional illness
   Dementia
   Total
	2.5-3/1000	0.17/1000
		2.5-3/1000
		2.67-3.17/1000

Day Hospital places:
   Functional Illness
   Dementia
   Total
	0.65/1000
	2-3/1000
	2.65-3.65/1000
		0.65/1000
		2-3/1000
		2.65-3.65/1000

Community Psychiatric Nurses	-	1/5000
Occupational Therapists	-	1/10,000
Psychologists	-	1/20,000
Physiotherapists	-	1/20,000

Sources: 1 Department of Health and Social Security (1971, 1972).
                 2 Royal College of Psychiatrists (1987).

The Hospital Advisory Service report 'The Rising Tide' (1982) reflected the concern expressed in the previous two circulars and set out the principles on which services should be planned. In 1987, the Royal College of Psychiatrists issued a set of guidelines to be used by college regional advisors in assessing the acceptability of service provision associated with new consultant posts (see Table 3). As can be seen, these were virtually unchanged from the figures published in 1972. Recently, the section of old age psychiatry within the Royal College of Psychiatrists has proposed that full-time consultants in teaching hospital districts (i.e. most of London) should be responsible for a *maximum of 10,000* over 65 year olds.

As Cooper (1991) has pointed out, the norms given above were largely based on 'contemporary standards of provision rather than … any independent estimation of the scale of need'.

(iv) Joint Facilities
The report 'Psychogeriatric Assessment Units' (DHSS, 1970) advocated the setting up of wards managed jointly by geriatricians and psychogeriatricians. The concept was that patients with delirium and acute onset or deterioration of dementia, or those in whom mental and physical problems were interrelated would benefit from joint management. The reality has been that in spite of successful examples (at St. Pancras and Goodmayes Hospitals which did not survive the 1980s) these joint facilities have not been developed in most districts.

'Organisational and Management Problems of Mental Illness Hospitals' (Hospital Advisory Service, 1980), usually known as the 'Nodder Report', drew attention to the difficulty of admitting elderly people to general psychiatric hospital units. The authors suggested that the 'long-stay demented' did not need hospital care and could be looked after in small nursing-home units, such as those in the Lewisham domus scheme (Lindesay et al, 1991) but not, on the whole, taken up in other parts of London where larger units have been favoured (for example, Handysides, 1993).

(v) Professional issues
In 1979 the Royal College of Psychiatrists and the British Geriatric Society issued 'Guidelines for Collaboration between Geriatric Physicians and Psychiatrists in the Care of the Elderly'. These were updated in 1992 (Murdoch and Montgomery, 1992) but remained essentially the same. The principles outlined were that liaison between specialities should be programmed into job descriptions and plans, procedures for quick and easy access to assessments with 'smooth' transfer of patients if necessary, co-operation and collaboration which should include all members of the multi-disciplinary team, reciprocal training in each other's speciality and joint involvement in service planning. These are issues of some importance as disagreements about whose clinical responsibility an elderly person might be can lead to disruption of care and be a source of frustration to outside agencies.

5.1.3 The development of a mixed economy of care
(i) Service organisation
Informal enquiries suggest that all London districts now have at least one specialist old age psychiatry consultant post and that the care of the elderly mentally ill is increasingly carried out by single-speciality doctors rather than those whose clinical time is split between old age and general psychiatry. However, as of 1/10/96, 20% of the posts in south London were either vacant or filled by long-term locums.

Most services cater for patients over the age of 65 years (in some cases, over 70 or 75 years). The age boundary is important as it alters the resultant case-mix: the later the boundary, the greater the proportion of cases of dementia. Given the lack of any biological reason for accepting the 65 year mark as the definition of old age some have made the case for reviewing this boundary (Mann, 1995).

Methods of service delivery vary greatly. This is sustainable because of the lack of any comparative evaluation (in terms of effectiveness and cost) of the different models of care. Services also differ because of the variation in local authority social services between boroughs. The majority of the elderly with depression or dementia have no contact with old age psychiatry but are maintained at home or in residential settings by their families, friends, neighbours, primary health care teams, social services, and private and voluntary care providers. This matrix changes by area. Old age psychiatry services need to be tailored to local circumstances, but there are common elements. Services generally include an in-patient assessment/treatment unit, long stay accommodation, day care and some form of non-hospital assessment and support. It is within these broad groupings that variation occurs.

(ii) In-patient assessment/treatment units

In-patient assessment/treatment units are increasingly sited in district general hospitals (DGHs) rather than mental hospitals (Shulman and Arie, 1991). This may improve access to medical help that may be needed given the high level of physical co-morbidity in the elderly mentally ill. However, when old age psychiatry is the only psychiatric speciality in a DGH there may be difficulties in maintaining 24 hour on-site psychiatric cover. A judgement needs to be made as to whether it is more important for elderly psychiatric in-patients to have on-site access to medical or psychiatric staff. Physical separation of old age psychiatry from the rest of psychiatry can lead to isolation and marginalisation, and may be more costly. Local circumstances should dictate local solutions.

In-patient units may be divided into organic (dementia and sometimes delirium) and functional wards or be based on geographical catchment areas. Units vary in their integration with geriatric medicine. The effectiveness of liaison appears to depend on the mutual willingness of consultant teams to cooperate. However, there is a case to encourage formal links.

(iii) Long-stay accommodation

Long-stay provision varies widely, even within London. Older patients requiring such psychiatric care fall into the three groups: those with dementia complicated by behavioural disorder, those with treatment resistant functional disorder first occurring after the age of 65, and 'graduates' with early onset functional disorder who grow old. (The latter group are generally cared for by general psychiatrists and will not be further considered here). Long term care may be provided in mental hospitals, DGHs, NHS community units, in collaborative ventures between health services and housing associations, by social services, and by the voluntary and independent sectors. Over the last 15 years government policy and funding have favoured an increase in independent sector care while NHS long stay beds and, to a lesser extent, social services provision have decreased.

Recently, Bebbington and Darton (1995) discussed the long-stay facilities for elderly people in London. Unfortunately, their report does not separate those with mental illness from those with chronic physical disabilities, but some general points remain relevant. Very old people (over 75 years) are frequently admitted to hospital (22% per year in London compared with 17% in the rest of England and Wales). This excess in London may represent a differential availability of hospital and long stay independent sector beds (Table 4). Over the last 10 years the number of local authority owned residential beds has fallen, particularly in London compared with the rest of the country. In the rest of England and Wales this loss has been compensated for by the growth in the independent sector. However, in London there was a net loss between 1985 and 1993 of 500 beds (Bebbington & Darton, 1995). The authors estimated that given the relatively slow growth of private sector beds in London (about 1000 beds per year) it would take 30 years for the private sector alone to meet the present levels of provision.

Table 4 Service levels for elderly people in London and England, 1985 and 1993

	Inner London		Outer London		Rest of England	
	1985	**1993**	**1985**	**1993**	**1985**	**1993**
Persons over 75 years (thousands)	163.6	151.6	284.4	294.9	2603.9	2964.0
Available beds on wards for elderly patients	18.5	15.4	15.6	11.5	18.3	11.6
Occupied beds by over 75s	-	18.3	-	15.1	-	15.7
Beds for elderly in registered nursing homes	6.5	13.6	7.9	18.7	11.8	46.5
Places in local authority residential homes	44.6	28.2	32.9	18.5	37.5	22.2
Places in registered voluntary homes	15.3	14.7	15.8	14.4	9.4	10.3
Places in registered private homes	6.1	7.5	13.0	21.4	28.8	51.9

Source: Bebbington and Darton (1995)

In London, as in other parts of the country, the geographical distribution of independent sector homes is uneven, depending on the availability of large, cheap properties for conversion rather than on local need. It can be difficult to find appropriate residential places in some inner city areas leading to the 'export' of elderly people to outer London boroughs. This not uncommon outcome seems to defeat one of the major purposes of the closure of distant mental hospitals, the maintenance of individuals in their own communities. It may also lead to greater social isolation and, in the case of people with dementia, greater functional impairment.

The closure of the large mental hospitals resulted in a decanting of assessment units either to general hospitals (for example, from Bexley to Greenwich District Hospital in

1983) or to smaller specialist hospitals (for example, from Cane Hill to North Dulwich Hospital in 1985). This left an opportunity for innovation in the provision of long stay accommodation. The first joint nursing home venture between a mental health service and the voluntary sector for people with severe dementia was opened in 1987 by Age Concern and the Maudsley Hospital after the closure of beds at Cane Hill Hospital. Novel units have also been developed in the grounds of old hospitals if they were in their catchment area. An example is Becket House (a hospital ward in the community) in the grounds of the old New Cross Hospital, opened in 1986. Knight's Hill, a similar unit, not on a hospital site, has received particular attention for its effective use of architectural and structural innovation for people with dementia (Handysides, 1993).

Another line of development originating in London has been the creation of 'domuses' in Lewisham and North Southwark, the first of which was opened in 1990. In these there is an attempt to create a home for individuals with severe dementia and challenging behaviour in the community maximising autonomy and privacy while providing high quality support (Lindesay et al., 1991). While the innovative approaches described above may provide a far higher standard of care than the back ward they replace, this quality reprovision is more expensive (Beecham et al., 1993).

(iv) Day hospitals

Day hospitals have been advocated as a means of providing effective monitoring, rehabilitation and relapse prevention for patients with late onset psychiatric disorders including dementia (Howard, 1994). Unfortunately, there is no direct evidence that this is the case and recently day hospitals have come under attack as costly, inflexible institutions that breed chronic symptomatology and dependence (Ball, 1993; Fasey, 1994). The National Audit Office (1994) examined the performance of 22 day hospitals (including 10 psychogeriatric day hospitals) in three health regions. They found that the review and monitoring of patients' progress was often patchy and that very few services could determine the true costs and effectiveness of the care provided. Until the utility of day hospitals has been properly tested their provision will remain an act of faith.

(v) Out-patient or community assessment/management

The maintenance of the elderly in their own households, if possible, is the paramount aim of the NHS and Community Care Act. As noted above this may require a complex web of support, and community old age psychiatry is part of this system. All services provide some sort of non-hospital assessment, but the nature of this varies greatly. The more traditional form of service delivery is the GP-requested consultant domiciliary visit (Donaldson and Hill, 1991) followed by out-patient assessment, or first assessment in an out-patient clinic. Out-patient assessment may be particularly inappropriate for the elderly for four reasons: the difficulties they have attending hospital due to disability, the disorientation imposed by transporting elderly people with dementia to unfamiliar surroundings, the inability to assess functioning within the home, and the decreased access to informants such as neighbours. Many services, such as that in north Camden, have almost entirely abandoned hospital-based out-patient assessments.

One interesting development in old age psychiatry, the growth of community teams (CTs), originated in London in the past 15 years. The way these teams function has been identified as a controversial issue in old age psychiatry (Dening, 1992). Usually the only team members common to both in- and out-patient services are the medical staff. CTs may consist only of CPNs, but many now have involvement from social workers, occupational therapists, psychologists, physiotherapists, case managers and speech therapists as well as doctors.

Teams may have more or less open access (i.e. the acceptance of referrals from 'non-traditional' sources) or may restrict referrals to other doctors. Restricted access may be particularly inappropriate for the elderly given the important role played by families and social and voluntary services. Fears that open access may swamp services or lead to inappropriate referrals have not been borne out by research evidence (Macdonald et al., 1994; Gupta et al., 1996). An area for concern is the somewhat perverse incentive to retain GP-to-consultant requests for home assessments introduced by the fee paid to the consultant for completing a domiciliary visit (Donaldson and Hill, 1991).

Another area of debate is the question of who is competent to carry out initial assessments and to formulate management plans. One view is that only doctors can do so, while another view holds that with appropriate training and supervision, a standardised assessment of new referrals by any team member followed by the CT formulating the management plan is more efficient and cost-effective. The former assertion is unsupported by research evidence but there is evidence that non-doctor CT members are as accurate in assigning psychiatric diagnoses to new cases as medical team members (Collighan et al., 1993). However, in some circumstances, it is possible that specialist skills will be neglected in favour of 'generic' assessment and treatment activities. It is of interest that the service which pioneered this model of team-work (the Lewisham and Guy's Mental Health Trust) is planning to develop further and devolve the functions of screening, full assessment and intervention to separate teams. Detailed study of the work of a CT is given in von Abendorff et al. (1994) and Brown et al. (1996).

The Lewisham care management scheme was set up in 1990 as a joint venture between Lewisham social services department, the local psychogeriatric service and the Gatesby Trust. The scheme has been evaluated by the PSSRU at the University of Kent. This was a randomised controlled trial of the use of intensive case management against standard clinical care in the management of patients with severe dementia living at home. Care managers, with their own devolved budgets, were responsible for co-ordinating and purchasing social care for elderly people with dementia with the aim of maintaining their lives at home for as long as possible and minimising stress to carers. This involved the creation of a unique package of care (for example, paying neighbours for services) which complemented that provided by the statutory sector. Case loads were low enough to enable very complex cases to be handled individually in this way. Results can be summarised as follows: at two year follow-up in the care managed group there were significantly fewer patients in institutional care, carer stress/burden was lower, and measures of personal care and levels of stimulation were higher. The cost of care management was higher than for the control group's care, but in spite of this care management has become widespread for this patient group in Lewisham (R von Abendorff, personal communication).

5.1.4. Changes in service use over the last ten years

(i) Routinely collected data

As discussed above the HES system replaced the MHE in 1987, and the data for the financial year 1988-1989 are too flawed to be used. Table 5 presents published data on all mental illness admissions and age specific rates of admission for England for the years 1989-90 to 1991-92 (Department of Health, 1995) and the recently analysed but as yet unpublished data for 1994-95 (Department of Health, personal communication).

Table 5 All mental illness admissions to NHS hospitals 1989-90 to 1991-92 by age group

	All admission (thousands)				Age-specific rate (per 100,000)			
	1989-90	1990-91	1991-92	1994-95	1989-90	1990-91	1991-92	1994-95
0–64	121	121	125	139	432[1]	438[1]	452[1]	327
65+	62	65	68	74	-	-	-	-
65–74	23	23	24	26	545	557	572	590
75+	39	42	44	48	1,175	1,232	1290	1411
Total	183	186	193	213				
% 65+	34	35	35	35				

Data refer to finished consultant episodes from the Hospital Episode Statistics system (Department of Health, 1995). Data separating first admissions from readmissions are not available.

[1] Age specific rates are for the 25-34 age group (the next highest after 65–74) rather than the 0–64 age group.

It can be seen that the proportion of all referrals over 65 years has remained stable at just over a third of all admissions and there is the same dramatic increase in age specific rates as noted above. However, the change to finished consultant episodes for the calculation of admissions may have introduced an important bias. The data only include patients discharged from hospital so that there may be a degree of age-related statistical bias if older adults are more likely to be admitted for longer periods.

The 1994-95 HES data also show interesting differences in age-specific rates of admission between inner London, outer London, other large cities and the rest of the country as shown in Table 6.

The admission rates for the 'younger-old' age group (65-74 years) mirror that of the general psychiatry population in being relatively higher in inner London and other large cities whereas this pattern is reversed in the over 75 year old group. The reasons for this may be related to local admission policies, the greater availability of long-stay beds in the rest of the country, the lack of intensive social support in rural areas or the 'export' of frail elderly people – particularly those with dementia – to residential and nursing

Table 6 Age-specific rates of admission during 1994–95 by area of residence

	Inner London	Outer London	Other large cities	Rest of the country
0–64	513	334	425	301
65–74	701	504	643	587
75+	1125	1018	1339	1478

homes outside London. Certainly, age-specific admission rates for dementia show differences when analysed by area of residence which need explanation (see Table 7).

Table 7 Age-specific rates of admission (FCEs) for senile and presenile organic psychotic conditions by area of residence for 1994–95

	Inner London	Outer London	Other large cities	Rest of the country
65–74	146	172	227	210
75–84	620	639	872	869
85+	1306	1247	1592	1680

(ii) Patient activity from a single mental health trust

The Lewisham and Guy's mental health trust psychogeriatric service (and its pre-trust forerunners) has maintained an annual statistical database since its inception in 1984. Minor changes in the catchment area and data collection methods have occurred but since 1989 it is possible to compare trends in referral and admission patterns from year to year. Summary statistics for all community referrals and details of their source and diagnosis are given in Table 8.

The number of community referrals has steadily increased since 1984. The initial rise can be attributed to increasing awareness among GPs and others of the existence of the service. During late 1993, the care of people with dementia was the focus of the Lewisham Mayoral Project and there was multi-agency collaboration in organising theme days in the borough, public meetings and comprehensive information, packages for carers and professionals which may have led to the 25% increase in referrals that year. However, this is only a partial explanation as the biggest increase in referrals occurred in north Southwark which was not involved in the project. The changes took place against the background of a fall in the elderly population from 51,648 in 1981 to 46,535 in 1991.

The service has an open access policy and only 55% to 65% of referrals come directly from GPs. The proportion of referrals from patients or their relatives has remained at about 4 to 6% although this figure is doubled in re-referrals. In spite of the gradually ageing population (there has been greater migration of the younger old, i.e. 65 to 74 year olds, presumably to outer London areas) the proportion of referrals with organic

Table 8 Community referral rates to Lewisham and North Southwark Community Teams 1984–94

	1984a	1988	1989/90	1990/91	1991/92	1992/93	1993/94
New referrals	275	-	660	616	579	613	735
Re-referrals	0	-	221	250	289	322	428
Total referrals	275	745	881	866	868	935	1163
Referral source (as % of total referrals)							
GPs	17	67	60	57	59	56	56
Self/relative	4	1	4	7	6	6	6
Diagnosis (as a % of total referrals)							
Organic disorders	50.0	45.4	46.5	44.8	43.4	48.3	45.4
Affective disorders	29.0	24.3	24.3	26.4	28.5	21.8	22.6
Other disorders	18.0	18.8	20.1	18.4	18.2	18.9	18.6
No psychiatric disorder	3.0	11.5	9.1	10.4	9.9	11.0	13.4

Source: Lewisham & Guy's Old Age Psychiatry Service: Annual Reports, 1984, 1988-1994.
NB: data is presented for the academic year (October to September).

psychoses has remained remarkably stable at between 45 and 50% while there has been a variable rate of 'no psychiatric diagnosis', a group which may include inappropriate referrals.

Acute psychogeriatric admissions to wards at Hither Green and Guy's Hospitals are shown in Table 9.

Table 9 Admissions to acute assessment wards, Lewisham and Guy's MHNHS

	1988	1989/90	1990/91	1991/92	1992/93	1993/94
Number of first admissions	227	187	173	203	190	-
Number of readmissions	57	43	56	73	77	-
Readmission (as % of total admissions)	20	19	24	26	29	-
Total admissions	284	230	229	276	267	295
Mean length of stay (days)	54	58	40	43	36	55

Source: Lewisham & Guy's Old Age Psychiatry Service: Annual Reports, 1988–1994.

Although the number of referrals to the service has increased, admission rates have remained relatively stable with a slight increase in the proportion of readmissions in recent years. This is matched by (and may be the consequence of) the gradual fall in mean length of stay during the period until the last year for which figures are available when length of stay increased by about 50%. Changes resulting from the Community

Care Act and greater delays in processing applications for residential care may have contributed to this increase.

5.1.5 Adverse events related to London Services

To our knowledge there have been no serious adverse events related to old age psychiatry *per se* during the past few years. However, complaints concerning what were considered inadequacies in planning the move of continuing care patients from hospitals destined for closure to new accommodation have led to inquiries involving at least two health providers (Southwark Community Health Council, personal communication). National concern was aroused by the practice of at least two provider units in transferring elderly patients with dementia to nursing homes hundreds of miles away from their original neighbourhood. Lastly, perceived professional boundary issues between old age psychiatry and geriatric medicine which were indirectly believed to have led to a patient's death (Southwark Community Health Council, personal communication) underline the importance of a good working relationship between the specialties as mentioned in section 5.1.2 (v).

(i) Published reviews of recent problems

The service provision envisaged within the policy initiatives outlined in section 2 can only occur with sufficient local funding and the agreement of all agencies to make it work. Abas and Silverman (1996) have drawn attention to difficulties encountered with community care in one London borough, Lambeth, which are largely caused by problems within the local authority. They point to delays in the residential placement of patients from acute assessment units, the continual threat of under-funding for care packages, delays in carrying out social work assessments of elderly people in the community and the lack of monitoring of private residential and nursing home provision. Shortly after the article was submitted for publication Lambeth Council announced substantial cuts in the social services budget leading to compulsory redundancies of social services staff, increasing the problems described by Abas and Silverman (1996). This is probably the most extreme example of difficulties so far documented and it is not known how far these problems may be generalised across London.

5.1.6 Reviews and inspections of London Services

The Health Advisory Service has generally commented on a number of issues including the need to close old-style long stay facilities and replace them with small purpose-built units in the patient's original community, to improve the quality of the environment in acute treatment facilities and occasionally increase the number of beds, to develop closer liaison between psychogeriatricians and geriatricians and in some cases general psychiatrists, and to introduce joint commissioning of services at every level.

The Mental Health Act Commission has echoed some of these concerns but has no major comments about the specialty as a whole (William Bingley and Elaine Murphy, personal communication).

5.1.7. Priorities for the future in London's services for the elderly

1) To develop the role of 'trained' carers (employed by the health service) to assist the practical, day-to-day support of mentally ill elderly people at home.

2) To expand the use of care management (as exemplified by the Lewisham care management scheme, see section 5.1.3 (v)), possibly by diverting part of the budget identified for residential and nursing home placements.

3) To develop the use of multi-disciplinary teams along the 'Guy's model' (see section 5.1.3. (v)).

4) To discourage the use of domiciliary visits by incorporating home assessments into the job plans of consultants while using the funds released to contribute to the development of community teams.

5) To set up reporting systems which would enable the collation of data relevant to service provision and service comparison across London (This would be best organised by commissioning authorities).

6) To commission evaluative research into old age psychiatry provision so that service development is evidence-based, not led by dogma.

Chapter 5.2

Child and adolescent services in London

Veira Bailey

Summary

- High levels of social disadvantage, a large refugee population, growing numbers of young people among the homeless, and high rates of children being 'looked after' by local authorities or on child protection registers indicate that needs for child and adolescent services in London are likely to be at the upper end of the national spectrum.
- Patterns of service provision are particularly complex for children and adolescents and the danger of fragmentation is especially great with the involvement of multiple agencies (child mental health, paediatrics, social services and education), between whom co-ordination is often poor. The internal market may have further increased this complexity, and in London, withdrawal of social workers from many child mental health units and the abolition of ILEA are likely to have had negative effects on resources available and on inter-agency working. The effects of fundholding remain uncertain.
- Despite evidence of considerable unmet need among children and adolescents and the great importance of effective intervention at this stage for prevention of later health and social problems, child and adolescent mental health still seems to be a 'Cinderella service', with very patchy services and levels of resources and staffing which are very low compared with other European countries.

The following are potential solutions to the current difficulties in meeting needs for child and adolescent mental health services in London:

- An agreed categorisation should be developed of children with mental health problems across health, education, social services and youth justice, so that databases with standardised information about these children and adolescents may be developed. Overlaps and fragmentation in care should be investigated, so as to improve joint planning between agencies.
- The proportion of the mental health budget spent on child and adolescent services and levels of staffing in these services should be reviewed. Local, high quality out-patient services should be developed, rather than allowing patients to be referred to distant in-patient units, and perverse incentives for in-patient treatment should be removed by adequate resourcing of mental health services in the community and by allowing cost-shunting between agencies.
- The effects of a primary care-led NHS on strategic planning for child mental health services should be monitored. Primary care staff training in detection and treatment of child mental health problems should be improved, with training for health visitors in behaviour modification and parent management techniques and multiprofessional training in child protection.

Recent national policy developments affecting child and adolescent services are outlined in this section, along with trends specifically affecting London. Provision for children and adolescents with mental health problems is complex, with the health service, social services and education authorities all making complementary major contributions: recent changes and the current status of provision in each of these sectors will be described.

5.2.1 Limitations to information available about London provision

A number of significant obstacles have made it difficult to obtain specific information on some aspects of London service provision. These include:

*   In the **Health sector**, spending on child and adolescent mental health services at a national and local level is hard to estimate as many purchasers have difficulty in separating spending on these from general spending on mental health or from general spending on children (Kurtz et al, 1994).

*   In **Education**, because of the pressure on schools of recent legislation, the Department of Education has initiated a no burdens policy which means that any non-essential work, such as requests for data, is given a low priority. There also seems to be a lack of clarity within the Department about how information should be obtained or even whether it should be made available to academic enquiry; discussions with academics in education suggested that this was a widespread experience. Further, since the Education Act (1981) classification of the precise nature of difficulties experienced by children in special schooling has been avoided because of a concern about labelling. It is therefore now impossible to track the local development of services in any specific category, for example, for autistic as opposed to 'emotionally and behaviourally disturbed' ('EBD') children.

*   In **social services**, clients are also classified in a way that does not allow the specific identification of the mental health component of their needs (Kurtz et al, 1996).

5.2.2 Needs for child and adolescent services

With the NHS reforms of 1991 and the purchaser-provider split, there has been a gradual increase in emphasis on purchasing child and adolescent services which are an appropriate response to local need and which are evidence-based. Child and adolescent mental health services have been among the areas for which the NHS Executive has commissioned a review of the evidence on health care needs (Wallace et al, 1996).

Estimates of overall prevalence of child psychiatric disorder give a crude guide to local prevalence (Light and Bailey, 1992). This can be refined using a graded overall prevalence rate based on epidemiological studies (Rutter et al, 1970; Rutter et al, 1975), multiplied by a factor derived from the local Jarman scale (Kurtz et al, 1996; Department of Health, 1993). This method warrants further refinement, but will leave unanswered questions such as whether all children with a psychiatric disorder should have child and adolescent mental health services input, and what level of support from child and adolescent mental health services is needed by paediatricians, who are the clinicians to whom the largest number of children with behavioural problems are referred (Kurtz et al, 1994).

As discussed elsewhere in this report, levels of social deprivation in many London areas (according to indicators such as the Jarman UPA score) are high, and would thus be expected to be associated with rates of child and adolescent psychiatric disorder higher than those encountered in most other areas of the country. Delinquency and pervasive hyperactivity have each been found to be twice as common in urban children compared with rural children (McArdle et al, 1995).

There is some evidence that in general needs for child and adolescent mental health services may be rising. A recent assessment of whether or not the apparent rise in anti-social behaviours and psychosocial problems in young people is real has confirmed that there is indeed a rise in rates of crime, substance abuse, depression and suicide in adolescents (Rutter and Smith, 1995). This study also concludes that there is evidence to suggest an increased vulnerability of young people to psychosocial disorder. It is likely that increased family pathology and particularly marital conflict may explain some of these increases. Social disadvantage and unemployment are unlikely to have contributed, as increases in adolescent problems have occurred when these factors were showing a general improvement.

Increased awareness of child abuse among all agencies and an increasing concern for proper assessment as required by the Children Act 1989 have led to increasing referrals for assessment by child psychiatrists of child abuse, particularly child sexual abuse. Forensic work is frequently difficult to integrate into a clinical timetable and highly labour intensive for experienced child psychiatrists and other senior members of multi-disciplinary teams who act as expert witnesses. In London, child sexual abuse may have become a particularly prominent issue because of the development of expert services at postgraduate centres, such as Great Ormond Street and the Tavistock.

Another factor with particular significance for needs for services in London is that the Refugee Council reports that 89% of the 29,000 refugee children of school age in the UK live in London. Many of these children suffer from post-traumatic stress disorder, do not speak English and, in a significant minority of cases, are unaccompanied. Helping these children is a time-consuming business involving consultation with several different agencies and sometimes work with interpreters. This makes large demands on a child and adolescent mental health service. On the other hand, many children come from families self-selected for drive, resourcefulness and a high regard for education.

A further recent London phenomenon is the presence of young people among the homeless in London. Many of the young homeless have recently left care, run away from home or been victims of abuse.

5.2.3 Matching needs to service responses

Both the HAS review (1995) and the Assessment of Needs and Unmet Need (Kurtz et al, 1996) give helpful advice on prioritising those at high risk of severe disorder such as children looked after by the local authority, children who are substance misusers, young sex offenders, children with a statement of special educational need or on a disability register, those on child protection register, and those who are absent from or excluded from school. However, this prioritising should not disguise the major shortfall in resources for child and adolescent mental health services and the need to develop appropriate services in all tiers. Tiers of need have been identified (HAS, 1995; Kurtz et al, 1996; Wallace et al, 1996), with different levels of service response appropriate to each:

Informal carers – in the family or community.

Tier 1: Primary care by professionals for those with mild disturbance – estimated prevalence 15%. For these less severe psychiatric disorders, a recently proposed innovation is the provision of child mental health workers, with a role bridging primary and secondary care (Hall and Hill, 1994).

Tier 2: Child and adolescent mental health services care by professional working alone for those with moderate/serious disorder – prevalence 7%.

Tier 3: Child and adolescent mental health services multi-disciplinary care for those with severe disorders – prevalence 1.85%

Tier 4: Supra-district specialist multi-disciplinary care for those with most severe problems – prevalence 0.075%

Kurtz et al (1996) found a relationship between predicted prevalence rates, adjusted on the basis of epidemiological studies (Rutter et al, 1970; Rutter et al, 1975) and of deprivation scores (Department of Health, 1993), and numbers of children actually known to both health and local authority services. However, this does not by itself demonstrate that children are being seen at the appropriate tier for their needs. Children and adolescents may arbitrarily or appropriately find themselves in contact with different services. At present, information about overlaps and discontinuities is lacking, and an overview needs to be produced of the complex networks with which children have contact. Evidence from the four districts studied by Kurtz et al (1996) suggested that services had become less coherent since the introduction of the NHS internal market. Further, even if children are being seen at an appropriate tier, this does not necessarily indicate that their needs are being met. While the majority of child and adolescent mental health problems are seen in primary care, it is not clear that they are adequately treated (Adams, 1991). Efforts have been made to increase awareness of child psychiatric problems among general practitioners by the provision of a booklet (Hughes et al, 1994) but few vocational training schemes include useful experience in child psychiatry in their rotations.

5.2.4 Providing evidence-based responses

The new management culture in the NHS has also led to an emphasis on the purchasing of services which are of proven effectiveness for the comprehensive mental health care of local populations. Idiosyncratic and single treatment services have been required to broaden their skills. Change has been slow as purchasers have developed knowledge and skills in how to purchase an effective service that is linked to their population needs (Vanstraelen and Cottrell, 1994; Kurtz et al, 1996a), but may accelerate as responsibility for monitoring performance management moves to the new regional offices (Jezzard, 1996). The reports by Wallace et al (1996) and Kurtz et al (1996) each make recommendations on the range of treatments which should be available, based on reviews of methodologically sound research studies.

There is an increased use of behavioural treatments generally and of medication for Attention Deficit and Hyperactivity Disorder. Simple, practical and valid outcome scales are being developed, such as the Health of the Nation outcome scales, child and adolescent (HoNOSCA), an adapted version of the adult Health of the Nation outcome scales. However, some well established treatments with good evidence for effectiveness are under-used, and treatments that have been evaluated very little or with inconclusive results are widely used. More research into treatments is needed, as is work on how far clinicians choose treatments on the basis of evidence, and how their practice might be improved (Graham, 1996).

An idiosyncrasy of treatment in London is that the city has a high proportion of analytically trained psychotherapists compared with the rest of the country. They provide highly tuned services to a relatively small number of children and engage in teaching and supervision. It has been suggested that their substantial presence in London has impeded the development of parent training techniques for children with conduct disorder and the appropriate use of medication for ADHD, both of which appear to be more widespread elsewhere.

5.2.5 Historical development of child and adolescent mental health services

Child and adolescent mental health services in the UK have developed by two main routes: child guidance clinics run by local education authorities, and hospital-based child psychiatric departments within the NHS.

The child guidance clinics were frequently based in education department owned premises, and included local authority employed staff, social workers and educational psychologists. Their theoretical approach aspired to a psychoanalytic model and was often deeply opposed to a medical model.

Hospital-based child psychiatric clinics were in closer contact with services such as paediatrics, accident and emergency and adult psychiatric services. They tended to develop expertise in serious psychiatric disorder and the disorders associated with physical illness. Their multi-disciplinary teams more often included junior medical staff in training, nurses and clinical rather than educational psychologists. Hospital services were also the basis for the development of academic child psychiatry, which occurred with the slow expansion of university departments from the 1970s and an impressive growth in good quality research.

In London, child guidance units were particularly well developed as part of the support services for the Inner London Education Authority (ILEA). These support services included home tuition services, off-site units, remedial teaching and residential and day special schools including schools for 'maladjusted' children now categorised as 'emotionally and behaviourally disturbed' (EBD).

The Court Report in 1976 recommended that child guidance clinics and hospital departments of child psychiatry should be 'recognised as part of an integrated child and adolescent psychiatric service, which involves clinics in a variety of settings and with varying emphasis, all of which apply the same body of knowledge'. It was recommended that all services should be health service based, multi-disciplinary and able to respond to the demands and needs for paediatric liaison, consultation with social services and schools, and interdisciplinary and preventive interventions, as well as providing a general clinical service.

The child and adolescent specialist section of the Royal College of Psychiatrists published a report in 1978 on the role, responsibilities and work of a child and adolescent psychiatrist, which was revised in 1986. In the eight years between these two reports there had been major changes in the roles of other professionals in the multi-disciplinary team. Educational psychologists were working independently with much of their time taken up by special educational needs assessment procedures after the Education Act 1981. In many districts social workers were withdrawn from clinics in order to concentrate on child protection work due to the increasing public concern about child death inquiries. Increasingly teams included clinical psychologists and community psychiatric nurses.

The broader based curriculum and improved training standards for child and adolescent psychiatrists appear to have had a positive effect on their professionalism, morale and self esteem. However, spending on child and adolescent services in the UK remains low in an international context, despite a more rapid rate of increase in the 1990s than in the 1980s (by around 2-3% per year rather than the previous 1%). This is reflected in levels of staffing. For child and adolescent psychiatry, European Union and EFTA countries have an average of 4.76 psychiatrists/100,000 under 21; in the UK, including senior registrars, there are 3.6 psychiatrists/100,000 (Hill, 1996). A specific staffing issue for child and adolescent mental health services in London is that problems of recruitment may be greater because of the high cost of living and the perception of stressful working conditions.

5.2.6 Recent changes in health service activity

There has recently been a national reduction in bed availability for child mental illness, from 636 in 1992/93 to 603 in 1993/94 to 551 in 1994/95 (Department of Health, 1995). In a similar period there was a reduction of 705 medical beds for children; and of 7 beds for children with learning difficulties. London was previously a high user of specialist therapeutic communities such as Peper Harrow, Chaldington and Kilworthy House, all of which have now closed.

The increasing effectiveness and helpfulness of modern child and adolescent mental health services have led to major increases in referral rates to departments. Evidence from an assessment of needs (Kurtz et al, 1996) suggest that there is incoherence and a lack of complementarity in services offered and that this is greater than before the introduction of the NHS internal market (Rea Price and Pugh, 1995).

In London, a particular obstacle to comprehensive planning of coherent services is that there appears to be a greater purchaser-provider split than elsewhere, with less working together than is evident in other parts of the country (Ham, 1996). Market competition between providers may cause further stress among stretched services who need to tender for services and feel concern about a lack of continuity in the service. On the other hand, tendering may produce innovative development and improvement in service. There is also concern in London that 'Tomlinson' money for community projects in London is tapering off and may not be replaced by health authorities with large overspends, often brought about by overspend on acute services.

5.2.7 Recent trends in provision by social services

Child and adolescent mental health services are closely affected by changes in social services and education. Local authorities have always been more sensitive to political change whether because of central policies, such as rate capping, or local political pressures. Social service departments are responsible for the care needs of children and adolescents, including child protection.

In London, in addition to the withdrawal of social workers from clinics, there is a high rate of agency social workers and cases are frequently unallocated. This makes for difficulties in joint working with social services over complex cases, with health services filling a social services gap, for example, using community psychiatric nurses to do preventive social work.

The national review of services for the mental health of children and young people (Kurtz et al, 1994) reported that between the years 1990 and 1993, social workers had been lost in 30% of child mental health units. Lessons learned from enquiries following child deaths and the emergence of concern about child sexual abuse in the 1980s led to the Children Act 1989, which aimed to provide a comprehensive legal framework dealing with these issues. The legal rights of children were stipulated and their welfare identified as paramount, and greater partnership between local authorities and parents was encouraged. Local authorities were charged with ensuring that support services for children 'in need' were provided, which raised thresholds for the identification of significant harm. Recently, 'Messages from Research' (Department of Health, 1995g) emphasised the importance of focusing on the needs of children and families rather than a narrow concentration on alleged incidents of abuse, although official Department of Health guidelines have not been revised to accommodate this 'lighter touch'. The report also stressed how very damaging emotional abuse may be for children.

In 1995, the Association of Directors of Social Services and The Royal College of Psychiatrists published a joint statement on an integrated mental health service for children and adolescents. They saw the past secondment of social workers and educational psychologists to child and adolescent psychiatric departments as being effectively a way of purchasing child and adolescent mental health services. Although they recognised difficulties in overcoming the different conceptual, resourcing and statutory positions of the agencies, they firmly opted for moving towards establishing joint or collaborative commissioning of a unified mental health service for children.

Revelations of abusive regimes in children's homes and residential schools led to the Utting Report, a review of residential child care (1991). The report recommended children's services plans. These are strategic planning documents similar to community care plans (LAC 1992/18), and became mandatory in 1996. Local authority social services departments are the lead agency for their production, and are required to consult with health and education authorities, NHS trusts, housing authorities and voluntary organisations. However, health has been variably involved so far (Rea Price and Pugh, 1995; Kurtz et al, 1996). In north Thames (west) only one out of 16 child psychiatrists asked had been consulted by their local authority.

5.2.8 Children 'looked after'

The number of children in care (referred to as 'looked after' since the implementation of the Children Act in 1991) has been declining nationally. In 1978, there were 95,791 children in care, whereas the number 'looked after' in 1993 was 51,000 (Department of Health, 1995d). Although fewer children are being fostered, the proportion has increased, whilst the proportion in community homes has fallen. Local authorities report that as numbers of children in care have declined, those remaining are found to be more disturbed. 58% of the children looked after in 1993 had been in care for two years or more, with approximately 25% having been looked after for more than five years. As indicated in Table 1, London has a rate of children looked after substantially above that for England as a whole:

Table 1 Regional variations in rates of children 'looked after'

	Children under 18 'looked after' – **rates per 10,000**		
	Started to be looked after between Oct 1991 and March 1992	Ceased to be looked after between Oct 1991 and March 1992	Looked after at 31 March 1992
England	12	13	50
Shire Group A (Audit Commission classification)	10	11	38
Shire Group B	12	12	41
Shire Group C	12	15	59
Metropolitan Districts	14	15	60
Inner London	17	17	102
Outer London	11	10	46

Places approved in secure units have fallen from 341 in 1986 to 266 in 1995. During that time, the occupancy rate has risen from 77% to 88%. The majority of children accommodated are boys (81%), 14–16 year olds amounted to 83%, 10% were under 14 and 7% over 16 years. These proportions have remained largely constant since 1984, although the number aged over 16 in 1995 was somewhat lower than in each of the previous years (Department of Health, 1995f).

5.2.9 Child protection

Reports from area child protection committees (ACPCs) comment on rising work loads in child protection, although there is no uniformity in terms used, which makes comparisons difficult (Department of Health, 1995e). Many ACPCs are operating in an environment of change and pressure from the various policy inputs. There are increasing referrals, pressures on professionals and a high turnover of staff. While the Audit Commission report (1994b) has played a significant part in achieving a shift towards preventative work, there are difficulties in allocating resources and planning coherent strategies. A continuing problem is the low level of engagement of general practitioners in child protection and the weaknesses in the training they receive.

In March 1995 there were 34,954 children and young people on child protection registers in England, representing a rate of 32 children per 10,000. It should be noted that registers are **not** records of levels of child abuse, as some children on the register will not be victims of actual abuse while other children who have been victims will not be placed on the register if there is no need for a protection plan. For example, a child who is dead or looked after will not be on the register. Sometimes registration has even been used as an entry criterion for scarce family support services.

While the proportion of children on the register allocated to 'physical injury' has been decreasing, the proportion of children listed under 'emotional abuse' has increased. The proportion of new registrations which are for 'sexual abuse' has fallen, but the overall proportion on the register in this category remains constant. The proportion where the risk is classified as 'neglect' has increased for both registrations and those on the register. These changes in proportions of categories are unlikely to be due to real changes but represent a change in emphasis following enquiries, policy shifts and increasing awareness of the damaging effects of neglect and emotional abuse.

The number of children on the register reached a peak of 45,300 in 1991 before falling to 32,500 in 1993, and increasing to 34,900 in 1994. Again there is regional variation in rates, with the highest levels in inner London, as indicated by Table 2:

Table 2 Regional variations in numbers of children on child protection registers

Region (Audit Commission definitions)	Children on child protection registers: rates per 10,000 children under 18 years		
Region	All Children	Boys	Girls
England	32	31	32
Shire Group A	23	23	23
Shire Group B	30	29	32
Shire Group C	34	33	34
Metropolitan Districts	38	37	40
Inner London	58	60	55
Outer London	29	29	29

5.2.10 Recent trends in provision by education authorities

The role of education departments is to provide educational facilities for all children, including those with special educational needs.

Recently, there has been a worrying increase in the numbers of exclusions from school at both primary and secondary level and even from special schools (Parsons et al, 1994). Even with discrepancies in the figures collected, it is clear that there have recently been major increases from 2910 in 1990-91 to approximately 11,000 in 1993-94 (Abrams and Ashton, 1995). This has been linked to the introduction of local management of schools (LMS) in 1990. This market-based system links funding to the ability to attract pupils and educate according to the demands of the national curriculum, greatly reducing the incentive for schools to work with difficult pupils. Thus exclusion becomes an attractive option (National Children's Bureau, 1995).

Of particular concern are the children looked after by local authorities, approximately 12% of whom do not attend school regularly. This figure rises to 25.6% of 14–16 year olds looked after (Joint Report SS1 and Ofsted, 1995).

A major change for education in London has been the transfer of educational responsibility from the Inner London Education Authority (ILEA) to 13 inner London boroughs, covering areas with a wide range of inner city urban problems. These 13 London boroughs are required to submit educational policy plans directly to the Secretary of State. In contrast with the ILEA's centralised policy, there are widely different conceptualisations and ideological differences in terms of education policy and practice.

Although changes in support services for children experiencing difficulties in schools are widely reported, there is no systematic information on changes following the 1988 Education Reform Act. ILEA was the provider of many support services and Pennell et al (1988) concluded that decreased spending after the abolition of ILEA had a profound effect on discretionary areas of the education budget. However, no precise differentiation of changes in services has been possible. This is partly because of the avoidance of specific 'labels' since the 1981 Education Act, so that the precise nature of children's 'special needs' now remains unrecorded. In many authorities, the process of statementing for special educational needs in itself makes major inroads into the special educational needs budget, and this further reduces funding available for support services.

In the decade 1973–1983, there was a 30% increase in residential provision for 'maladjusted children' regarded by some as an 'out of sight, out of mind' policy (Cole, 1986). Placements rose in maintained and non-maintained schools from 4101 in 1973 to 5367 in 1983, but placements by LEAs in independent schools (mainly boarding) reduced from 3515 to 2376. Reduction in boarding school placement to approximately 4,500 in 1994 has been a product of several factors including a view that children should be educated within their locality, publicity about the scandals and abuse in some boarding schools, and a view that boarding school placements did not lead to an overall good outcome.

In January 1994, there were 38 registered EBD ('emotionally and behaviourally disturbed' order) schools run by 25 London boroughs, 11 of which provided residential accommodation. Occupancy rates of the residential schools varied from 100% to under 40%. They were able to accommodate 1917 pupils, 401 of whom were boarders (Cole, 1996). Further work is necessary to separate London LEA placements in 1983 for comparison with present provision.

Parsons (1995) in a study of children educated out of school showed there was provision for approximately 7000 excluded children, many of whom might be said to have emotional and behavioural disorders. Many of these numbers are difficult to clarify. Educationalists consulted did not know of work which disaggregated figures for London children. There is general agreement that there has been a massive reduction in hospital schools; there are more children with statements now attached to mainstream schooling; some boarding school provision was very poor and had high unit costs per child as the numbers were low; some schools were closed because of abuse; often agencies who set up fostering homes needed then to establish their own schools because LEAs do not have any or enough EBD provision. More work is needed to clarify these areas, particularly the overlap with health and social services provision. The Department of Education circular, Pupils with Problems (1994) stresses early and effective liaison between education and social services; how well this is happening is unclear.

5.2.11 Provision for adolescents

There is widespread concern that with an overall reduction in places for disturbed adolescents (in health, education and social services provision) and a failure to implement recommendations of the Health Advisory Service report on disturbed adolescents (1986) the needs of this particular age group, in spite of public concern about delinquency, substance misuse and violence, are not being sensibly resourced.

5.2.12 Conclusion: the unmet needs of children and adolescents

However needs for services for children and adolescents are estimated, it remains clear that there is very significant unmet need. Provision for children and adolescents appears to be a Cinderella service, which does not have demanding or articulate clients, and receives a small proportion of the overall mental health budget or child health budget. Both the Audit Commission (1994b) and Kurtz et al (1994) recognised that services were frequently disjointed and uncoordinated, and that there were particular difficulties over services for children with conduct disorder. Contracts for services may not include consultation with education or social services, and youth justice services are very rarely involved. The degree of overlap, discontinuity and lack of coherence with other agencies is unknown because it is unmapped.

Different agencies have different priorities, and difficulties in working together may become more marked when all agencies are overworked and defensive about the quality of the work they do. The complex network within which child and adolescent mental health services are placed includes not only education and social services, as discussed above, but also the youth justice system, family courts and voluntary agencies. Joint commissioning of services by health, education and social services may accelerate under the pressure on all services to consider the urgent unmet needs of those in high risk groups.

The trend away from residential placement both in social services and education arguably increases the pressure on community-based services without a commensurate increase in resources. Within health authorities, there may be perverse incentives which discourage the development of high quality, local secondary child and adolescent mental health services and encourage referral to inpatient units.

At the primary care level, although first and second wave GP fundholders may have been keen to develop close links with secondary services, the overall impact of GP fundholding on strategic planning is unclear. Better training is required for primary care staff in the detection and treatment of child mental health problems. In particular, health visitors should be trained in behaviour modification and parent management techniques. All primary care staff, including general practitioners, should be trained in child protection. Such training should be multidisciplinary and involve social services, education and local specialist child mental health services.

Services which have endeavoured to provide good quality and appropriate care for their catchment area have found themselves overwhelmed by referrals and are particularly susceptible to pressures from over-stretched education or social service departments, with consequent cost-shunting. More work is needed on cost benefit analysis of psychiatric interventions, in particular on the cost of health interventions which produce benefit to education, social services and criminal justice budgets. A strong case can be made for investing in child mental health services, in that it is likely that they not only produce immediate health gain but also reduce long term social and financial costs (Light and Bailey, 1993).

Chapter 5.3

Substance misuse services in London

Michael Farrell, Jane Marshall and John Strang

Summary

- Substance misusers are highly concentrated in London, with evidence from regional databases suggesting that about a third of people starting contact with drug misuse services in the UK are in the capital.
- There has been substantial growth in community drug services over the past two decades, but this has not matched the inexorable growth in numbers of people with drug problems. Waiting times for services are often long. The availability of in-patient services has decreased, and the availability of funding for specialist residential care has become very patchy with the shift from central to local authority funding.
- Despite the high prevalence of alcohol problems, service development in this area has been limited and there have been few policy initiatives concerned with alcohol treatment.
- Substance misusers are a highly mobile population who tend to have contact with a variety of different agencies. Lack of co-ordination across services and across areas within London is a significant problem in their management.
- The needs of people with multiple problems, such as homeless substance misusers or people with a dual diagnosis of substance misuse and severe mental illness, and those of women with children, people from ethnic minority backgrounds and young people are often not well met by current services.

The following solutions are suggested to some of the problems arising in service provision for substance misusers in London:

- Rapid access services should be developed, with minimal waiting times for treatment.
- Services should be centrally co-ordinated on a pan-London basis.
- Comprehensive provision of methadone maintenance services is needed across London, with a co-ordinated approach between primary care and specialist services.
- Adolescents and young people involved in substance misuse, homeless people and people with dual diagnosis should be high priorities for future service development.
- Further development of prison services is required, with clear links between these services and community substance misuse teams.
- Comprehensive provision of hepatitis B vaccination is needed among drug users.

5.3.1 Historical development

Before the 1960s there were no specialist drug services in London. There was a handful of general practitioners and private practitioners involved in prescribing. The first drug dependency units were established in 1968, with a heavy concentration of units in London (Strang & Gossop, 1994). At the same time as the drug dependency units were established, a number of residential rehabilitation and street agencies were started. During the 1970s the number of advice and counselling agencies increased. During the 1980s services expanded and there was a change in the pattern of provision.

There was no similar development of alcohol services. The number of in-patient alcohol services fell, with a push towards non-statutory community based services and the development of community alcohol teams (Clements and Stockwell, 1988).

5.3.2 Policy initiatives

In 1982, the report 'Treatment and Rehabilitation' by the Advisory Council on the Misuse of Drugs recommended the expansion of community based services. The 1984 Central Funding Initiative (MacGregor et al, 1990) resulted in a major expansion of services, with over 50% of the funding going towards community based services, as shown in Figure 1.

Figure 1 Drug Service Developments 1982 to 1992

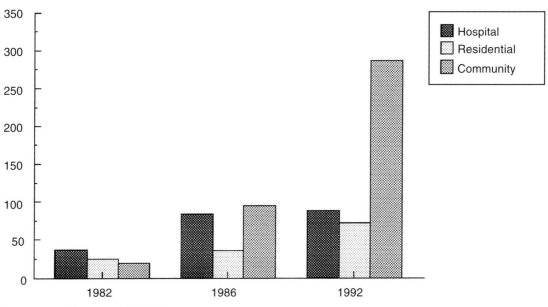

Source: MacGregor et al, 1990

Sixty-two per cent of this expenditure was for statutory services and 38% for non-statutory services. In London, North West Thames was the region most successful in bidding while South East Thames was the least successful.

The expansion of services mirrored a major increase in drug problems. There was an initial growth in heroin injecting in the mid to late 1960s, with a second wave of more drug problems including heroin injecting in the late 1970s. The mid 1980s saw the development of needle exchange schemes, as part of a policy on HIV and AIDS prevention. There are now over 300 schemes.

In the late 1980s and 1990s, cocaine and other stimulant-related problems have increased, with a concentration of cocaine problems in major metropolitan areas, as shown in Figure 2.

Figure 2 Metropolitan Police seizures

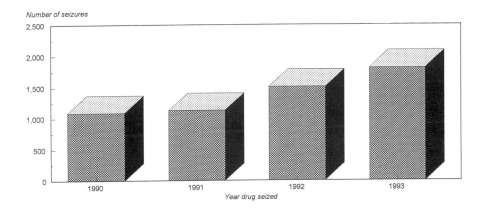

Metropolitan police seizures
Number of seizures of cocaine 1990-1993

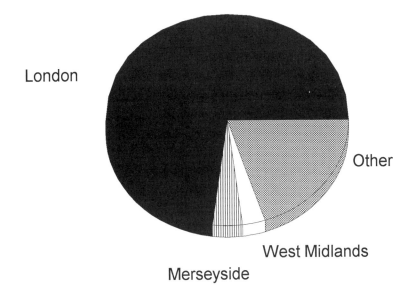

Police seizures of cocaine by region

A new government drug policy, 'Tackling Drugs Together', was published in 1995. The Department of Health has completed a review of the effectiveness of services for drug misusers (Task Force to Review Services for Drug Misusers, 1996) and made recommendations on the benefits of services.

Despite the scale of the problem, with the exception of the Alcohol Specific Grant there have been no major policy initiatives in the field of alcohol treatment..

5.3.3 Recent trends: the development of a mixed economy of care

Substance misuse services have traditionally had a substantially mixed economy of service with provision by the voluntary and statutory sectors. Recently there has been some debate about the advantages that the purchaser-provider division has given to the different sectors but there is no evidence to indicate whether one has developed in preference to the other. Indeed the distinction between voluntary and statutory sector seems less relevant in the new culture of contracting.

Drug services have continued to grow, with a mixture of statutory and non-statutory residential and community based schemes and with a major emphasis on primary care provision of services. A recent mapping exercise reported that specialist drug services are delivered by 475 providers in England, about half in the statutory sector and the rest in the voluntary sector (Task Force Review of Services to Drug Misusers, 1996). This task force has recommended that there be a continued expansion of shared care services with primary care.

Alcohol Concern has managed the distribution of funds through the Alcohol Specific Grant to the voluntary sector.

5.3.4 Changes in service use over the past ten years

In London, numbers of new admissions to services (residential or community-based) have increased by between 10% and 20% per year over the past 10 years. In 1994 the number of addicts notified to the Home Office from the North and South Thames Regions was 10,182, accounting for 30% of the total of 33,952 for England and Wales, an increase of 21% from the year before, as shown by Figure 3.

In 1994 the number of drug offenders in the Metropolitan Police Authority area increased by 24%, and accounted for 24% of all offenders in the UK (Home Office, 1995). The Drug Misuse Database statistics for the London health regions showed that 35% of people starting contact with services in the UK were reported in London. There are now long waiting lists for in-patient services ranging from three to 12 months and significantly shorter waiting times for community services, as indicated by Figure 4 (Task Force report, 1996).

There is considerable mobility in London's drug using population, with large numbers of users travelling to London from elsewhere in the UK and from other European and non-European countries. One study in London reported that 26% of a sample of injecting drug users had been born outside the UK, and 29 different non-UK countries of birth were represented (ACMD, 1993).

HIV prevention and treatment have been a major impetus to service development. Overall rates of HIV infection in English drug users remain very low by international standards at less than 1%. The London figure for HIV infection among injecting drug users is estimated at 6% (ACMD, 1993).

Figure 3 All drug addicts notified in London to the Home Office, 1989–1994

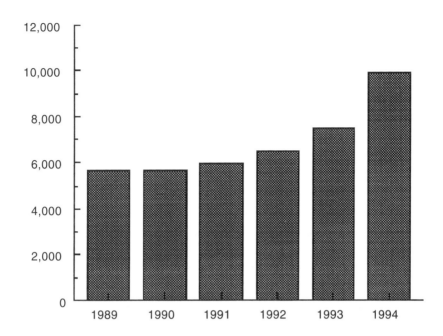

Figure 4 Waiting times for access to drug services in England

Agency Type	Number of Agencies Responding	Numbers With Waiting List	Percentage	Average Weeks Waiting
Residential Services	50	32	64%	8
Drug Dependency Clinics	28	17	61%	8
Advice/ Counselling/ Daycare & Information	112	33	29%	2

Source: Task Force 1996

5.3.5 Adverse events related to London services

The inexorable growth in drug problems over the last decade has not been matched by a growth in drug services. There has been a major emphasis on the expansion in community services and there has been a decrease in the availability of specialist in-patient services. The residential care sector has shifted its funding base from central funding to local authority funding and has experienced major difficulties in adapting to this change in funding base. There is a push to integrate alcohol and drug services in order to make up for the shortfall in alcohol service provision.

5.3.6 Reviews and inspections of London services

The Drug Advisory Service has conducted a series of reviews at district level across many districts in London but no pan-London assessment has been made. The Advisory Council on the Misuse of Drugs (AIDS and Drugs Misuse Update, 1993) reported on the absence of an overview or any co-ordination of services in London. In particular it noted the unique problems in London in relation to the size of the problems and the number of drug users moving there. In general the government white paper 'Tackling Drugs Together' reported on the lack of co-operation between health and social services, probation, the police, and housing and education authorities in dealing with drug misusers. It recommended the establishment of drug action teams which would have the chief executives of the constables, probation officers and prison services and representatives from local voluntary drug services to enhance the co-ordination of drug services. Across London there will be 28 drug action teams but no pan-London mechanisms for strategic planning above this. A number of health authorities, in particular Lambeth, Southwark and Lewisham, have been involved in joint commissioning between social services and health authorities for drug and alcohol services and there is also some joint commissioning with probation services.

Lambeth, Southwark and Lewisham health authority conducted a detailed needs assessment of drug and alcohol services and outlined a five year development plan, which for drug services included:

- the development of a more community orientated and less hospital centred service;
- the development of process and outcome measures and health targets for the population;
- the development of a mixed economy of statutory and non-statutory services.

For alcohol services, it included

- the development of a more community orientated service
- the transfer of resources from providing intensive services for a small number of people to having less intensive services for a larger number of people
- the development of jointly agreed plans for alcohol misuse service provision with local authority social service departments
- the establishment of community alcohol teams

Prisons contain large numbers of drug misusers, and recent prison initiatives have looked at developing services for drug misusers in custody. However, given the overall demands on community services there remains a gap in the provision of services within prisons and in the continuity of services between prisons and the community. The recently published Department of Health Task Force Report reviewing the effectiveness of services for drug misusers describes the positive impact of services for drug misusers and recommends that a wide range of services be made available. In particular it recommends the abolition of waiting times for drug services and the provision of a range of flexible treatment options.

5.3.7 Overview

Substance misuse services, in particular drug misuse services, have expanded considerably over the past two decades reflecting the growth in drug problems.

The problems of substance misuse in the homeless populations, the prison population and the general psychiatric population have not been adequately addressed.

The needs of women with children, young people and ethnic minority populations require specific initiatives.

The push for community based services requires greater development of liaison and consultation with other community based services.

5.3.8 Priorities for change in substance misuse services

- There is a need to develop rapid access services with minimum waiting times.
- There is a need for the co-ordination of services on a pan-London basis, particularly for the residential and in-patient substance misuse services.
- There is a need for the comprehensive provision of methadone maintenance services, with a co-ordinated approach between primary care and specialist services.
- There is a need for further development of services for adolescents and young people involved in substance misuse.
- The problems of dual diagnosis patients with substance misuse and severe psychiatric problems need to be addressed.
- The multiple needs and problems of the homeless strongly overlap with the dual diagnosis patient group.
- There is a need for the development of prison based services which are properly linked to community based services.
- Comprehensive provision of hepatitis B vaccination is needed among drug users.

Chapter 5.4

Consultation-liaison psychiatry services in London

Tom Sensky, Amanda Ramirez, Simon Wessely and Peter White

Summary

- There is substantial evidence supporting the need for liaison psychiatry services in all acute hospital settings, as well as research showing the benefits to patients and to acute services of adequately resourced and trained liaison psychiatry teams.
- Despite this evidence, liaison services have been slow to develop in London. This may result from liaison psychiatry's unusual position, straddling mental health and acute services and forced to compete with other very pressing priorities within each field.
- In a survey of 52 London hospitals, only 4 (8%) met the minimum resource requirements stipulated by the Royal College of Psychiatrists. Even using less stringent requirements – having at least five consultant sessions dedicated to liaison psychiatry plus ten sessions of other staff time – only 12 hospitals (24% of the sample) reported adequate resources.
- 14% of London hospitals reported no liaison services whatsoever.
- Although some growth had taken place since publication of the Tomlinson Report in 1992, relatively few of the services responding reported any anticipated growth in liaison psychiatry services in the foreseeable future.
- The development of adequate liaison services in all of London's general hospitals needs to be a priority in future service development, with implementation of agreed minimum standards of provision. Purchasers may exert pressure for this development by stipulating that the acute services which they purchase must include adequate and appropriate liaison services.

5.4.1 Background

Consultation-liaison psychiatry

Consultation-liaison psychiatry (alternatively described as general hospital psychiatry) is that branch of psychiatry providing psychiatric services, training and research in general hospital settings (medical, surgical obstetric, and other settings). For brevity, consultation-liaison psychiatry will be referred to in this report as *liaison psychiatry*.

The importance of liaison psychiatry within the NHS

A recent joint report of the Royal College of Physicians and the Royal College of Psychiatrists (1995), *The Psychological Care of Medical Patients*, reviewed evidence for the efficacy and effectiveness of liaison psychiatry services, their role within services in acute hospital specialties, and models of service delivery. This report also identified some of the special clinical skills relevant to the assessment and management of psychological problems in the general hospital setting. Specialists in liaison psychiatry have argued that these clinical skills particular to their work indicate that liaison psychiatry is appropriately regarded as a subspecialty within psychiatry.

The importance of liaison psychiatry to patient care and staff training can be illustrated by brief reference to four specific areas of work.[1] Relevant bibliographic references can be found in the Joint Colleges' Report (Royal College of Physicians and Royal College of Psychiatrists, 1995).

(1) *Prevention of suicide*: Approximately 11 % of acute admissions to London hospitals are for deliberate self-harm. Following deliberate self-harm, the risk of subsequent suicide rises substantially, accounting for an estimated 25% or more of completed suicides. Effective management of cases of deliberate self-harm is essential not only as part of the appropriate service provision to patients but also to help to meet the specific Health of the Nation target for suicide reduction. Even though admissions for deliberate self-harm are usually brief, a large number of bed-days is involved because of the numbers of admissions. Prompt psychosocial assessment of such patients, even if it only reduces each admission by a few hours, is likely to have a significant impact on overall admission rates.

(2) *Comprehensive patient care*: 20-40% of patients in acute medical settings manifest psychiatric morbidity to some degree, and an even higher percentage may show symptoms of psychological or emotional distress. Such morbidity is important not only in its own right but because it is known to have adverse effects on the outcome of interventions for physical illness, and on patients' perceptions of wellbeing. There is ample research evidence that such morbidity rates can be significantly reduced by appropriate psychiatric interventions. Conversely, unless such interventions are widely available and readily accessible to patients, it is not possible to provide a good quality, patient-centred health service in keeping with the aims of Health of the Nation.

(3) *Effective use of health service resources*: Research evidence (see Joint Royal Colleges Report, 1995) indicates that recognition and appropriate management of psychiatric morbidity among physically ill inpatients can improve the effectiveness of health care, for example by improved rehabilitation and reduction in lengths of stay in hospital. In addition, some patients are referred to specialists with somatoform disorders – a range of psychiatric syndromes presenting in predominantly or exclusively somatic form. In some medical specialties, such patients constitute a significant minority of total referrals. In the absence of liaison psychiatry input into their management, such patients are commonly given more investigations than they should have, and take up more staff time in the medical clinic than is appropriate. Over-zealous investigation of such patients can not only be hazardous for the patients themselves (as some of the investigations are invasive, and all have costs to the patient as well as benefits) but also leads to this patient group inappropriately consuming a disproportionate share of resources.

---

[1] Some of this material has been adapted from a letter submitted by the authors and several other liaison psychiatrist colleagues in 1993 to the London Implementation Group

(4) *Training*: Liaison psychiatrists are the only medical specialists whose training, clinical work and research manifestly focuses on the relationship between (physical) disease and the psyche (in its broadest sense). Evidence such as that outlined above clearly demonstrates the importance of this relationship, which is at the heart of the holistic approach to medicine, which is widely espoused by doctors and patients alike, but not consistently achieved in the absence of appropriate training. While such training may include input from disciplines other than medicine eg health psychology, behavioural medicine, medical sociology, the liaison psychiatrist is in a unique position to contribute to such a multidisciplinary approach by virtue of his/her medical training. In medicine, such training must begin at undergraduate level. The General Medical Council has long recommended changes in the training of medical undergraduates, including a reappraisal of training priorities to focus on training graduates to become better house officers and assigning specialist training to postgraduate courses, and a shift from teaching 'blocks' within isolated specialties towards integration between specialties. Some medical schools have already acted on these recommendations, but others (including most of the London medical schools) are currently revising their undergraduate courses to attempt to meet them. The integrated approach envisaged, as well as aiming to equip junior doctors with knowledge, skills and attitudes to manage their work more effectively, suggests an increasingly prominent and important role for liaison psychiatrists in all teaching hospitals.

Development of liaison psychiatry services in the NHS

In some countries, liaison psychiatry is well established. In the United States, for example, it is clearly recognized as a specialty in its own right. In Germany, every medical school has a unit specializing in psychosomatic medicine.

Despite the evidence for its importance and effectiveness, liaison psychiatry in Britain has seen no systematic development. Clinical services and training in liaison psychiatry vary markedly from one hospital to another. Many liaison psychiatry services owe their existence to either the research interests of Academic Departments or to the enthusiasm of individual psychiatrists committed to liaison work. From such origins, wider clinical services have sometimes developed, although often without systematic planning and almost always without increasing resources.

Elsewhere, general adult psychiatrists who work on the same site as their medical and surgical colleagues have provided an 'informal' liaison psychiatry service, in most cases without specific resources, and sometimes without special training. Liaison psychiatrists argue that this practice fails to acknowledge the specialist skills and knowledge of the liaison psychiatrist. This argument is accepted in other countries where liaison psychiatry is a specialty in its own right but has yet to be fully accepted by psychiatrists in Britain. Furthermore, in the absence of new resources, liaison psychiatry must compete with other aspects of psychiatric care for those limited resources available. It is therefore extremely difficult, if not impossible, for liaison psychiatry to achieve priority status. However, such competition is wholly inappropriate; it is equivalent to a hospital aiming to provide a comprehensive health service to its community being told that it can provide a service in general medicine or one in general surgery, but must choose between these. Under such circumstances, it is hardly surprising that the development of liaison psychiatry does not have the unequivocal support of all psychiatrists.

Obstacles to the development of liaison psychiatry

Recent NHS reforms have had an adverse impact on liaison psychiatry in several ways.

(1) *Transfer of psychiatric resources into the community*: Most psychiatric services are appropriately moving from the hospital into the community. A liaison psychiatry service which is not based in the general hospital is likely to be unsuccessful in meeting the needs of patients and non-psychiatric clinicians alike. On the other hand, liaison psychiatry has developed to date in many hospitals by taking a share of the overall resources available to psychiatric services. Recent trends have made such resources far less accessible.

(2) *The relationship between purchasers and providers*: Many psychiatric services have formed NHS Trusts of their own, separate from the Acute Trusts with whom they used to share hospital facilities. Nationwide, very few Acute Trusts either 'inherited' their own liaison psychiatry service, or made the development of such a service of their own a major priority. If therefore Acute Trusts wish to have a liaison psychiatry service, this must be purchased. Even if it were possible to resolve the question of the best provider of such a service (a specialist within the Acute Trust, or linked to the now separate Mental Health Trust), in most hospitals, where liaison psychiatry did not have previously earmarked resources, this would be a new service. This new provision must compete with existing demands for resources. Such existing demands and the services already established to meet these have, furthermore, been the main determinants to date of purchasers' decisions on mental illness service provision.

(3) *Relationship between NHS and academic resources*: A prominent academic component to liaison psychiatry is appropriate, given its importance in medical education at all levels. However, some liaison psychiatry services have been developed within Academic Departments from specific research interests, such as oncology or AIDS. The funding for such research, and/or the use of established Academic Department staff, have effectively subsidized the provision of the service to the NHS. Where this has occurred, it is extremely unlikely to continue. There is now a considerable risk of liaison psychiatry failing to find adequate resources by falling between the two stools, academic and NHS.

These difficulties and others were identified in the Joint Royal Colleges' Report, referred to above.

Needs for special consideration of liaison psychiatry

Because of the obstacles noted above to the development of liaison psychiatry, liaison psychiatric services require special consideration and support. This was acknowledged in the Tomlinson Report (Department of Health, 1992b), which stated that *[liaison psychiatry] services are sometimes neglected, or transferred to specifically psychiatric units which ... are not always adequately provided or well sited. We recommend that facilities for "liaison psychiatry" should be included in the review of specialties ...* Despite this recommendation, there was no specific mention of liaison psychiatry in the document *Making London Better* (Department of Health, 1993c).

Resources required for liaison psychiatry

The Royal College of Psychiatrists' (1992) report responding to the *Health of the Nation* recommended 0.5 whole-time equivalent consultant psychiatrist posts in liaison psychiatry (including postnatal psychiatry) per 100,000 total population. The Liaison Psychiatry group of the Royal College of Psychiatrists has recommended that a *basic* team to set up a liaison psychiatry service should include at least 5 sessions of consultant time, a full-time equivalent psychiatric trainee, two liaison psychiatric nurses and five sessions of clinical psychologist input (House and Hodgson, 1994). The Joint Colleges' Report recommended that an adequate liaison psychiatry service requires *at least one consultant psychiatrist whose main (ie not less than five weekly sessions) clinical commitment is to this work*, and that *a large hospital with several specialist units requires a full-time consultant liaison psychiatrist*. This report also stressed the need for a multiprofessional team, including liaison nurses, clinical psychologists and specialist social workers as well as psychiatrists.

5.4.2 Survey of London liaison psychiatry services

Method

Trusts in the North and South Thames Regions with catchment areas approximately within the M25 were identified from Regional directories [North Thames Regional Health Authority, 1995; South Thames Regional Health Authority, 1995]. No information was available on the range of services provided by each trust, but those known to have neither acute specialty services nor psychiatric services were excluded from the survey.

A brief questionnaire and a covering letter were sent to the chief executive or medical director of 66 trusts in March 1996. Those trusts which had not responded by May 1996 were sent a further questionnaire and covering letter. A total of 52 responses were received (80%). Of these, 13 replies indicated that the trust concerned either did not have a psychiatric service, or was an acute trust with a liaison psychiatric service provided by another trust included in the survey.

Profile of respondents

The 40 trusts which provided data for the survey covered 52 separate hospitals or specialist units.

Seven responding trusts (18%) were identified as providing both psychiatric and acute specialty services.

Since liaison psychiatric services provide a resource for acute specialty trusts, the survey enquired about the extent to which these services were funded by the mental health trusts which provided them and by the acute specialty trusts which received them. This was clearly not relevant to those seven trusts providing both psychiatric and acute services. Of the 33 trusts providing a mental illness service but no acute specialty services, 22 (67%) contributed 75% or more of the funding for their liaison psychiatry service. The service in a further 6 trusts (15%) was jointly funded by an acute and a mental health trust, each contributing at least 25% of the funding. Only 3 respondents reported that their liaison psychiatry service was funded predominantly by a non-psychiatric trust. Funding arrangements for 2 trusts were unknown.

The remainder of the results below summarize services at the 52 hospitals covered by the survey.

Profile of services

The type of hospital, and provision of psychiatric services for Accident and Emergency Department, are summarized in Table 1.

Table 1 Description of hospitals in survey

		N	%
TYPE OF HOSPITAL	District general	24	46
	University	10	19
	Teaching	12	23
	Specialist[a]	6	12
A&E DEPARTMENT ON SITE		42	81
ON-SITE PSYCHIATRIC SERVICE FOR A&E DEPT		30	58

[a]   *Specialist hospitals* include specialist units and postgraduate teaching hospitals

Of the 42 hospitals which had an Accident and Emergency Department, 12 (29%) did not have a psychiatric service for the A&E Department on site. Among these, the distance of the mental health unit from the A&E Department was up to 10 miles (median 2.5 miles).

Liaison psychiatry staffing

Table 2 reports the number of sessions of staff time devoted to liaison psychiatry, broken down by type of hospital. A more detailed summary of the configuration of services is shown in Table 3. Staff resources were not provided for one hospital, therefore these data are based on returns for 51 hospitals.

Of the hospitals included in the survey, 12 (24%) had no consultant sessions in liaison psychiatry. University hospitals and teaching hospitals were least likely to have no consultant sessions at all. Only 14 hospitals (28%) had at least one full-time psychiatric trainee, with 27 hospitals (53%) having no psychiatric trainee sessions dedicated to liaison psychiatry. The majority of hospitals (65% – N=33) had no liaison psychiatric nurses. Again, university or teaching hospitals were more likely than others to have some liaison psychiatric nursing provision. Clinical psychologists attached to liaison services were mainly confined to teaching hospitals, with 38 hospitals in the survey (75%) having no clinical psychology input. Only 5 hospitals (10%) had social work input to the liaison psychiatry team.

Table 2 Frequency of weekly staff sessions by type of hospital

Column percentages in parentheses		Type of hospital				
	Sessions	DGH	University	Teaching	Specialist	TOTAL
Consultant	None	8 (35)	1 (10)	-	3 (50)	12 (24)
	<=2	10 (44)	4 (40)	2 (17)	1 (17)	17 (33)
	3-5	4 (17)	4 (40)	3 (35)	1 (17)	12 (24)
	>5	1 (4)	1 (10)	7 (58)	1 (17)	10 (20)
Psychiatric trainee	None	15 (65)	4 (40)	2 (17)	6 (100)	27 (53)
	<10	4 (17)	2 (20)	4 (33)	-	10 (20)
	10	4 (17)	4 (40)	2 (17)	-	10 (20)
	>10	-	-	4 (33)	-	4 (8)
Liaison psychiatric nurse	None	21 (91)	3 (30)	4 (33)	5 (83)	33 (65)
	<10	2 (9)	-	2 (17)	-	4 (8)
	10	-	3 (30)	1 (8)	1 (17)	5 (10)
	11-20	-	4 (40)	2 (17)	-	6 (12)
	>20	-	-	3 (25)	-	3 (6)
Clinical psychologist	None	21 (91)	8 (80)	5 (42)	4 (67)	38 (75)
	<10	1 (4)	2 (20)	4 (33)	-	7 (14)
	10	-	-	2 (17)	1 (17)	3 (6)
	>10	1 (4)	-	1 (8)	1 (17)	3 (6)
Social worker	None	22 (96)	9 (90)	9 (75)	6 (100)	46 (90)
	10+	1 (4)	1(10)	3 (25)	-	5 (10)

Only four hospitals (8%), all of them teaching hospitals, had services which met the minimum standards recommended by the Royal College of Psychiatrists' Liaison Psychiatry Group. Even adopting a much lower threshold for an adequate service (at least 5 consultant sessions dedicated to liaison psychiatry, plus at least 10 sessions of other staff), this standard was reached by only 12 of the hospitals in the survey (24%). Of these, 6 were teaching hospitals and the other 4 were university hospitals. Of the 23 district general hospitals, only 2 reached these minimal requirements. The specialist units were particularly poorly provided for in their liaison psychiatry services.

Service changes since the Tomlinson Report

Changes since the Tomlinson Report to date are summarized in Table 4. Anticipated future changes are summarized in Table 5.

The majority of hospitals have seen no change in their liaison psychiatry services since 1992. Of the 20 hospitals (39% of the total) which have seen their liaison psychiatry services expand since 1992, 16 (80%) were either teaching hospitals or university hospitals. While 26 hospitals (51% of the survey) did not expect their liaison psychiatry service to expand, 14 (27%) anticipated some expansion. However, from the questionnaire responses, in only 8 of these hospitals had funding apparently been secured for these developments.

Table 3 Summary of liaison psychiatry service provision by type of hospital

Type of service	Frequency of services by type of hospital				
Column percentages in parentheses	DGH	University	Teaching	Specialist	TOTAL
None	4 (17)	1 (10)	-	2 (33)	7 (14)
Less than adequate A	14 (61)	1 (10)	2 (17)	3 (50)	20 (39)
Less than adequate B	3 (13)	4 (40)	3 (25)	1 (17)	11 (22)
Less than adequate C	-	-	1 (8)	-	1 (2)
Less than adequate (all)	21 (88)	6 (60)	6 (50)	6 (100)	39 (76)
Adequate	2 (9)	4 (40)	2 (17)	-	8 (16)
Comprehensive	-	-	4 (33)	-	4 (8)

Key to service categories in Table 3

None	No staff dedicated to liaison psychiatry service
Less than adequate A	Some sessions of consultant *or* trainee *or* nurse *or* psychologist
Less than adequate B	<5 consultant sessions *plus* sessions of psychiatric trainee *or* nurse *or* psychologist
Less than adequate C	5+ consultant sessions *plus* <10 sessions of psychiatric trainee *or* nurse *or* psychologist
Adequate	5+ consultant sessions *plus* 10+ sessions of psychiatric trainee *or* nurse *or* psychologist
Comprehensive	5+ consultant sessions *plus* some psychiatric trainee sessions *plus* 10+ nurse sessions *plus* some psychologist sessions

Table 4 Service changes since publication of the Tomlinson Report by type of hospital

Column percentages in parentheses	Frequency by type of hospital				
	DGH	University	Teaching	Specialist	TOTAL
Reduction	3 (13)	-	-	2 (33)	5 (10)
No change	17 (74)	1 (10)	5 (42)	3 (50)	26 (51)
Growth	3 (13)	9 (90)	7 (58)	1 (17)	20 (39)

Table 5 Anticipated future service changes by type of hospital

Column percentages in parentheses	Frequency by type of hospital				
	DGH	University	Teaching	Specialist	TOTAL
Reduction	3 (13)	-	1 (8)	-	4 (8)
No change	6 (26)	7 (70)	6 (50)	3 (50)	22 (43)
Growth	6 (26)	2 (20)	5 (42)	1 (17)	14 (27)
Unknown	8 (34)	1 (10)	-	2 (33)	11 (22)

5.4.3 Discussion

The number of responses received indicates that the results of this survey probably reflect the state of liaison psychiatry services in London. Among the different types of hospital, the poorest response rate was from postgraduate teaching hospitals. Anecdotal evidence suggests that in general, these have particularly inadequate liaison psychiatry services. However, given the low response rate from this group of units, the data on specialist hospitals above must be interpreted with particular caution.

This survey confirms that the provision of liaison psychiatry services in London is grossly inadequate. Of the hospitals surveyed, 7 (14%) had no liaison psychiatry service whatsoever. 12 (24%) had no consultant psychiatrist sessions dedicated to liaison psychiatry, and a further 8 hospitals (16%) had a skeleton service provided by other staff without any consultant sessions on site. In two cases, there appeared to be psychiatric trainees working in liaison psychiatry without dedicated consultant sessions on the same site. Even where hospitals had an Accident and Emergency Department, this did not guarantee the availability on site of psychiatric staff. In nearly one-third of hospitals with A&E Departments, there were apparently no psychiatric staff on site.

Most liaison psychiatry services are led by a consultant. There is widespread agreement among liaison psychiatrists that it is impossible to set up and develop an adequate liaison psychiatry service with less than 5 consultant sessions per week dedicated to liaison psychiatry, plus some other staff in the team. Thirty-eight of the hospitals surveyed (74%) failed to reach this minimum standard. Only 4 hospitals (all of them teaching hospitals) had a service with at least five consultant psychiatrist sessions, a full-time psychiatric nurse plus some input from psychiatric trainees and clinical psychologists. Thirty-three of the hospitals (67%) had no psychiatric nurses as part of the liaison psychiatry team, and 38 (75%) had no clinical psychology input. Only 5 hospitals (10%) had any dedicated social work input to the liaison psychiatry service.

As already noted above, considerable differences were found in service provision between the different types of hospital. Teaching hospitals and, to a lesser extent university hospitals, tended to have better liaison psychiatry services than district general hospitals. This was also reflected in the reported service developments since 1992. However, given the inadequacies in overall service provision, it is disappointing that only 14 services (27%) anticipated new developments in the foreseeable future.

5.4.4. Priorities for future development

Despite evidence of their benefits to patient care and overall service provision, liaison psychiatry services have not been adequately developed in London, as elsewhere in the United Kingdom.

Liaison psychiatry can certainly hold its own in justifying its call for resources. Liaison psychiatry services are well used, and popular with staff and patients alike – the former because of the nature of the services offered, the latter because of the proximity of the service to where it is needed, avoiding the stigma of treatment in a 'mental hospital' or other specialized treatment setting.

As in other branches of psychiatry, liaison psychiatrists are called upon to help in the management of disorders covering a wide range of severities, including a significant proportion of cases which are certainly severe, in terms of their impact on the patient's psychological state, physical illness, family and the health service. Not only do psychiatric disorders contribute significantly to impaired quality of life of physically ill people, but there is growing evidence that their presence can influence significantly the outcome of physical illnesses, in some instances increasing the risk of death. Although such risks have been demonstrated convincingly in research studies, it has been difficult to date to take them into adequate account in planning clinical services. To give just one example, recent work, quoted in the Joint Colleges' Report has shown that symptoms of depression following a myocardial infarction are associated with an increased risk of death (mainly from cardiac causes) in the subsequent 12 months (relative risk approximately 3). On this basis, and assuming a very conservative prevalence rate (10%) for depression post-infarct, depression is expected to contribute to approximately 4,400 *excess* deaths annually in the United Kingdom as a whole. If even 10% of these deaths are avoidable by more effective management of the depression, this would still represent an important contribution to reducing mortality. Until now, such details have been lost in the overall mortality statistics attributable to cardiac disease.

Within mental illness services, there has developed an increased focus on *severe mental illness* defined not by severity but by diagnostic category. Increasingly resources are being shifted away from the general hospital towards so-called SMI services, not least because of increasing public and political concern over the apparent failure of community care to prevent homicide by the mentally ill. This shift of resources has resulted in the relative neglect of services for patients with psychiatric disorders arising from physical illnesses such as cancer or myocardial infarction, for those presenting to hospital with deliberate self-harm and for those with mixed physical/psychiatric disorders such as irritable bowel syndrome and chronic fatigue syndrome.

Pressure for development can come from purchasers stipulating that the acute services which they purchase must include adequate and appropriate liaison psychiatry services, as recommended by the Joint Royal Colleges' Report. Specific funding should be made available to provide these liaison psychiatry resources, either through mental health services or through acute services, depending upon local circumstances at each district general hospital.

Acknowledgements

We thank Mrs Sheila Davidson for her help in sending out the questionnaires and in collating the results.

Chapter 5.5

Services in London for HIV/AIDS-related mental health needs

Jose Catalan

Summary

- A range of mental health problems is associated with HIV infection, including adjustment disorders, major depression, mania, hypochondrial disorders and a form of dementia. Carers also often need substantial support.
- Needs for services for HIV/AIDS-related mental health problems are concentrated in London, with more than two-thirds of AIDS cases notified in the UK being in the two Thames Regions.
- Specialist services for HIV-related mental health problems have developed in a number of centres, but are generally funded to provide out-patient services only. Where psychiatric admission is required, substantial difficulties have been encountered in treating this group on London's over-crowded in-patient wards, particularly as they often have complex medical problems as well as psychiatric illness.
- Ring-fenced moneys for HIV services are being reduced, and any reduction in funding for the mental health element of these services is likely to lead to substantial difficulties in meeting the high demand for such services.
- People with HIV-dementia have particularly complex needs for clinical and social needs, and the care received by this group is currently patchy and sometimes uncoordinated.
- Concerns have been expressed that people with severe mental illness may be a group at substantial risk of HIV infection.

The following are identified as current priorities for HIV/AIDS-related mental health services:

- Funding for these services needs to be maintained at least at current levels for mental health needs related to HIV/AIDS to be met.
- Service provision for HIV-dementia needs to be reviewed, with a view to establishing a well-coordinated and comprehensive system of services throughout the city.
- HIV-related mental health services need to become more closely integrated with both liaison psychiatry units in general hospitals and community mental health services.
- The prevalence of HIV infection in psychiatric populations needs to be monitored over the next few years to ensure that mental health services identify individuals with special needs, and that education strategies are implemented for both patients and staff.
- A small but worrying group of individuals have difficulty in initiating and maintaining behaviours that reduce the risk of HIV infection. Mental health specialists may have a role to play in helping these individuals to reduce the frequency of their risk behaviours, and strategies for doing this should be considered.

5.5.1 Historical development

London has been particularly affected by the AIDS epidemic, and this has resulted in the development of services and initiatives to deal with the psychiatric consequences of the disease.

At the end of 1995, 11,872 cases of AIDS have been reported in the UK since the beginning of data collection in 1982 (CDR, 1996a). The two Thames regions account for almost 70% (8 281) of AIDS cases. Since 1984 when reporting started, 25,689 cases of HIV-1 infection have been identified, with more than two thirds in the Thames regions. Projections regarding the incidence and prevalence of AIDS in England and Wales for 1995 to 1999 (CDR, 1996b) suggest this pattern of distribution will continue, with over 70% of people with AIDS or severe HIV-1 disease in the South East, in particular within London. In practice this is likely to mean about 5,600 people with AIDS/severe HIV disease alive and in need of care each year until the end of the decade.

Initiatives for the development of mental health services for people with HIV infection and their relatives and carers came from the medical units involved in their treatment, rather than from the mental health services, which in general were slow to appreciate the psychiatric implications of HIV infection. At first, mental health input was linked to genitourinary medicine (GUM) units, mostly in relation to the provision of support for people with AIDS, and later as part of the pre and post HIV test counselling. Psychologists played a crucial part in raising awareness about the psychological consequences of the infection, and were actively involved with GUM physicians, nurses and health advisors in the education and training of other staff and the general public. Full and part-time posts for clinical psychologists were developed in the main GUM clinics in London dealing with HIV patients, and in the newly developed in-patient medical services attached to them.

As the epidemic progressed, other problems became apparent. Psychiatric syndromes, including major depression, mania, and hypochondriacal disorders were recognised, and more disturbingly, a syndrome of dementia was described, which at first was thought likely to affect the majority of people with AIDS. Psychiatrists with an interest in HIV were appointed, usually on a sessional basis, but occasionally full-time. The involvement of psychiatrists led to a strengthening of psychiatric liaison services in some centres, and to the development of multidisciplinary teams, including psychologists and psychiatric nurses, the latter sometimes being involved in community-based work.

HIV-related problems spread among injecting drug users and other users of illicit drugs, and the risk for drug users of HIV infection also meant that considerable efforts were made to develop outreach services and other modalities of care, usually covered by the concepts of harm minimisation and risk reduction. Drug services have experienced major changes to a large extent in response to the HIV crisis (see section 5.3).

Most of the clinical work carried out by mental health workers has been on an out-patient basis or involving medical in-patients, with some community work. In addition, a number of people with HIV infection who develop severe mental health problems require in-patient psychiatric treatment which has not always been easy to achieve. As a rule, the overcrowded acute psychiatric units in London have not been the ideal place to treat individuals with complex medical problems who are also psychiatrically ill. Staff in psychiatric units have sometimes experienced difficulties caring for people with AIDS because of fears of infection or problems with confidentiality. Specialist funding for mental health services for HIV patients has usually been restricted to out-patient care, so that patients requiring admission have had to be referred to their district of residence, often far from the centre for HIV care.

Psychiatrists, psychologists and psychiatric nurses may be involved in the care of people with HIV-dementia at the stage of assessment and planning a package of care, and also in offering support for carers. Most people with HIV-dementia are cared for at home, with the assistance of respite and hospice care provided by independent agencies, and with medical in-patient care when required. Only one centre has been specifically developed for the care of people with HIV-dementia – this is Patrick House, in west London which is run by an independent organisation (see below).

Recently, concern has been expressed about the risk of HIV infection in people with severe psychiatric disorders, and about the need to monitor the prevalence of HIV in psychiatric patients in the capital (Stefan & Catalan, 1995).

5.5.2 Policy initiatives

(i) Funding:

Funding for HIV prevention and care services has been allocated to health regions on the basis of the number of cases of AIDS reported, although it was recognised that many patients with HIV would not be resident in the area where they received care. Funding for mental health services for HIV patients was only obtained through a complex process of bid submissions to the local health district on an annual basis. AIDS monies were ring fenced at first, although after 1994/5 only HIV prevention monies have continued to be ring fenced. Funding for HIV care is being reduced in 1996/7, and this process is likely to continue in future years, leading to difficulties meeting what is now a high demand for mental health services.

(ii) Professional standards:

The General Medical Council (GMC) issued guidelines in 1988, revised in 1993, about consent for HIV testing, and the duties of doctors regarding confidentiality and the duty to treat, all of which have had an impact on the development of services. The Royal College of Psychiatrists has endorsed guidelines for the psychiatric care of people with HIV infection (Catalan et al, 1989).

(iii) Legislation:

The AIDS (Control) Act, 1987 has required providers to give details of their activity and use of resources on an annual basis.

5.5.3 The development of a mixed economy of care

The history of the psychological and social care of people with HIV infection only started about 10 years ago, and existing services are the result of developments prompted by the AIDS epidemic. From the start, independent organisations have played an essential part in the provision of services for people with AIDS, in addition to the contribution made by statutory services. Unfortunately, figures are not available about the funding of the different sectors.

The mental health component of care has been relatively small compared with the general medical and social services costs, and has essentially been aimed at the provision of psychiatry, psychology and psychiatric nursing time. Most provision has been hospital based, attached to GUM departments and HIV/AIDS in-patient units, although some psychiatric nursing time has also been devoted to community work. While much of the work has being focused on care, prevention of the spread of infection through sexual contact has also been a target.

The contribution of independent organisations has been invaluable. They have been funded both by government money (direct contributions as well as via local health authorities) and through private donations and charities. People with HIV infection are actively involved in these organisations. The following are examples of such organisations and their functions:

(i) The Terrence Higgins Trust (THT): education and public awareness; legal and financial advice; provision of "buddies", volunteer personal carers for practical and emotional support; individual and group support for people with HIV and carers.

(ii) Residential: a) London Lighthouse: Residential care, both respite and palliative; individual and group counselling and therapy; day care; education and campaigning. b) Mildmay Mission Hospital: respite and palliative care; day care; support.

(iii) Counselling and support: There are many organisations including the Red Admiral Project, CARA, Body Positive, Positively Women. Some are targeted for certain groups such as women, ethnic minority groups and drug users.

(iv) Care of people with HIV-dementia: Patrick House: Small residential unit for people with HIV-dementia.

The role of general practitioners has been rather limited, although in recent years there has been a determined effort to involve them in the care of patients with HIV. Several factors have contributed to their lack of involvement. First, HIV was initially identified among GUM attenders, and the need to ensure confidentiality, as well as the historical absence of links with GPs in this speciality have tended to perpetuate the status quo. Second, GPs initially seemed unwilling to care for stigmatised patients about whom they themselves had negative feelings. Third, the complexity of the condition has tended to make patients seek specialist advice for health problems, rather than visit their GPs. However, in the last few years, many GPs have started to take on the day-to-day care of their patients with HIV, provided they have easy access to the hospital specialist. An advantage of this change for mental health workers in HIV has been the possibility of involving GPs in the care of the patients and their relatives.

5.5.4 Recent trends in service use

There are no central figures available, but some local units such as the author's have data available.

Our mental health team is based at the Chelsea and Westminster Hospital, where about 25% of all AIDS cases have been reported. We have a team which includes, psychologists and psychiatric nurses. We see for mental health assessment/care about 30% of all the HIV/AIDS patients looked after in the unit, which represents about 3 000 attendances per year. This has increased by around 10% per year over the last two years. More than three quarters of patients referred for mental health care are suffering from AIDS or have symptomatic disease. At the time of referral, two thirds are out-patients, while the rest are severely ill in hospital at the time of assessment. Table 1 shows the distribution of problems referred:

Table 1 Mental health problems in people affected by HIV infection

Patients experiencing psychological distress at some stage in their illness	most patients
Patients referred to services	30% of those in contact with specialist medical services
Psychiatric diagnosis of HIV patients referred to mental health services	30% adjustment disorder 30% depressive syndromes 15% organic brain disorder 10% sexual dysfunction 5% mania
Partners and informal carers	most carers experience some degree of psychological distress

Source: Catalán et al. (1995)

The most common psychiatric diagnosis is adjustment disorder (30%), followed by depression (29%). Organic brain syndromes occur in about 15%. A small number of patients (5%) require in-patient psychiatric treatment, usually as a result of mania or major depression, or against a background of poor coping and personality problems. The increasing number of patients with dementia referred for mental health care requires the involvement of psychiatrists and neuropsychologists, and often results in many case conferences and meetings with carers in the community and in other organisations. People with severe personality disorders, often complicated by substance misuse, usually require the continuing involvement of senior mental health staff in partnership with physicians and other workers. This group includes probably the most demanding patients seen by mental health workers. There is evidence of an increased risk of suicidal behaviour in people with HIV infection, and referral for an assessment of suicidal ideas is common (Catalan et al, 1995).

5.5.5 Adverse events related to London services

No such events are reported.

5.5.6 Reviews and inspections of London services for the speciality

The following reports are relevant to the current state of London's services:

(i) Bond, T. (1991) HIV Counselling: Report on National Survey and Consultation 1990. British Association for Counselling and Department of Health Joint Project.

Although not specifically about London this report involves a number of local members. It outlines some of the difficulties in providing psychological care, and gives examples of good practice.

(ii) Catalan, J. (1993) HIV infection and mental health care: implications for services. World Health Organisation, European Office, Copenhagen.

This is a survey of European professionals, including a substantial number from London. It describes the mental health needs of people with HIV infection and highlights the need to develop general hospital mental health services and for community support.

(iii) Higginson, I., Mallandain, I., Butters, E., Wilkins, S. (1995) What services are needed to care for people with HIV/AIDS encephalopathy in North Thames? Estimates of need and the views of clients, carers and professionals. Health Services Research Unit, London School of Hygiene and Tropical Medicine, London.

The report estimates the number of people with HIV-dementia, and the nature of services they require. It highlights the need for an adequate mix of services, awareness of the needs of carers, and further provision of neuropsychological assessment services and research.

(iv) Catalan, J., Meadows, J., Baldeweg, T. (1995) Epidemiology of HIV-associated dementia in London 1991–1994. Department of Health.

This is a detailed study of the prevalence of HIV-dementia in the London regions in 1991, and the incidence and prevalence in west London, 1991-1994, showing a significant increase in the incidence and prevalence figures. It reports the needs of carers, and describes the pattern of referrals to Patrick House.

5.5.7 Current priorities for HIV/AIDS-related mental health services

There is a danger that existing mental health services for HIV patients will be reduced over the next few years as a result of the slowing down in the number of new AIDS cases each year. However, any reduction in funding would be undesirable, as new cases of HIV infection continue to occur and patients with symptomatic HIV disease continue to live longer, with an increased risk of having psychiatric and social difficulties.

The prevalence and needs of individuals with HIV-associated dementia and other brain disorders require continuing monitoring. The provision of services for this group of patients and their carers is patchy and needs better co-ordination.

There is a need for the integration of HIV-related mental health services with both liaison psychiatry units in general hospitals and community mental health services.

The prevalence of HIV infection in psychiatric populations needs to be monitored over the next few years to ensure that mental health services identify individuals with special needs, and that education strategies for both patients and staff are implemented.

There is a small but worrying group of individuals who have difficulty initiating or maintaining behaviours that reduce the risk of HIV infection (i.e. sexual behaviour and injecting drug use behaviour). Mental health specialists may have an important role to play in helping these individuals reduce the frequency of their risk behaviours.

Chapter 5.6

Services for mentally disordered offenders

Hilary Guite and Vida Field

Summary

- London is markedly over-represented both among the population of the high security Special Hospitals (54.5 Special Hospital in-patients per million for London health authorities, 29.5 for England and Wales as a whole), and among medium secure unit patients (total medium secure bed use 58.3 per million for London, 31.1 for the country as a whole).
- Rates of use of these facilities are particularly high for Inner London health authorities, with close correlations between secure bed use and local unemployment rates. Expenditure on private sector medium secure places for London health authorities is currently about £15 million per year. This expenditure is largely a new development which was not required five years ago, and Health Authorities have no obvious source for funding it.
- London services have led in the development of court diversion, which has been associated with a doubling of numbers of people transferred from prisons to psychiatric in-patient units. Less attention has been paid to mental health care in prison, where current services appear very patchy.
- A severe shortage of forensic staff of all disciplines is an increasingly significant problem for London services.
- The Black population is markedly over-represented among mentally disordered offenders in London (for example, 40–50% of those diverted from prisons into psychiatric care are Black Caribbean, Black African or Black Other according to Census categories). Possible explanations include police and/or members of the public responding differently to Black people, the tendency for members of these ethnic groups not to reach psychiatric care by voluntary routes and the difficulties services have in engaging them effectively, and the high prevalence of schizophrenia which has been reported in these groups.
- Unemployment and lack of a permanent address are other characteristics strongly associated with mentally disordered offenders as a group. Previous convictions and previous psychiatric admissions are both frequent.

Possible solutions to problems currently encountered in these services include:

- Funding formulae need to be reviewed to reflect London's need for secure services, particularly for those inner city areas where use of secure facilities is very high. Ring-fenced mental health funding would be helpful to protect it from pressure from other sectors.
- The capital and revenue funding possibilities for supported housing for mentally disordered offenders no longer needing hospital care should be re-examined. Decisions on Housing Corporation funding and housing benefit are likely to have a major impact on the ability of such vulnerable groups to obtain and retain housing.
- More accessible and appropriate services for ethnic minorities are required to prevent young Black men with severe mental illness presenting via the criminal justice system at a late stage in the onset or relapse of illness.
- Attention needs to be paid to the training of staff in a variety of agencies in risk assessment and in management of mentally disordered offenders.
- Since London health commissions are the major purchasers of private medium secure places, they need to become concerned with better monitoring of the quality of care provided in these institutions.

5.6.1 Introduction

The Reed Report, a Department of Health/ Home Office (1991) review of services for mentally disordered offenders, states clearly that the majority of mentally disordered offenders are appropriately dealt with by local general adult psychiatric services. However, media attention, recent enquiries and cost pressures all focus on those people with mental illness who commit very serious offences. The particular pressures in London with high psychiatric morbidity and levels of offending mean that developments have targeted those with the most pressing needs and that those who commit petty offences and whose mental illness does not yet justify statutory intervention do not get access to services.

The focus in this review is on the state of London services for this small but important minority who have committed or are at risk of committing serious offences. The term 'mentally disordered offender' is widely used to describe those with a mental disorder whose behaviour is difficult, dangerous and often against the law, and includes more people than come under the remit of forensic psychiatry. However, it should be noted that some would argue that the use of the term 'mentally disordered offenders' is problematic, disadvantaging both those whom it is intended to describe and the services which might offer them care and treatment.

5.6.2 Historical development of services

a. The Special Hospitals

The first secure hospital was built at Broadmoor in 1863 to house 500 "criminal lunatics", Rampton Criminal Lunatic Asylum opened in 1912 and Moss Side in 1919. Moss Side merged with Park Lane Hospital to become Ashworth in 1989. These three special hospitals serve the whole of England and Wales but there is no one hospital which serves the whole of London. Broadmoor serves South East and SW Thames, Ashworth NW Thames and Rampton NE Thames, but Rampton has developed a specialisation in mental impairment and severe mental impairment and Broadmoor only very exceptionally admits mentally impaired people. The catchment area relationship is further complicated by historic patterns of admission and more recently by the admission of patients to Rampton because Broadmoor has no available beds.

In 1989, as a result of concern about standards of care, the Special Health Services Authority was established to run the hospitals along NHS general management lines. The system of management then changed again in 1996 to bring it more nearly in line with the rest of the health service. Each Special Hospital is now a Special Health Authority, and the High Security Psychiatric Commissioning Board, with representatives from all the regions, is now responsible for contracting for high security services.

The population of the Special Hospitals has fallen from 2350 in the early 1970s to approximately 1520. Londoners are over-represented in their population, with 375 of Special Hospital patients having originated from Greater London at February 1996.

The Report of the Working group on High Security and Related Psychiatric Provision (Department of Health 1994b) recommended that high security services should be more widely dispersed and should cater for no more than 200 high security patients each. The

Orville Blackwood Inquiry (Prins, 1993) found that the cultural and ethnic differences between the staff and patients in Broadmoor made it difficult to provide an appropriate service for the Black Caribbean inner city young men being admitted from London.

A Department of Health needs assessment exercise conducted in 1995 estimated that 32% of current Special Hospital patients would be more appropriately placed in long term medium security and a further 10% need longer term low security. If these proportions hold true for London patients then approximately 120 London patients need long term medium secure accommodation and 37 longer term low security. The study of a 20% sample of Special Hospital patients by Maden et al. (1996a) found similar proportions needing long term medium secure but stressed that their treatment needs would vary considerably and their security needs might vary over time. Longer term facilities need space for day time occupation, leisure, privacy etc. and need also to be culturally appropriate, which raises issues about where they might be sited. Space, planning permission and staffing problems would raise practical difficulties in London even if there were a model of good practice to implement. Currently patients in Special Hospital are not a charge on local Health Authorities. Health Authorities question whether it will be possible to reprovide for these patients within the budget which will be devolved from the High Security budget. Any development would need to be integrated with existing facilities to prevent isolation and institutional practice.

Although most of the emphasis is on reproviding for those who need a lower level of security there are those within the prison service whose need for high secure psychiatric care is not always met. Gunn et al. (1990) found that about one third of male sentenced prisoners needing transfer to NHS hospitals required high security care. About 8-15 beds in maximum security are needed by the remand population in maximum security.

Table 1 shows numbers of patients in Special Hospitals from London districts. The number of patients in Special Hospitals per million resident population correlates highly with the number of MSU beds commissioned by districts.

Figure 1 shows how numbers of Special Hospital beds vary with unemployment rates:

Figure 1 Special Hospital beds and unemployment

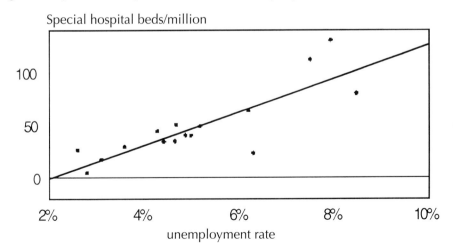

Unemployment rates in Figure 1 are from Department of Employment data, and give % of total population unemployed – not adjusted for numbers who are economically active.

Table 1 Patients in the Special Hospitals (Broadmoor, Rampton and Ashworth) from London districts 1996

District	Number of patients in Special Hospital	Number in Special Hospital per million resident population
Barking, Havering and Harrow	11	29.1
Barnet	7	23.0
Bexley & Greenwich	15	34.5
Brent & Harrow	22	48.4
Bromley	5	17.14
Camden & Islington	40	112.1
Croydon	11	34.0
Ealing, Hammersmith & Hounslow	26	40.1
East London & The City	47	80.0
Hillingdon	1	4.2
Lambeth, Southwark and Lewisham	95	130.3
Kensington, Chelsea & Westminster	17	50.3
Kingston & Richmond	8	26.2
Merton, Sutton & Wandsworth	27	44.0
New River	30	63.3
Redbridge & Waltham forest	18	40.0
Total Greater London	378	54.5
England & Wales	1520	29.5

Thus SHA bed use appears closely associated with local unemployment rates: the correlation between the two variables is 0.84.

b. Medium secure units

The development of less restrictive care within general psychiatry made psychiatric hospitals much less able to deal with those needing some level of security. As locked wards disappeared fewer mentally disordered offenders were admitted to psychiatric hospitals and numbers of hospital orders fell throughout the 1970s. It was recognised that there was a gap in provision between the high security special hospitals and the psychiatric hospitals for both very disturbed psychiatric patients and mentally disordered offenders.

Despite the recommendations of the Glancy report (Department of Health and Social Security, 1974) and the Butler Report (Home Office and Department of Social Security, 1975) that there should be 1000/ 2000 medium secure beds respectively and the earmarking of special funding, progress was very slow and the Reed Report (1992) noted that even the lower Glancy targets had still not been met. Latest figures from DH indicate that there will be about 1200 NHS medium secure beds by the end of 1996 and a further 400 provided in "interim secure units". The private sector has not been slow to offer services to meet the gap in provision and there were over 400 private medium secure beds available in 1995.

Following the Glancy report the government allocated capital to Regions on a formula of 20 beds per million population. As shown in Table 2, progress in relation to the allocation was very different in the Thames regions:

Table 2

	Allocation	**open 31/1/92**	**open mid 1995**
North West Thames	69	46	62
North East Thames	74	14	46
South East Thames	72	85	96
South West Thames	58	0	30
TOTAL THAMES REGIONS	273	145	234

The different rate of development of medium secure beds reflects not only relative speed in making progress but also different philosophies and models of care. The former North East Thames Region historically used placements in the private sector. Although it still has fewer beds than the other three former Thames regions, it is now looking to develop further facilities. The old South West Thames took a different approach to the recommendations of the Butler report and opted for an integrated approach involving the development of close supervision units within each district with plans for only a small medium secure unit. The former South East Region originally developed a central unit on the Bethlem site with four other satellite units around the region. Increasingly the differences between these four areas have disappeared as the South West and North East Thames have developed more local medium secure beds at Springfield Hospital and Hackney Hospital and the South East Thames has moved to 5 catchment area services. North West Thames developed the Three Bridges medium secure unit as the core of its forensic service, but with a range of other wards to prevent blocking of the medium secure beds. The addition of the Bentham Unit, a remand ward, has demonstrated the potential of such a facility but this has now encountered difficulties with continuing funding. The close supervision units remain in the South West and the Bethlem and Maudsley Trust has an open forensic ward, up to now as part of their national service. Increasingly, medium secure units as the core of the forensic service are developing community outreach functions although the debate about parallel and integrated services (Gunn and Taylor, 1993) continues to exercise minds. Whatever the theoretical or pragmatic solutions to this debate the interface between the forensic and general psychiatric services and between different levels of security must be agreed at local level.

Despite the increase in NHS medium secure beds during 1995 and 1996 there has also been an increase in the use of private sector beds. (E.g. LSL HA used 6 private medium secure beds in 1990 and about 50 in 1995). Table 3 shows the current levels of Medium Secure bed use in each London district.

Table 3 Use of medium secure unit (MSU) services in London, 1995–1996

District	Population '000s (mid year estimates 1993)	Number of beds commissioned 1996	Commissioned MSU beds/million population	Number of Extra-contractual (ECR) medium secure beds in June 1996 (NE Thames, June 1995 South Thames)	Total MSU beds including ECRs/million resident population
Brent & Harrow	454.3	11	24.2	0	24.2
Ealing, Hammersmith & Hounslow	647.6	28	43.2	0	43.2
Kensington, Chelsea and Westminster	337.9	11	32.6	9	32.6
East London & City	590.7	27	45.7	53	120.2
Camden & Islington	356.9	18	50.4	45	50.4
Lambeth, Southwark and Lewisham	728.9	47	64.5	47	129.0
Merton, Sutton & Wandsworth	614.1	15	24.4	0	24.4
Barnet	304.7	3	9.8	0	9.8
Hillingdon	239.6	0	0	2	8.3
Barking & Havering	377.7	7	18.5	8	39.7
Redbridge and Waltham Forest	452.5	2	4.4	0	13.3
New River	473.7	12	25.3	21	25.3
Bromley	291.8	7	24.0	0	24.0
Bexley and Greenwich	434.7	10	23.0	7	39.1
Croydon	323.3	2	6.2	0	6.2
Kingston & Richmond	304.6	7	23.0	1	23.0
Total Greater London	6933.0	207	30.0	197	58.3
England & Wales	51439.0	1200	23.3	400	31.1

Figure 2 shows the relationship between total medium secure unit bed use (including extra-contractual referrals) and unemployment.

Figure 2 Medium secure bed use and unemployment

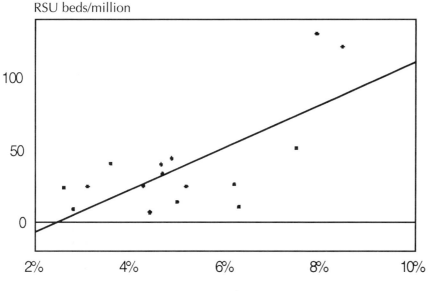

Thus use of medium secure beds is also closely associated with unemployment rate: the correlation between proportion of the total local population who are unemployed and use of RSU places (including extra-contractual referrals) is 0.71.

c. Low secure units/intensive care wards

Wards with lower levels of security have at least two functions: intensive treatment for acutely ill people requiring short term intervention before returning to the acute ward, and longer term treatment and rehabilitation for challenging behaviour.

The lack of an agreed definition of low secure provision makes statements on the supply of local provision difficult to make. However, an NHS Executive (1996a) paper to the Inner London Mental Health Purchasers estimates however that North and South Thames contain approximately 40% of the nation's low secure services.

Low secure bed numbers have fallen with the closure of long stay hospitals. Reed estimated that there were 1176 beds in locked or lockable wards in 1986. The Department of Health needs assessment of July 1995 estimated that 2320 current clients need longer term (>24 months) lower security placements nationally. The increasing pressure on both medium secure beds and acute psychiatric beds in London is likely to have led to a bottleneck at the low secure level.

d. Diversion schemes

The case for major improvements to the system of liaison between the criminal justice system and mental health services was made largely by London psychiatrists (Bowden, 1978; Taylor, 1986; Coid, 1988; Fahy, 1989; Herridge, 1989; Gunn, 1990 & 1991; James 1991). The disproportionate number of people with severe mental illness involved in the criminal justice system, the needs for support in managing prisoners with mental illness and the long delays accessing help were recorded. Patients remanded to prison for a psychiatric opinion often suffered one of two fates: i) spending longer in prison waiting for a psychiatric opinion than they would have served if convicted and managed in the usual way (James, 1991); ii) waiting in prison for a psychiatric opinion only to be rejected for psychiatric treatment (Coid, 1988).

The effect of these reports, encouragement from the Home Office (1990) and the Reed report (1993) led to a doubling of the number of people transferred from prisons to psychiatric hospitals between 1991 and 1994, as shown in Table 4:

Table 4

Year	1974	1985	91/92	92/93	93/94	94/95
Transferred to psychiatric hospital	1209	546	390	648	774	715

Source: Bowden (1990) and HM Prison Service (1996)

The Reed report advised that schemes should be set up to divert mentally disordered offenders to health and social services from four main points in the criminal justice system:

a) at first contact with the police, the arresting officer may decide that the offender is suffering from a mental illness and is in need of immediate care and control;
b) while held in custody, the arresting officer, the forensic medical officer or, where there is a police station diversion scheme in operation, the Community Psychiatric Nurse or psychiatrist may advise diversion;
c) at court where a court diversion scheme is in operation;
d) in prison where either the offender is seen as a result of being remanded by the court for psychiatric assessment or are identified by the prison medical service or the prison diversion scheme.

By 1993 15 out of 18 inner London courts either had their own psychiatric assessment scheme or access to one at a nearby court whereas in outer London 8 of 18 courts had a scheme (Burney 1995). By the end of 1995 the vast majority of courts in London had formal court diversion arrangements, though the amount of time available to the courts and the grade and professional discipline of the staff vary considerably (Table 5).

The interface between the Home Office and the Department of Health is particularly important when court diversion is being considered. The Home Office circular 12/95 which updated 66/90 placed much greater emphasis on public safety issues and lays more stress on psychiatric assessment than diversion.

Arrangements for psychiatric care in London's prisons still vary from a few sessions a week from a visiting psychiatrist to a multi-agency team providing assessments within 48 hours for all patients referred by admitting officers (personal communication; H.M. Prison Service Health Care).

Table 5 Magistrates Court diversion schemes in London

Health Authority	Courts	Delivered by	Days per week
EL&C, C&I	Clerkenwell, Hampstead, Highbury, Old St	Psychiatric referrals are sent from the four courts to Clerkenwell to be seen by a forensic psychiatrist. A CPN visits Old St and Highbury Corner to provide screening	n/a
EL &C	Newham	CPN and consultant psychiatrist on call 2 mornings a week to undertake assessments	2 x 0.5
EL &C	Thames	Voluntary agency- Homeless Health East London Project in addition to a psychiatric senior registrar	n/a
C&I	Highgate	CPN funded by a charitable trust, and involving collaboration with the Inner London Probation Service and the Mental After Care Association. Referral of relevant cases to Clerkenwell Court for consultant psychiatrist assessment.	full time
LSL, B&G	Tower Bridge, Greenwich, Woolwich, Bexley	Psychiatrist and CPN from Bracton medium secure unit to three courts. Woolwich remanded defendants requiring a psychiatric opinion to Greenwich court. Social worker from Lewisham Social services attends Tower Bridge. Bexley & Greenwich social services provide on-call service only.	one day in each court
LSL	Camberwell	Psychiatrist and CPN from Cane Hill	0.5
MSW, K&R	Wimbledon, Richmond, Kingston, Sutton	Psychiatrist (0.5 days), clinical nurse specialist (1 day)	1
MSW	South Western	Forensic psychiatrist (1 day), CPN from St George's (2 *0.5 days)	2
EHH, KCW	Horseferry Rd, Bow St, Marlborough, Marylebone, West London	All psychiatric referrals are remanded to Horseferry Rd. Service provided by forensic psychiatrist, CPN and ASW	daily
Bromley	Bromley	Nurse and social worker from Cane Hill medium secure unit	0.5-1 day
Croydon	Croydon	General psychiatrist with a special interest in forensic psychiatry, forensic CPN and ASW	0.5
NR	Tottenham Court, Enfield	Staff from Camlet Lodge. Defendants from Enfield court referred to Tottenham Court	one day
B&H	Barking, Havering	n/a	0.5 each
Br & Har	Brent	Staff from Central Middlesex Hospital	0.5
Br & Har	Harrow	CPN every morning, psychiatrist when needed	0.5 * 5
RWF	Waltham Forest	Staff from Camlet Lodge	0.5
RWF	Redbridge	CPN from Goodmayes	daily
Barnet	Barnet	n/a	n/a

Source: South Thames Regional Office and Revolving Doors Agency

e. Staffing

With the development of new medium secure facilities in London, the shortage of forensic staff predicted by the Reed Report has become apparent. The Report of the Staffing and Training Advisory Group provisionally identified minimum needs for :

- at least 80 additional consultant forensic psychiatrist posts, plus 175 other consultant posts and 10–15 consultant posts for academic work, supported by additional senior registrar, registrar and junior posts. Enhanced input from GPs would also be needed;
- over 2,000 nursing posts to be filled if medium secure provision is increased to 1,500 places;
- as many as 80 new NHS clinical psychologists;
- enhanced provision of occupational therapists, speech therapists and physiotherapists;
- some 125 with additional social workers for work on medium secure units and court diversion schemes, with additional needs for a range of social services staff working in a multiplicity of settings.

The lack of these additional staff is beginning to have an impact on many of the units in London and the shortage of trained forensic staff is exacerbated by the difficulties of recruiting any psychiatric staff in London. As the pressure on services increases, comparative cost of living and quality of life are no longer offset by the attractions of working in a centre of excellence as academic departments are established outside London.

The increasing need to work in the community with discharged patients has highlighted the need for multi-disciplinary and interagency working. Not only is there a need for greater professional training in working within the forensic service but people working within the general psychiatric services need training to enable them to work with mentally disordered offenders.

5.6.3 Prevalence of mentally disordered offenders

a. Arrest

About 1 in 40 to 50 people arrested are found to have a mental disorder – estimates range from 1.85% to 3.95% depending on the definition of mental disorder (Cherrett 1996, Revolving Doors Agency 94, 1995a, 1995b). This represents about 10,000 people with mental health problems dealt with each year by London's Metropolitan Police, a rate of 1.39/1000 resident population (Revolving doors agency 1995b).

b. Section 136

Whether someone who has committed a breach of the peace is charged, diverted at point of arrest or transferred under a section 136 tends to be determined by the availability of psychiatric services and social services (Fahy 1989, Robertson 1995). In 1986 in London there were 1,322 section 136 applications which accounted for 87% of all section 136 applications in the UK.

c. Court

Hudson (1995) found that about 0.5% of all custody cases were referred for a psychiatric opinion, an estimated 0.53/1000 population/year.

d. Prison

Gunn (1991 a & b) found that 37% of men and 56% of women sentenced prisoners had a psychiatric disorder (including drug abuse and personality disorder). Overall 3.5% of men and 4.0% of women required transfer for inpatient psychiatric treatment.

A report is due later this year from work in progress by the Forensic Department at the Institute of Psychiatry on the prevalence of mental disorder among remand prisoners.

5.6.4 Demographic, clinical and social characteristics of mentally disordered offenders

There are marked similarities in the demographic, clinical and social characteristics of patients diverted at point of arrest from police stations, at courts, or from prisons. There are differences in the type of offence and the outcome of referral at different points in the system. The following summary of the characteristics of mentally disordered offenders derives from studies of London's criminal justice system and court and prison diversion schemes (Taylor, 1985; James, 1991; Dell, 1993; Joseph, 1993; Revolving Doors Agency 1994; Exworthy, 1994; Banerjee, 1995; Hudson, 1995).

The mean age of mentally disordered offenders is between 30 and 34 years at police stations, courts and prisons. Mentally disordered offenders are principally male – typically about 90%. As shown in Table 6, the Black populations (Black Caribbean, Black African and Black Other) are over-represented amongst mentally disordered offenders making up 40% to 50% of patients diverted from prisons. 50% of the variation between districts' demand for MSU beds is accounted for by the variation in the proportion of the population who are black, but it is also worth noting that there is a similar correlation with unemployment.

Table 6 Rates of diversion to psychiatric in-patient care and use of in-patient beds following diversion from courts and prisons by ethnic group

Type of ward	Black (Black African, Black Caribbean, Black Other)	White	Other
OPEN WARDS Number of mdos diverted/100,000 residents aged 16-64 years	25	6	17
Number of occupied bed days used/1000 residents aged 16-64 years	56.04	14.56	101.7
LOCKED WARDS Number of mdos diverted/100,000 residents aged 16-64 years	34	5	8
Number of occupied bed days used/1000 residents aged 16-64 years	9.76	6.75	22.0
MEDIUM SECURE WARDS Number of mdos diverted/100,000 residents aged 16-64 years	28	4	17
Number of occupied bed days used/1000 residents aged 16-64 years	150.94	10.85	69.06

Source: Guite et al. (unpublished), Diversion from courts and prisons to psychiatric in-patient care in an inner city district.

The majority of patients are known to local psychiatric services and between two thirds and three quarters have had a previous psychiatric admission. A similar proportion have a diagnosis of a psychotic disorder. Up to a half had lost contact with services prior to offending. Approximately one third of patients have a secondary diagnosis of alcohol or drug misuse, while 10% have a primary diagnosis of drug or alcohol misuse. Between one third and one half of all offending by people with mental disorder is judged to be directly related to active psychotic symptoms. Of those with psychosis the majority (93%) were found to be ill at the time of their offence.

Most court and prison diversion schemes depend on staff who are not psychiatrically trained to identify patients for a psychiatric opinion. At police stations 25% of patients were missed by arresting officers and 40% were missed by prison officers.

The majority (83-90%) of mentally disordered offenders are unemployed. Between 40% and 50% have no permanent accommodation. For at least 29%, it was recorded in their psychiatric notes that they had been in residential care of local authorities, mostly as a result of bereavement or parental illness (Guite, 1996). Around 50% of patients in Special Hospitals have a history of being in care as a child (Taylor 1995, inaugural lecture).

Table 7 shows the correlation between census variables and admission to medium or high secure care. The Jarman UPA8 score explains 56% of the variation between districts. Single variables (% Black population and % unemployed) provide similar explanations of variability of use of medium secure beds.

Table 7 Correlation of census sociodemographic variables with admission rates for medium and maximum secure beds (combined)

Census variable	Spearman's rank correlation coefficient
Under privileged area 8 score	r=0.75
Elderly alone	r=0.27
Children under 5 years	r=0.29
One parent families	r=0.49
Unskilled workers	r=0.50
Persons unemployed	r=0.64
Overcrowding	r=0.66
Moved house last year	r=0.41
Ethnic minorities	r=0.51

Source: Coid J. Unpublished data based on admissions to medium secure (NHS and private) and maximum secure units in North East Thames 1989-1993.

5.6.5 Forensic characteristics of mentally disordered offenders

The type of index offence and severity of any violence tend to increase with the level at which diversion takes place, from point of arrest to diversion from prison. Over half of mentally disordered offenders identified in police stations were charged with public order offences. In contrast over 50% of those diverted by the courts were charged with violent or aggressive offences. Two thirds of these violent and aggressive offences involved violence against the person and one third involved criminal damage. About one third of those identified by prison diversion schemes have assaulted, of which 40% were serious violent offences.

The majority of victims are known to the mentally disordered offender, with complete strangers accounting for 20% of victims (Guite, 1996).

In general psychotic populations one third have a recorded history of previous conviction, (PRISM unpublished data), while the majority (77%–80%) of mentally disordered offenders have previous convictions.

5.6.6 Current pattern of service use by mentally disordered offenders and factors affecting demand for services

Over two thirds of mentally disordered offenders transferred to in-patient care are managed solely by general adult psychiatrists (Guite, 1996). One third (36%) of all patients diverted from courts and prisons are cared for entirely on open wards, one third (34%) spend some time in a locked ward and otherwise are on open wards and just one third (30%) of mentally disordered offenders spend time on medium secure wards (Guite, 1996).

a General adult open psychiatric wards and low secure wards
Patients diverted from courts account for between 1.7% (Exworthy, 1994) and 5% of all general psychiatric admissions (Joseph, 1993).

b. Medium secure wards
The current provision of medium secure beds in Greater London districts has been shown in Table 3. Including extracontractual referrals London's rate of use of these beds is nearly double that of the country as a whole. Lambeth, Southwark and Lewisham Health Authority and East London and City Health Authorities uses about four times as many medium secure beds as the National average.

c. Special Hospitals
Table 1 has shown the number and population based prevalence of patients in the Special Hospitals. The rate of use of Special Hospital beds for Greater London is 80% above that or England and Wales as a whole.

d. Outcomes of diversion
Mentally disordered offenders are more likely to have cases against them discontinued or proceedings dropped than non-mentally disordered offenders. In 40% of those identified in police stations no further action was taken while 29% of cases were not proceeded with in court compared to 4.6% generally (Hudson, 1995). Only around one quarter of those referred for psychiatric opinion in court are admitted for in-patient care (Exworthy, 1994; Joseph, 1993).

Overall, court diverson schemes appear to reduce prison stays on remand for mentally disordered offenders substantially. As late as 1993 Hudson reported that their mean length of stay on remand was 50 days. Court and prison diversion schemes can reduce these periods to between one to two weeks (Joseph, 1993, Exworthy, 1994)

e. Outcomes of hospital treatment
Joseph (1993) reported that 23% of patients received no benefit – most of these absconded or were discharged because of unacceptable behaviour. Thirty two per cent derived some benefit and improvement in their mental state, but only 4 out of 21 attended subsequent follow up appointments. 45% benefited markedly showing both improvements in mental state and successful rehabilitation.

Robertson's (1994) follow up of 101 men who received a hospital order in 1989 found that 23% absconded at some time during their stay, 11% discharged themselves or were discharged after absconding. Nearly all hospitals (93%) recorded that the admissions were appropriate. 53% were still in-patients at 3 months, 16% were violent towards people. 91% showed at least some improvement, and 59% reported marked improvement in the patient's condition.

f. Reoffending
It has been argued that assessing the effectiveness of services in reducing offending behaviour is inappropriate for mental health services who should concentrate on treating the patient's mental illness. No London based studies report rates of reoffending. Cooke (1992) in Glasgow reported that within 31 months of assessment at a forensic clinic 15% of those accepted for treatment had reoffended compared to 41% of those not treated. When selection factors were controlled for there was a trend which suggested treatment had an effect but it failed to reach statistical significance.

5.6.7 Inquiries and reports

Within the field of mentally disordered offenders there have been four highly influential reports which have received both public and professional attention. In 1990 Stephen Tumim's report into prison suicides described appalling conditions in which reception to the prison occurred and in which medical assessments took place. In 1993 the Reed report set out the UK strategy for the development of services for mentally disordered offenders and the two reports from the Confidential Inquiry into Homicides (1994 and 1996) were extensively reported in the media.

In the decade from 1978 to 1988 there was only one independent inquiry into a homicide in the UK by someone with a mental illness. During 1988 to 1996 there have been at least 26 published independent inquiries in England, 11 of which were in London. The inquiries published in the 1990s have been summarised in Section 4.4. The published reports are a biased group but still provide valuable information in the form of detailed accounts of how systems of care can work or fail in practice. These case histories can help to focus on the difficult and sometimes abstract issues of causation of these rare tragedies. The accessibility of these reports and the work of relatives of victims have meant that some have received a very high profile. The Ritchie report (1994) is probably the best known of these and, as discussed in Section 6.8, data from South London seem to suggest that the report may have been responsible for a rapid increase in demand for acute inpatient care in each of three mental health trusts. There was anecdotal evidence an increasing orientation towards risk aversion in clinical behaviour (Guite et al, 1995).

The major themes of these inquiries are discussed more fully in Chapter 4, but important emphases throughout are on the importance of explicit assessment of risk, communication between agencies, the need to record clearly previous histories of assault and to take their severity seriously, and the lack of continuity of psychiatric care characterising many of the histories of these mentally disordered offenders. It is striking how closely the recommendations of subsequent inquiries resemble those of one of the earliest, the 1988 inquiry into the care of Sharon Campbell, where the homicide victim was a social worker. In 1988, recommendations included improvements in care planning, keyworker allocation and multi-disciplinary review, better risk assessment training, clearer recording of risk, training in managing people from differing cultural and ethnic backgrounds, and the development of a register of patients who are vulnerable and require special supervision. All these recommendations required restatement six years later in the inquiry into the care of Christopher Clunis.

5.6.8 Current key issues

a. Personality disorder

Different views are taken in different services about the appropriate response to people with personality disorder/ psychopathic disorder. When the Butler Committee reported in 1975, specialist units within prisons were envisaged for those with psychopathic disorder who posed a grave risk to the public. No such units have developed and the special prison unit in Parkhurst Prison which might have met a similar need has now closed.

Since the passing of the 1983 Mental Health Act there has been increasing concern about risk to the public especially where Mental Health Review Tribunals discharge patients on the basis that their psychopathic disorder no longer makes it appropriate for them to be detained in hospital. The Report of the Department of Health and Home Office Working Group on Psychopathic Disorder 1994 literature review concluded that there was insufficient evidence to determine whether or not those with psychopathic disorder could be successfully treated.

The working group recommended that a range of services be developed so that their effectiveness could be evaluated. It also recommended that the concept of a hybrid order should be more widely discussed and there is now proposed legislation from the Home Office. This would extend to all those with a mental illness for whom a new disposal would be available to the Crown Courts which would combine a hospital direction and a fixed tariff. Offenders would be sent directly to hospital but in the event of them proving untreatable or no longer needing treatment they would be transferred to prison to serve the rest of their sentence. It is not clear how many people might be affected by this proposal if it became law and whether its main impact in practice would be to impose a harsher punishment on those currently deemed suitable for a hospital order or whether it might extend the possibilities of treatment to those currently sentenced to a prison term. The proposal has been widely condemned and is opposed by the Royal College of Psychiatrists.

b. Ethnicity

Burney (1995) has summarised the main factors which have been suggested as explanations of the striking excess of young Black men among mentally disordered offenders:

i) 'over-representation of Black people in the diagnostic category of schizophrenia'
ii) 'evidence from the British Crime Survey that white people are more likely to report minor acts of violence which led to no harm to the victim if these result from black assailants than if the assailant had been white';
iii) 'racial prejudice and negative stereotyping of black people within the police service mean that interactions between the police and public are significantly different at the point of arrest';
iv) the routes to care for Black people are more frequently through the criminal justice system than through primary care.

c. Women

Women are in a minority within the criminal justice system and are represented at low levels in forensic psychiatry, making up just 16% of the Special Hospital population. Women are less likely to have been before the courts, (44% of women in Special Hospitals are on civil sections as compared with 16% of men) and more likely to be unrestricted (47% of women as against 30% of men).

Service provision is geared to needs of male patients because they are in such a majority. It is difficult for women to feel safe especially as they are having to live in close proximity to men, many of whom have histories of domestic and sexual violence when so may of the women in secure care have been victims of physical and sexual violence by men. The proposal that there should be separate facilities for women has attracted some support and a London-wide approach would make it feasible, especially if such a facility had both high and medium secure services on site.

d. Homelessness, housing and aftercare

The fundamental role of housing in the spectrum of care for people with mental health problems has been increasingly recognised in recent years (Mental Health Foundation, 1994). Homeless people have been shown to have high levels of multiple special needs and many of them could be characterised as mentally disordered offenders. Housing breakdown has shown to occur in association with mental health problems and criminal behaviour by the Revolving Doors Agency in their study of people coming to the attention of the police. Unsuitable housing and lack of bail provision can mean that people are remanded to prison for psychiatric reports. Homelessness, shortage of affordable rented housing, and unemployment leading to loss of tenancies are all problems which have increased at the same time as pressure on psychiatric beds, including secure beds, has risen.

There is also a shortage of appropriate housing for people ready for discharge from medium secure units. There is a lack of high support accommodation which can provide for people with serious offending histories and can meet the need for supervision in the community. Access to housing, support in maintaining tenancies, and greater facilities for long term high levels of support would all increase the potential for mentally disordered offenders to remain safely in the community. Local authority housing departments and housing associations need to be involved in the care planning process and to be given the information they need to provide safe and suitable housing.

e. Funding crises

Nationally £30 million pounds per year is being spent on private sector places for mentally disordered offenders (source: briefing paper for the Inner London Purchasers

Group 1996). About £15 million of the expenditure on private medium secure places comes from London which as shown in Table 3 uses half of all UK private medium secure beds. Most of this is additional expenditure which was not required five years ago, and there is no obvious funding source. Since the NHS reforms, funding has been allocated to Health Authorities on the basis of a weighted capitation formula. The factor within this formula which has the greatest impact on the amount of money each health authority receives is the size of the population. Many of London's inner city health authorities have falling populations which means that their overall target budget will be reducing year on year. In order for Regional Health Authorities to provide strategic and secure funding rather than crisis funding for mentally disordered offender services they would need to devolve so much money to some inner city districts that it would push them off course for reaching their target under the weighted capitation formula.

f. Interagency working

One of the central conclusions of all recent inquiries and government guidance has been that there is a pressing need for better co-operation across agency boundaries. There are now a number of multi-agency working groups, usually Borough-based, which can contribute to cross-agency needs assessment leading to joint (or at least co-ordinated commissioning) protocols for interagency referral, joint policies and strategies and greater understanding of the roles and responsibilities of health, social care and criminal justice agencies. Of course, each agency will have its own priorities but when fully discussed in this forum the tensions induced are likely to be creative. Joint training has been found to be useful in improving inter-agency working on the ground.

5.6.9 Potential for prevention

There is currently no direct evidence to support the idea that the development of severe mental illness can be prevented. Similarly there is no rigorous evidence to support the notion that people with severe mental illness can be prevented from committing criminal offences as a result of receiving health care. There are however several areas where there is the potential for prevention of offending and early identification of the risk of offending.

i) Early prevention

Taylor (1996) has summarised areas for early prevention of mentally disordered offenders where we might cautiously expect prevention could occur. These include a reduction in perinatal factors such as low birth weight, Homestart programmes and support for abused children. Children particularly at risk are those who show damaged processing of social information evidenced by an increased attribution of intent to harm. They often have a limited repertoire of responses to perceived threats.

ii) Services for young people leaving care

Those leaving care are about 30 times more likely to become mentally disordered offenders than the general population (Guite, 1996). Local authorities are only required by statute to provide services to young people leaving care until the age of 21 years (Bonnerjea, 1990). Psychological support and long term aftercare to this group jointly from health and social services could potentially prevent breakdown and provide for early identification.

iii) Services for people who are homeless and in hostel accommodation

Mentally disordered offenders who are homeless or in temporary accommodation are another group who would benefit from additional support and services since they form nearly half of this group.

iv) Active support following significant life events

Preliminary results of the Revolving Doors Agency study of people with mental illness in police stations found that half had experienced a major life crisis (loss of home, friend, relationship etc.) within the 6 months prior to the offence (personal communication). Improved recognition and response to crises may help.

v) Routes to care

Patients from Black populations are more likely to enter psychiatric care through the criminal justice system and at a later stage of their illness. The development of services and structures to improve access to care which is more acceptable to young Black male populations could increase the numbers who access care directly from health and social services.

vi) General adult services – reduction in rates of relapse

An increase in the use of measures shown to reduce relapse rates such as psychosocial interventions in families with high expressed emotion and cognitive training to improve use of anti-psychotic medication would be expected to reduce offending related to mental state.

vii) Improvements in the working environment

The development of effective call and response systems, improved information and communication would be expected to reduce episodes and severity of violence (Taylor, 1996).

viii) Training in diversion and calming techniques (Taylor, 1996).

ix) Reduction in numbers of temporary staff and staff turnover (James 1990).

x) General adult services – care for carers

Carers are the victims of half of recorded offences (Guite, 1996). Training for carers in the management of aggression may be indicated where there has been aggression in the past.

xi) General adult services – care for other patients/ residents

Other patients and residents are victims in about one quarter of violent offences (Guite 1996) suggesting that facilitation of the relationships between residents and training for patients who are frequent victims could be beneficial.

xii) General adult services – care for staff

Sheridan (1990) has shown that there are fewer violent incidents on wards where staff stress is lower, roles and responsibilities are clear, and staff use a range of approaches to diffuse situations.

xiii) Probation services/prison service

The Prison service has identified from meta-analysis of correctional evaluations the key components of programmes effective in reducing offending behaviour (personal communication David Thornton). Programmes should be based on a sound theoretical model of offending; use cognitive or behavioural approaches; be skills orientated; be multi-modal rather than narrowly focused; provide sufficient time (over 18 months or at least 100 hours of treatment); be provided in a community setting with arrangements for through care; be designed with the support of a researcher and have adequate quality control measures to ensure programme integrity; be integrated into the routine management of the establishment.

Studies are required to assess whether these components also apply to mentally disordered offenders or what modifications may be necessary. Joint approaches from Health, Social and Prison services would be required.

If effective, each of these possible preventive measures promises to be very cost-effective, as none requires in-patient care.

5.6.10 Possible solutions

The expenditure of London purchasers on services for mentally disordered offenders is currently very high, yet significant problems continue to arise in their management. The following are proposals for change in this system of care:

There is a need to review funding formulae to reflect London's need for secure services, particularly for those inner city areas where usage of secure facilities is very high.

It would be helpful for mental health funding to be ring-fenced to protect it from the increasing pressure from other sectors and to allow research into outcomes in forensic psychiatry, which will enable authorities to move towards evidence based purchasing.

The capital and revenue funding possibilities for supported housing for mentally disordered offenders no longer needing hospital care should be re-examined. Decisions on Housing Corporation funding and housing benefit are likely to have a major impact on the ability of vulnerable groups to obtain and retain housing.

More accessible and appropriate services for ethnic minorities are required to prevent young black men with severe mental illness presenting via the criminal justice system at a late stage in the onset or relapse of illness.

Attention needs to be paid to the training of staff in a variety of agencies in risk assessment and in management of mentally disordered offenders.

Attention needs to be paid to finding ways of making working conditions and environments more attractive to professionals, so as to attract more staff to London.
Since London health commissions are the major purchasers of private medium secure places, they need to become concerned with better monitoring of the quality of care provided in these institutions.

Chapter 5.7

The homeless in London

Dinesh Bhugra

Summary

- Although substantial difficulties arise in precise definition of homelessness and in enumeration of the homeless population, it is clear that London is at an extreme on the national spectrum for homelessness. 47% of 'rough sleepers' counted in the 1991 Census were in London, and it has been estimated that in total there are around 100,000 individuals experiencing various types of homelessness in London.
- Compared with homeless populations elsewhere, the homeless in London are more likely to be from ethnic minority backgrounds, tend to be younger, and are more likely to be in relationships and to have children.
- There are high rates of psychiatric morbidity among the homeless in London. Psychosis and substance abuse are frequent problems, and homeless individuals are more than 5 times as likely as the general population to report experiencing symptoms such as depression and anxiety.
- Homeless people tend to have complex needs, as they commonly experience a combination of mental health, physical health and social problems.
- A variety of obstacles currently impede effective delivery of care to this group by statutory services, including rigid catchment area boundaries, a tendency to discharge patients from in-patient care as soon as acute symptoms have subsided, lack of services which can meet multiple needs for care of different types in a co-ordinated way, and difficulties experienced by homeless people in trying to register with a GP.
- Specialist teams have been set up targeting single homeless people with severe mental illness in inner London Boroughs. The services they provide appear to be highly valued by other local agencies.

Strategies suggested for improving care for homeless people with mental illnesses include:

For purchasers:
- Purchasers should lead in developing databases for accurate enumeration of homeless individuals, based on clear definitions of types of homelessness.
- Joint commissioning between voluntary agencies and statutory services should be encouraged, to provide adequate, appropriate and accessible services that meet the needs of the community. Joint initiatives should be encouraged, and these should be monitored, reviewed and rewarded.
- At a local level, joint working groups should be set up to ascertain levels of needs and provisions for mentally ill homeless individuals.

For providers:
- An assessment of numbers of homeless individuals and their needs should be the starting point. Joint planning with local primary care services, housing departments and voluntary organisations is essential.
- The providers of mental health services must work closely with GPs and develop effective models of joint working.

Specialist mental health services:
- There remains a need for identifying a consultant in each Trust whose multi-disciplinary team will be clearly responsible for assessing and meeting the needs of homeless, mentally ill individuals. The teams should have the skills and the capability for assertive outreach and flexible approachable provisions of service.
- These teams should act as leaders in liaising with other agencies – voluntary or statutory, and should also be the source of information on the extent of homelessness and the special needs of the homeless for that geographical area.

5.7.1 Introduction

Mentally ill individuals who also experience homelessness endure a double jeopardy, and the associated stigma affects their help seeking and accepting help if offered. A majority of those who suffer from mental illness have circumstances somewhere along the continuum of poverty: homelessness is the extreme and most marginalised end of this continuum, where a disproportionate number of the mentally ill are found (Timms 1996).

5.7.2 Definitions of homelessness

There are many varieties of homeless individuals and many definitions of homelessness. The word 'homeless' may be used as a category, as a description of one of many complex needs, as a legal definition or as a self-ascription relating to the quality of individual's accommodation. The Royal College of Physicians Working Party (RCP1994) proposed that the homeless can be divided into three groups:

- the 'official' homeless, including families with children
- hostel dwellers and rough sleepers who do not appear in official statistics
- those who have inadequate housing and a significant housing need.

However, serious problems remain in the classification of homeless individuals. Bhugra et al (1992) proposed using a simple classification of the homeless which included as categories single homeless, young homeless and homeless families. To be homeless certainly means that an individual lacks access to regular and customary access to a conventional dwelling unit, yet there remain considerable ambiguities in trying to define 'regular and customary access' and a 'conventional dwelling unit' (Wright 1989). Wright (1989) draws a distinction between the 'literally homeless' and the 'marginally housed'. The former have nowhere to go – no rented rooms, no hostels, no friends to live with, and they either live on the streets or avail themselves of space like shelters hostels, whereas the marginally housed have a 'more or less reasonable claim to a more or less stable housing situation of more or less minimal adequacy, being closer to the 'less' rather than the 'more' on one or all criteria' (Wright 1989).

Leach (1979) proposed a simple classification of 'intrinsic' and 'extrinsic' homeless people – for the former, mental or physical disability was the cause of their homelessness, whereas the latter were homeless because of external factors. Morse et al (1991) suggest using a system which focuses on current psychiatric or physical impairment and on whether such an impairment was the original cause of homelessness or not: this distinction is better at identifying needs for service. No one definition is universally accepted, and without such a consensus it remains difficult to compare different bodies of research, based on different sample groups as well as different categories of mental illness. Researchers often study relatively accessible groups of individuals and generalize their needs to other groups. Whatever definitions are used, the central focus in research and service planning needs to be on the ways in which being roofless, shelterless or homeless prevents individuals gaining full access to social, physical and mental health care.

5.7.3 A history of homelessness in London

A link between homelessness and psychiatric disorder is often assumed to have been observed only in recent decades, and in discussions of hospital closure and care in the community, it is often suggested that with the closure of hospitals, large numbers of ex-patients have been thrown out onto the streets. However, history and literature give ample evidence that the homeless were visible at a much earlier date and institutions existed to deal with the poor and indigent (Timms 1996). The first statutes regarding homeless people were passed in the 14th century, but the devolution of responsibility to the local level did not occur till much later, when individual parishes were asked to respond to the demands placed upon them, but without any clear financial support.

The Poor Law Amendment Act of 1834 combined all but the largest parishes into Unions, thereby reducing the number of workhouses from 15,000 to 650, resulting in the building of the Camberwell 'spike', which closed down in 1985. In 1889, only 2% of London lunatics were accommodated in workhouses. Over the next hundred years the debate about numbers of mentally ill individuals among the homeless population has continued, but without clear conclusions being reached. In successive surveys in hostels, prisons, night shelters and among those of no fixed abode in the hospitals, substantial rates of severe mental illness have been demonstrated, but strikingly few individuals with milder symptoms such as anxiety and depression have been identified (see below).

5.7.4 Current levels of homelessness in London

Problems with definitions and methodologies for enumeration make it difficult to ascertain precisely the level of homelessness in London. The available figures should be viewed as rough estimates, which will generally be under-estimates. They often do not take into account people who are living in temporary accommodation or do not meet criteria for acceptance as statutorily homeless. Data are collected on statutory homelessness (which covers the activities of local authorities and housing associations under the 1985 Housing Act), but these are confined to information on households rather than individuals. This means that actual numbers of homeless individuals rehoused is much higher than the recorded number of 'acceptances' of households. In the last year for which figures were available (1992) the 143,000 homeless acceptances under this Act actually represented more than 400,000 individuals (Standing Conference on Public Health 1994:18).

Rough sleepers: A street survey of rough sleeping in 17 London boroughs on a single night in 1989 found 751 people sleeping out on the streets or in railway stations (Carter et al 1989). The Census in 1991 enumerated 2703 people sleeping rough in England and Wales of whom 1275 were in London (OPCS 1991). As Craig et al (1995) caution, significant numbers of people sleeping in abandoned buildings or less accessible sites are likely to have been missed, since these figures were based on individuals sleeping at sites known to be popular with rough sleepers on a single night. The Central London Street Monitor (November 1995) found 359 people sleeping rough in areas known for such activity. There were ten times as many men as women, and only 7% of the sample were black. Three quarters of the sample reported sleeping rough regularly over a year. A lower figure of 270 was reported by the Next Challenge (1996).

Direct access hostels: Official figures for direct access hostel occupancy are also subject to errors of classification and missing data. In a parliamentary answer, the Department of Environment reported 22,383 hostel bed spaces for single people in February 1991.These hostels have a high rate of occupancy especially during cold weather. In November 1995 there were 2,823 people (2,124 men and 699 women) resident in direct access emergency night shelters and short stay hostels, but only 11 beds were available by 11.30 pm across London, none in central London, and the hostels reported 183 people whom they were unable to help (Crisis, 1995). The most recent figures for the five Winter Shelters (1994/5) indicate that 1,613 individuals were accommodated over 32,899 bed nights in 331 bed spaces (CRASH 1995).

Lodging houses and temporary accommodation: Based on DSS data, Randall (1992) reports that 11,694 single claimants were resident in board and lodgings in London. Data from the DSS indicate that in August 1995, there were 23,780 housing benefit recipient 'boarders' (single person or a couple) for all the local authorities in London (total of 3,480 local authority tenants and 20,300 private tenants).In 1994-95, 28,490 households were accepted as homeless in London Boroughs of London (LRC 1995/96).

Total homeless population: Health Action for Homeless People (1994) estimate that there are a total of 100,000 to 120,000 homeless individuals in London, including travellers. Peace and Quilgars (1996) give an estimate based on data for the last quarter of 1994 of 106,000, of whom 71% are statutorily homeless and 29% non-statutorily homeless or sleeping rough. Fisher et al (1994) estimated that there were 5,000 homeless people in the Borough of Westminster alone in 1993.

The geographical distribution of homeless populations varies: rough sleepers tend to aggregate in inner London and the statutory homeless in greater London boroughs (Please and Quilgars 1996). Levels of homelessness are particularly high in Hackney, Haringey, Newham and Brent, and non-statutory homelessness prominent in the inner London boroughs of Westminster, Camden, Tower Hamlets, Southwark, Lewisham and Lambeth.

There are some differences between characteristics of homeless people in London and elsewhere. In a study which compared homeless people in London and elsewhere, the London homeless were found to be generally younger, they tended to have children and nearly half were in relationships (Thomas and Niner 1989). The London Research Centre (1991) reported that in an exclusively London-based sample 25% were black, 15% Asian and 3% Irish, compared with 87-96% of U.K. White origin in Thomas and Niner's national sample. The much greater number of homeless households from ethnic minority backgrounds in London reflects the ethnic diversity of the capital.

Craig et al (1995) report that despite variations in survey methodology, there is substantial evidence that overall numbers of homeless people have grown considerably in Britain in the past decade. This is probably truer of London as many drift to the capital. The increase is accounted for by greater numbers of young people, women and people from ethnic minority backgrounds in the homeless population. The reasons for homelessness are many and changes in the benefit system made by the Government are important. The selling of public housing stock, and lack of cheap affordable housing and of employment opportunities are other important factors contributing to the increase in homelessness.

5.7.5 Rates of mental illness in homeless people

Although closure of UK mental hospitals has been blamed for the increase in numbers of (mentally ill) homeless, the evidence suggests that when discharged to appropriate accommodation, the numbers of people becoming homeless due to their illness are quite small (Dayson, 1992; Leff, 1993). Rates of mental illness among homeless populations vary dramatically for several reasons. Varying sites for sample selection, different methods of measuring psychiatric morbidity and different time frames contribute to producing variations in rates which are not always clearly interpretable.

a. The single homeless and mental illness

Only figures collected for single homeless populations in London are presented here. Several studies have identified high rates of severe mental illness in general and of comorbidity between severe mental illness and substance abuse in particular. It has been argued that an interaction between low quality community care and problems directly related to mental illness affects such individuals in a way that they cannot cope with ordinary life and become homeless (Craig and Timms, 1992). Such a pattern has also been identified in other cities (see Bhugra, 1993). Bines (1994) studied the single homeless in five London boroughs and reported that fits, depression, anxiety and nerves; as well as physical problems were between 2–20 times more likely when compared to general population. Self-reported mental health problems were between 6 and 8 times as likely as in the general population for men and between 9 and 12 times as likely for women. People sleeping rough were the most likely to have mental health problems and to have ever stayed in a psychiatric hospital. The physical and psychological health of people living on the streets is potentially at risk because of poor living conditions, risk infection, poor personal hygiene, lack of rest and sleep and lack of access to appropriate health services.

b. Young adults and young families

There has been a threefold increase in the number of households in England accepted as officially homeless, from 53,110 in 1978 to 145,800 in 1990 (Faculty of Public Health Medicine) – a similar threefold increase was seen in London. Reasons for family homelessness in this group includes break-up of relationship, poor work record, unavailability of work and of child care facilities, sexual abuse, eviction, domestic conflict and unsafe living conditions (Mills and Ota, 1989). In a study of 319 homeless households in North and West London, Victor (1992) found that 20% of her sample suffered from significant psychological morbidity on a standardised questionnaire, and 45% showed some evidence of mental morbidity, twice the rate for general resident populations. Utilisation of general practitioner services, accident and emergency departments and inpatient admissions was much higher than by the regional residents On the other hand, 92% of the sample were registered with GPs but the GPs were at a longer geographical distance for a number of individuals. The population was poor, young, often drawn from minority communities and consisted of parents with pre-school age children. In an earlier study Victor et al (1989) had observed that hospital admission rates for the homeless group in general and their children in particular were much higher when compared to local residents. These high rates may reflect either the increased morbidity or social circumstances or a mixture of the two. Overall 9% of the beds at St Mary's Hospital, Paddington were being used by the homeless.

American studies suggest that **children** in families in bed and breakfast or temporary accommodations do poorly in school, and tend to have developmental delay in one or more of the areas of language, gross motor skills, fine motor coordination and personal and social development. Whether these delays are due to physical undernourishment, lack of adequate parenting or available personal space or emotional problems due to poor environment is difficult to say. These children have been shown to be more aggressive, with poor attention span and impulse control and are more likely to be abused physically and sexually (see Bhugra 1996 for a review). The problems associated with adolescence and homelessness are discussed below.

c. Women

The proportion of women amongst the adult homeless population is currently estimated at between 10-25% (Marshall, 1996). The numbers of women suffering from mental illness has varied tremendously. Marshall (1996) cautions that the type of accommodation used may be a function of age – the homeless women are generally younger than men; and are also more likely to have completed schooling, to have married and be in contact with their families. Such factors obviously make it more likely that some of the women may remain hidden and – as Marshall and Reed (1992) had found – they were more likely to have been sleeping on floors at their friends'. Herzberg (1987) reported that in his sample, women were more likely to have been referred for admission on a section 136 by the police, whereas a man may be more likely to be taken to prison. In this sample 42% of women were diagnosed as having schizophrenia compared to 64% in Marshall and Reed's (1992) sample. These discrepancies may be explained by two different sources of sample recruitment and the age groups. Associated alcohol use was reported in 36% of women by Marshall and Reed (1992), although a much lower proportion (1%) had admitted to any problem with alcohol. In the older age group associated physical morbidity has varied between 0-27% of the sample. In addition to general factors reported above the pathways into homelessness for this group also include physical and sexual abuse or neglect when these women are pushed into leaving home.

d. Ethnic Minorities

For some time it was considered that ethnic minorities did not appear among the homeless because their families were able to look after them. Hinton (1992, 1994) at two different sites in London found that the black and minority ethnic groups were not visible, and overcrowding in Asian households was a way of dealing with homelessness amongst friends or relatives. A high number had reported that they had not had a home of their own in the last five years. In a recent study Bhugra et al (1996d) in a drop-in centre studied 70 homeless individuals and reported that one fifth of their sample belonged to minority ethnic groups. The black males were more likely to disagree with their clinical diagnosis and white men were more likely to have been in prison at some time. In the black group 4 out of 13 were females.

e. Refugees and Asylum seekers

Data on refugees and asylum seekers are hard to come by. Pleace and Quilgars (1996) report that during 1994, 1,345 households applied for rehousing under the homelessness legislation in London and were refused assistance on the basis that they were asylum seekers – on average 42 households per borough. Health care needs and access to primary care for this group are likely to be even more complicated.

f. Adolescents

Both adolescent boys and girls are likely to be attracted to the bright lights of the city. Abrahams and Mungall (1992) studied 4 police forces areas in England along with 5 of the 75 metropolitan divisions. The majority of the runaways were aged 14–16 and those in institutional care were more likely to run away. More than a quarter of 6,068 runaways were African-Caribbean and common reasons for running away were perceived danger to self. Other vulnerability factors were prostitution, pregnancy, sexual abuse and learning difficulties. Adolescents were defined as runaways, homeless or throwaways. Many of the adolescents ended up in prostitution (Benjamin, 1985), and substance abuse was another major problem. The risk of sexually transmitted diseases increases dramatically with prostitution as does the risk of violence, pregnancy and assault. Negative experiences with their families and schools are bound to compound these problems.

g. The elderly

Crane (1993, 1994) studied 190 individuals over the age of 60 and in a series of one night surveys Weller et al (1989) studied 319 homeless individuals and a subgroup of 55 men with a median age of 70 living in a direct access hotel to give a picture of the older homeless individual in London (see Cohen and Crane, 1996). The Irish were dramatically over-represented, and two fifths of the sample in Crane (1994) study reported substantial levels of depressive symptoms. In the same sample, moderate or severe cognitive disturbance was found in 39% of individuals. To make matters worse at a personal level, although 34% had children but no contact, 31% had siblings or relatives but contact with only 3%. The reasons for becoming homeless were found to be financial, breakdown of relationships, dissatisfaction with residence or eviction. Cohen and Crane (1996) conclude that structural forces outlined above contribute to homelessness and statutory regulations are necessary but not sufficient to provide housing and income support to older persons.

h. Dual Diagnosis

Wright (1987) has estimated that the rate of alcohol abuse is 3-5 times greater in the homeless. Drug abuse too is not uncommon and rates between 8-94% have been reported (see Table I). Although homeless women have a lower problem of substance abuse, again findings have varied widely from 4% to 36% (see Marshall 1996). In addition, often the homeless individual has physical illness which complicate not only the diagnosis of mental illness but also the management of both physical and mental illnesses, especially if the two are being managed by separate teams with limited contact with each other. From Baltimore, Breakey et al (1989) had reported that homeless women were marginally more likely to have physical problems including oro-dental, gynaecological and anaemias. Thus there is a need for services which can deliver multiple types of intervention to the homeless.

5.7.6 Service delivery and the homeless mentally ill

For the **rates of mental illness** are higher in the homeless population, the most likely explanation is that both mental illness and homelessness are related to an initial failure to develop adequate coping skills, which is compounded by a continuing downward drift as a part of the secondary handicaps of illness (Craig et al 1995). Even though the statutory services may offer some care often this is too little too late especially in areas where no specific targeting of homeless individuals is being carried out. Specialist teams targeting individual have their advantages but in the present climate of purchasing and providing services, how many individuals can be targeted remains a quandary.

Barriers to help seeking: The major emphasis on care provisions by the mental health statutory services is on the mental health of the individual, and if appropriate housing and social support is not available the individual is likely to be sent back to inappropriate or poor quality accommodation. Many barriers to help seeking and effective health care have been identified by various authors in literature.

- **Inflexible services**: With increased sectorisation of mental health services, limited resources and very narrow purchaser-provider agreements, only short term emergencies can be treated for out of catchment area patients. Often individuals who do not have a fixed address fall out of the safety net of post-discharge support and planning. In addition, the services are often seen as rigid, inflexible, inappropriate and the individuals may not seek help early enough or find the help they are offered appropriate (see below). Related to this factor is the major emphasis of modern psychiatric practice on providing intensive but brief treatment for the acute phase of a mental illness (Craig et al 1995), which means that due to pressure on beds few patients can stay in the hospital once the acute phase has subsided and a lack of inappropriate housing is often not a barrier to discharge. An additional problem is the inflexibility resulting from provision of community services only in office hours. There are very few targeted rehabilitation services in the community providing multifaceted services 24 hours a day. Thus those individuals who need community support may not get services they need.

- **Multiple Needs**: Multiplicity of needs in terms of health care alone means that these needs are not being met and homeless individuals are often discouraged from seeking help. Co-morbidity of physical and psychiatric illnesses means that both types need to be treated assertively and unless the two caring teams work together the health needs are not likely to be identified or treated. In addition housing and social needs such as benefits, occupation etc. need to be addressed, and pressures on beds, and lack of financial and staffing resources, often mean that the needs are often not assessed properly.

- **Responsibility**: The debate on whether poor inappropriate or inadequate house produced or contributed to mental ill health or latter led to former tends to ignore the individual. Such a debate in identifying responsibility between the health and social care services means that often the individual gets lost between the two. Where the two components of the multi disciplinary team work well together, they tend to increase the smooth functioning and successful placement of individuals. However, by and large the financial squeeze on both components means that a degree of suspicion and hostility remains.

- **Primary care:** Registering with a GP is also often problematic. Although the exact impact of fund holding on the registration of homeless individuals is not known, it is worth bearing in mind. Even though in inner city areas where the numbers of fund holding practices is unlikely to be very high this will create problems because of lack of fixed or permanent address, and disputes may arise over the 'ownership' of such cases. Victor (1992) reported that although 84% of her sample were registered with GPs, in a significant number of cases these surgeries were several kilometres away. This may simply reflect the fact that surgeries nearer to the individual's 'new' residence may be more reluctant to take patients on. An additional factor may well be the surgeries' reluctance to take on chronic severely mentally ill individuals, especially when the current fashion of management guides individuals towards counselling. There may be barriers in providing 'compulsory' treatments to such individuals and the prejudices of individual carers may contribute to the barrier.

• **Internal barriers to help-seeking:** The decision to seek help is a complex one involving individuals or those around them assessing their problems, their significance and the likely impact of the consultation. El-Kabir and Ramsden (1996) suggest that similar   factors affect the decision to seek medical advice amongst homeless people though other pressures like shelter or food may take precedence. Even when services are seen to be accessible and flexible some individuals may prioritise their needs completely differently when compared to others. Furthermore, internal barriers such as emotional factors also play a very important role in preventing help-seeking. Many patients may express guilt at their circumstances and lifestyle and seeing others who are not homeless and the stigma homeless individuals perceive and receive all contribute to effective early help seeking and complying with the help. In addition, the perceived roles of doctor and patient themselves affect their consultations.

Craig et al (1995) highlighted another barrier which is due to services failing to recognise the high care needs of homeless individuals who were previously in large direct access hostels.

Overall, **existing services for the mentally ill homeless** have the following structural barriers:

AVAILABILITY: As noted above, the hospitals provide secondary care for which the general practitioner is the acknowledged gate keeper. This means that if GP is not involved in the process of referral, the individual may use emergency services or the police may pick such individual up under section 136 thereby contributing to inappropriate admissions which may then go on to be unnecessarily long. Individuals who may be withdrawn or isolated may not come in contact with the services at all and others may refuse services because of poor insight, or cognitive impairment.

ACCESSIBILITY: Using medical models of services has meant that unless there is a clear medical/psychiatric condition, the individual may not get into the system. The attitudes of the staff as well as geographical accessibility of services are important factors in help-seeking. Prejudice of the staff including those in GP surgeries and the fear of treatment have both been identified as barriers to accessibility of services. In cases of the teenagers, women or those of ethnic minority groups additional factors play an important role in providing access to services.

APPROPRIATENESS: The perception of services as appropriate is crucial to their acceptance by the individuals. If the individual identifies housing, shelter or food as first priority, to try and treat them with neuroleptics as the first choice treatment is likely to create conflict and lead to rejection of the services.

5.7.7 Proposed solutions

In order to set up appropriate services which will be used by the individuals, each district with a homeless population needs to know the exact numbers, be clear about the definitions of homelessness and availability of local resources.

a. Catchment areas

The Royal College of Psychiatrists Working Party (Bhugra et al, 1992) recommended that each district should have a nominated consultant and a team for the engagement and care of homeless individuals which provides outreach services including links with local primary care services. Dedicated forms of care management for those with dual diagnosis may prove to be very helpful. The numbers of homeless individuals will vary in each health district but are likely to be much higher in London compared with rural districts. Multiple sources of information such as housing department figures, direct access hostel places, voluntary organisations, no fixed abode admissions and so on, can be used for this purpose.

General psychiatrists should remain the first port of call and, depending upon numbers, each district should have a nominated consultant and team for care of the mentally ill homeless (Bhugra et al 1995). Craig et al (1995) reports that five specialist teams in three Thames regions were working with voluntary and statutory agencies as appropriate to their local context and all these were valued by the majority of agencies they worked with. Essentially these were praised for their approach, flexibility, sessional work, crisis intervention and psychiatric input. Interestingly all these teams had targeted single homeless people who have severe mental health problems and were not in contact with mainstream services. The Community Care legislations and Care Programme Approach and Supervision registers do offer opportunities to keep a closer eye on mentally ill homeless individuals but often the homeless individuals are the first casualty of limited resources.

b. Flexibility of services

As mentioned earlier, Craig et al (1995) found that their specialist services were valued by the patients and other agencies as useful because of their flexibility and sessional work – maintaining a high level of direct client interaction. The teams had a key worker approach and had close links with inpatient psychiatric services as well as courts. In this survey, organisations which had had dealings with specialist teams were aware of the pressures under which these teams were working but they also had high expectations of the specialist teams. Thus a balance needs to be struck between the expectations and the ability to deliver. They were keen on flexible sessional input by members of the team and were aware that this was the most effective way to secure the targeting and engagement of all clients with serious mental health problems.

Those agencies who do not receive such a focused service will undoubtedly require an efficient referral system and the individuals who require help also see flexibility as an important characteristic of the service. A 24-hour service which does not rely on letters from GPs and responds promptly and appropriately is also more likely to be used appropriately. Thompson (1990) has described the flexibility of his local psychiatric services picking up mentally ill homeless individuals sooner rather than later.

c. Multiple needs, multiple services

There is no doubt that like most patients with mental illness, homeless individuals who have mental illness also have very complex needs. These are related to their mental illness as well as to physical environment. Reasonable quality housing, adequate levels of benefits and social support, and medical and psychological inputs for their physical and psychiatric needs are all essential components of the service. A close liaison with voluntary agencies should be encouraged and key workers from the community invited to attend multidisciplinary ward meetings and discussions of individual cases. Full follow-up arrangements should be made, including registering with GPs, and outreach services encouraged.

Innovative services for dual diagnosis individuals should be encouraged eg. providing rehabilitation services for chronic severely mentally ill in the community along with community management of substance abuse e.g. providing wet houses or wet floors (where drugs are allowed) and dry floors (where they are not) in the same accommodation. Multiple needs may require multiple services but it is important that these are met within the same team, otherwise the individual is more likely to fall out of the net, and the waiting and getting used to another team only compounds the problems. Thus as noted earlier if specialist homeless care teams are to be set up these have to be encouraged and supported in being innovative and providing a range of services within the team.

d. Housing & Health

With an increasing squeeze on the budgets of health and social housing services, joint initiatives to cater for the needs of homeless mentally ill individuals are rare. Furthermore, with increasing emphasis on care in the community has also led to increasing separation between health and housing. With reduction in the housing stock (especially for special needs) available, the pressures are immense and often housing associations or voluntary organisations are forced to step in. This has led to a feeling of mutual distrust on both sides.

Two kinds of beds may be needed – for treatment and for residence. Both of these do not have to be in the hospital. Respite care beds in the community or 'focused' treatment units may well encourage individuals to use these and stick with them. A reduction in hospital beds for mental illness may not necessarily have contributed to increase in numbers of mentally ill homeless individuals but at the same time closures of direct access hostels may have contributed to this increase and voluntary and local hostels may be reluctant to take mentally disordered homeless individuals.

With housing and health, two additional problems of poverty and unemployment need to be highlighted. With increasing cut-backs on social security benefits and changing patterns of unemployment, lack of a fixed address also adds to the difficulties of individuals in making any attempts at coming out of this vicious circle.

e. Primary care

Stone (1990) first brought the plight of bed and breakfast families and their poor physical and mental state to public attention. Ramsden and El-Kabir set up a primary care service for the homeless at Great Chapel Street Medical Centre (see El-Kabir and Ramsden, 1996) and found funding from a charity to support a psychiatrist. In 1984 these authors set up a sick bay to admit such patients, and to date 1400 patients have been treated – these individuals present with physical problems eg. leg ulcers, pulmonary tuberculosis and also psychosis and since hospitals are reluctant to admit those with 'social problems' this stigma is by-passed. Not only does this allow treatment of complex problems, but a thorough assessment of their needs also means that housing options after discharge are made available and up to 40% have remained in stable accommodation two years later. Such a model emphasises primary care – a model being put forward in the NHS. El-Kabir and Ramsden (1996) suggest that areas with high numbers of homeless individuals should have a clinic taking the lead in co-ordinating information, liaising with secondary care services, accident and emergency departments and emergency clinics. Fast track assessments need to be made available.

f. Voluntary Organisations

When 85 organisations were approached to get their views on each of the specialist homeless teams in the Thames regions, Craig et al (1995) found that the satisfaction for services varied from 68-85% and overall 95% of those surveyed were satisfied with their local teams. Voluntary organisations often have street credibility and know in much greater detail the needs of their clients and preferences. Joint planning especially while planning to set up services in the community is to be encouraged and welcomed. Voluntary organisations can offer day care facilities, outreach work, drug and alcohol support along with housing, in a way which is more likely to be accepted by the homeless individuals. As we had demonstrated, only one out of 70 clients interviewed in a drop-in project had felt unhappy with the services offered (Bhugra et al, 1996).

The ultimate success of any team depends upon its skills in identifying multiple needs and dealing with these multiple needs and linking up with local services which can be statutory (primary or secondary care) or voluntary.

5.7.8. Current priorities

A. **General**

1. There is a clear need for multidisciplinary teams in each health district with a homeless population, with clear responsibility for assessing and meeting the needs of homeless mentally ill individuals.

2. Such teams should act as leaders for liaising with other agencies – voluntary or statutory and also be the source of information on the extent of homelessness and the special needs of the mentally ill homeless for that geographical area.

3. The teams should have the skills and the capability for assertive outreach and flexible approachable provisions of services.

4. The teams should look after *all* homeless individuals be they adult, homeless families, from ethnic minorities as long as a locally agreed definition of homeless is applied.

B.   **For Purchasers**
1.   Joint commissioning between voluntary agencies and statutory services be encouraged to provide adequate appropriate and accessible services that meet the needs of the community.
2.   Adequate support to housing associations and special needs housing and joint working of primary and secondary services is to be encouraged. An opportunity for joint review and monitoring of housing and health services at the local level may encourage innovative developments in the area.
3.   Joint health and housing initiatives locally should be encouraged.
4.   At a local level joint working groups should be set up to ascertain the levels of needs and provisions for the mentally ill homeless individuals.
5.   Purchasers should take a lead in developing data bases for the accurate enumeration of homeless individuals, types of homelessness and defining homelessness clearly.
6.   The role of fundholding practices in the care of the homeless needs to be identified urgently.

C.   **For Providers**

(i) *Primary Care*
1.   The providers of mental health services must work closely with primary care and develop models such as those outlined above.
2.   Clearly identified team be responsible for providing secondary care services so that within the district primary care providers know who to contact.

(ii) *Joint Planning*
1.   An assessment of the numbers of homeless individuals and their needs ought to be the starting point. Joint planning with local primary care services, housing departments and voluntary organisations are essential.
2.   Internal management structures and referral procedures be as simple as possible.
3.   Joint steering groups in the district be set up to monitor and review the functioning of statutory services dealing with mental illness.
4.   Joint functioning with physicians and surgeons as well as other specialists eg. substance misuse will allow appropriate quick assessments of problems and acceptable management.
5.   The accessibility, acceptability and accountability of teams is a must and the barriers in services must be minimised.
6.   The services should devote health care resources to individuals proportional to their needs.
7.   Clinical and medical responsibility within the team needs to be identified and supported.
8.   Assertive outreach and follow-up are a must and special skills need to be developed for these.
9.   Engagement will depend on the quality and comprehensiveness of the services. Appropriate infrastructure and working partnerships should be encouraged.

Chapter 5.8

Mental health services in primary care in London

Shaun Kerwick, André Tylee and David Goldberg

Summary

- Compared with GPs in similarly deprived inner city areas outside London, GPs in inner deprived parts of London appear to be under-performing. Factors contributing to this are likely to include high mobility of patients, lower numbers of attached staff, a higher proportion of single-handed practices, and difficulty accessing services from multiple providers.
- There has been increasing awareness of the scale of psychological morbidity in primary care populations and the need to respond to this previously unmet need. Following the Tomlinson Report, money was made available to develop primary care services in areas of greatest need in the 'London Initiative Zone' (LIZ), and substantial numbers of the projects funded under this initiative have been in the area of mental health.
- Some examples of good practice do exist among London's practices, with initiatives including case registers and practice protocols. The great variation encountered between London practices may be explained partly by inadequate human resources, and also by lack of adequate skills and knowledge for detection and management of mental health problems in primary care.
- There are significant problems in communication and joint working between primary and secondary care, compounded by the fact that a single practice often has to deal with multiple providers and by lack of readily available information about non-statutory services.

Possible solutions to the difficulties currently encountered in this area include the following:
- Training of primary care staff is a priority, and needs to focus mainly on improving the skills of GPs and practice nurses in detecting and managing psychiatric disorders. A number of training packages of established effectiveness are available. Motivated tutors and protected time for educational activities are important factors for the success of such packages.
- There should be a more equitable distribution of counsellors and psychologists between general practice surgeries. These attachments are probably best administered from outside the practice, using professionals with appropriate qualifications. This would allow good referral policies to be put in place, autonomy for the therapists, and adequate supervision within a professional context.
- Development of shared care registers should be adopted as good practice and promoted by the Royal College of General Practitioners. Practice protocols based on best available evidence or consensus, developed internally or borrowed, would help foster a more systematic approach to clinical problems.
- Secondary care services would serve primary care in London better if catchment areas were aligned to general practice populations. In connection with this, a community-based mental health team could provide a liaison worker attached to a group of GP practices.
- It would be helpful to provide primary care teams with an updated resource directory of locally based statutory and non-statutory service providers. This has already been done in some places, but the practice should be generalised.

5.8.1 Introduction

> 'administrative and medical logic alike...suggest
> that the cardinal requirement for improvement of
> the mental health services is not a large expansion
> of psychiatric agencies, but rather a strengthening
> of the family doctor in his therapeutic role'
> **Michael Shepherd, 1966**

In the current context of debate about a primary care-led NHS and increasing awareness of mental health issues amongst the public, health professionals, and politicians, Michael Shepherd's words from his seminal work on psychiatric illness in general practice remain apposite (Shepherd et al, 1966). This piece of work highlighted a concern, important and relevant today as it was then, that there is considerable variation in general practitioners' ability to detect and manage mental illness, and that secondary care services would be overstretched if all cases of psychiatric morbidity were referred. Primary care and psychiatric services have developed considerably during the intervening period, yet there are still readily identifiable improvements that could enhance the provision of mental health services.

Whilst government reforms have affected the delivery of health services nationally, London has received particular attention regarding the transfer of resources from the acute to the primary care sector (Department of Health, 1992b). The provision of services in London will continue to be unique owing to its characteristics of having a large population, high levels of mobility, a large ethnic population, high levels of deprivation, a higher number of health and local authorities, and a greater number of service providers. With these considerations in mind, this report aims to provide an overview of the current mental health services in primary care in London, and consider options for the development of these services.

5.8.2 Existing services

a. Human resources available in general practice settings

Within the NHS, the majority of people with a mental illness come first into contact with a member of the primary care health team, be that the general practitioner, practice nurse or health visitor (Shah, 1992; Goldberg and Huxley, 1992). It is therefore appropriate to give an overview of available firstline services within primary care in London.

Table 1 shows the data available from statutory sources on London's general practices and their staff.

Table 1 General practice characteristics in London's sixteen Health Authorities

Health Authority	No.of patients	No.of GPs	No. of Practices	Practice size – No. of partners				Practice Nurse wte	Counsellor wte
				1	2–3	4–5	>5		
Barking & Havering	379939	193	99	57	30	8	4	60	0
Barnet	363466	208	84	37	30	13	4	66	1
Brent & Harrow	554572	323	125	52	54	13	6	119	2
Bromley	304648	170	57	19	21	12	5	55	0
Camden & Islington	442373	263	104	52	33	13	6	80	6
City & East London	710089	394	165	74	60	22	9	107	2
Croydon	336905	179	69	24	30	14	1	69	0
EHH	824818	408	194	94	75	21	4	156	2
Enfield & Haringey	563461	294	127	62	48	11	6	96	1
Greenwich & Bexley	432654	234	87	34	34	12	7	49	4
Hillingdon	243792	127	52	17	28	5	2	48	1
KCW	406658	240	105	58	40	6	1	104	30
LSL	847247	447	173	75	60	29	9	168	25
MSW	666734	352	132	42	56	28	6	123	2
Redbridge & Waltham	454507	249	123	66	44	12	1	64	1
Kingston & Richmond	337277	205	62	19	22	12	9	73	3
Totals	7.8M	4,286	1,578	782	665	23	80	1,437	80
Practice size/total number of practices – percent				50%	42%	1.5%	5%		

EHH – Ealing, Hammersmith & Hounslow
KCW – Kensington, Chelsea & Westminster
wte – whole time equivalent

LSL – Lambeth, Southwark & Lewisham
MSW – Merton, Sutton & Wandsworth
No. of patients – number of patients registered with GPs, not Health Authority population

The data presented in Table 1 are derived from the 1995 annual report of the Department of Health on general practice statistics. The Family Health and Services Authorities and Health Authorities have a statutory responsibility to report centrally data concerning primary care within their area. The first problem encountered is that the information is not current, and secondly there are questions over the reliability of the data. It is unlikely that there are no counselling services paid for through GMS[1] funds in three Health Authorities, and that the provision is so low in other authorities. The value of the data is limited by the fact that only GMS-funded counsellors are included: those mental health workers who work in a general practice setting but are employed by a different organisation are not included. It is possible that in some Health Authorities the requirement for 'counselling' is being met by health professionals of another category e.g. psychologists, funded by different means.

In preparing this report, a postal inquiry about local general practices was sent to all sixteen Health Authorities. Two months after writing, nine had failed to reply. The incomplete data from the seven who did reply are presented in Table 2.

---

[1]General Medical Services (GMS) funding is the portion of funds available from the Family Health Services expenditure for General Practice

Table 2 Data received from postal inquiry to Health Authorities

Health Authority	No. of GPs	No. of Practices	Practice size – No. of partners	Mental health workers			
			1	2–3	4–5	>5	
Brent & Harrow	na	na	na	na	na	na	6 counsellors
Bromley	156	58	17	25	13	3	4 counsellors
Croydon	163	70	24	32	13	1	5 counsellors (4.4 wte) 6 psychologists (5.5 wte) 15 CPNs (14.5 wte)
EHH	412	207	92	88	23	4	na
Hillingdon	118	52	17	28	5	2	4 counsellors
KCW	na	na	na	na	na	na	23 people carrying out 41 counselling sessions (3.5 hours = 1 session)
Redbridge & Waltham	209	121	69	42	9	1	na

na – not available

Two major observations may be drawn from comparing the data presented in Tables 1 and 2. The situation in general practice is constantly changing, especially with regard to staffing levels, and there is no standard way of reporting data across Health Authorities in an intelligible and comparable form. Given the rapid rate of change, this second observation is critical if an accurate picture of what is happening in primary care mental health services is required.

b. Description of variation between areas

Two health authorities, KCW and LSL are notable in having larger numbers of counsellors than others, although the reader will see from Table 5 that KCW has in fact reduced its numbers of counsellors recently. Other authorities employ none whatever. The total number of practice nurses now almost equals the total number of practices. Fifty percent of practices are still single-handed.

General practice fundholding was introduced in 1990. This gave general practitioners (GPs) their own budget with which to purchase secondary services. Nationally one practice in three is fundholding. Information specific to London about numbers of fundholders is not available, but it has been adopted more in suburban areas than in the inner-city. Debate about the effects of fundholding continues, and two recent Audit Commission reports indicate that patients may not be benefitting as much as they might (Audit Commission, 1996a, 1996b).

Mental health services which GP fundholders may purchase include out-patient treatment, counselling services, referrals to all members of mental health teams except psychiatric social workers, learning disabilities, and referrals made by community psychiatric nurses for other services included within the fund-holding scheme. A study in a fundholding area of Outer London (Ford and Sathyamoorthy, 1996) showed that fundholding had resulted in less severe mentally ill patients being referred to community mental health teams, a quarter of whom had no definite clinical symptoms. Most were not psychotic: the latter were not referred to the teams, for whose services the GPs had to pay. The patients seen by psychiatrists were likely to be psychotic but stable, while social workers were seeing the most disabled patients. Another study (Corney, 1996) highlighted the increased links being made by fundholding practices with mental health professionals. The authors comment that available services may favour patients with less severe mental illness.

5.8.3 Comparison of London inner city provision and non-London inner cities

By employing the statistical technique of cluster analysis on demographic and socio-economic characteristics, a tripartite taxonomy has been developed to allow comparison between health authorities (Boyle and Smaje, 1992; Benzeval et al, 1992). This divides Health Authorities into three groupings; inner deprived, mixed status, and high status. Routinely collected data including GMS performance indicators can thus be compared between areas of similar grouping and between different geographical locations. Table 3 compares performance on general practice targets between areas classified as inner deprived in London and outside London. Whilst the data do not directly pertain to mental health services available in general practice settings, they do inform about the difference in practice standards between inner deprived areas in London and elsewhere.

Table 3 Comparison of GMS data between inner deprived areas

	Inner deprived areas	
	London	Non-London
Child immunisations – % of target	44	85
Schoolage boosters – % of target	32	69
Cervical cytology – % of target	33	80
Child health surveillance – % provided	47	70
Practices with no practice nurse – %	26	8
Practices below minimum standards – %	37	3
Minor surgery list – %	39	65
Single handed GPs – %	22	13
Average list size	1700	2400

The data presented in Table 3 suggest that for a smaller list size, GPs in inner deprived areas in London are under-performing when compared to colleagues in similarly inner city deprived areas outside London. It is unlikely that there is a simple explanation for this, but factors such as high mobility of patients, lower numbers of attached staff, the many practices below minimum standards, the larger number of GPs working on their own, and increased difficulties in accessing services from multiple providers will all contribute. Where mental health is concerned, recent data confirm better figures for psychiatric case identification by GPs in Manchester than GPs in London: in Manchester (Warner et al, 1993; Kisley et al 1995) they identify approximately 61% of psychiatric cases, while in London only 45.5% are identified (Armstrong, 1996). Similar differences have been reported previously: Manchester 54% (Marks et al, 1979); against London 36% (Boardman, 1987).

Table 4 compares primary care staffing between inner deprived areas in London and outside London. Consistent with Table 3 is the evidence that more GPs are in single-handed practice in deprived settings in London than outside. Practice nurses are present equally between London and the other cities. Provision of counselling time is considerably higher in two of the London Health Authorities. The place of the counsellor within the primary care team is still a matter of controversy, as there is as yet no evidence that they produce better outcomes than GPs working on their own. Thus, their role may be to take pressure off those GPs who temperamentally dislike this kind of work, or who perceive themselves to be in overload. However, resources for counsellors should be found from within the primary care budgets, rather than from the mental illness budgets.

Table 4 Comparison of general practice data between deprived areas in London and outside London

FHSA	No. of patients	No. of GPs	No. of practices	Single Handed GPs	Practice Nurse wte	Counsellor wte
London						
Camden & Islington	442373	263	104	52 (19%)	80	6
City & East London	710089	394	165	74 (19%)	107	2
KCW	406658	240	105	58 (24%)	104	30
LSL	847247	447	173	75 (17%)	168	25
TOTAL	2.4M	1,344	547	259 (19%)	459	63
Outside London						
Leeds	731115	437	126	29 (7%)	154	2
Liverpool	496356	275	104	40 (15%)	80	4
Manchester	497516	297	116	49 (16%)	66	1
Sheffield	534369	352	111	25 (7%)	117	5
TOTAL	2.3M	1,361	457	143 (11%)	417	12

KCW – Kensington, Chelsea & Westminster
LSL – Lambeth, Southwark & Lewisham

5.8.4 Changes in service provision

There has been increasing awareness of the scale of psychological morbidity in general practice and of the necessity to respond to this previously unmet need. This has largely been addressed by increasing counsellor time within general practice and in some areas by developing stronger links with secondary services through community mental health teams. National publicity campaigns, offering information and training opportunities, such as the Defeat Depression campaign (Priest, 1991), have contributed to raising the profile of mental illness among health professionals and the public. This has been reinforced by the inclusion of mental illness among the five key areas in the government's Health of the Nation document (Department of Health, 1992a), and by the Royal College of General Practitioners creating a national mental health fellowship to produce educational materials for GPs (Turton and Tylee, 1995). After the Tomlinson Report on London's health services (see Chapter 3), money was made available to develop services in primary care in areas of greatest need within what has become the London Initiative Zone (LIZ). LIZ encompasses the following Health Authorities:

- Brent (excluding Harrow)
- Ealing, Hammersmith & Hounslow
- Kensington, Chelsea & Westminster

- Barking (excluding Havering)
- Camden & Islington
- City & East London
- Eastern Enfield and Edmonton area of Haringey
- Waltham Forest (exluding Redbridge)
- Greenwich (excluding Bexley but including Thamesmead)
- Lambeth, Southwark & Lewisham
- Wandsworth (excluding Merton & Sutton)
- Croydon (North only)

Table 5 presents data on changes in clinical staff in general practice within LIZ. These data are again from the Department of Health annual statistics and they present a mixed picture. Nearly all authorities have increased funding for practice nurses, who are now much more numerous. Half have increased counselling time, there being a marked increase in LSL balanced by a sharp decrease in KCW: the overall number increases only slightly.

Table 5 Variation in whole time equivalents of counsellors and practice nurses over time and health authority

Health Authority	Counsellor		Practice Nurse	
	1992	1995	1992	1995
Barking & Havering	0	0	56	60
Barnet	1.3	1	58.9	66
Brent & Harrow	2.9	2	106.3	119
Bromley	0	0	45.2	55
Camden & Islington	2.5	6	63	80
City & East London	4.7	2	91.4	107
Croydon	0.4	0	44.9	69
EHH	0.7	2	115.5	156
Enfield & Haringey	0.5	1	66.3	96
Greenwich & Bexley	0.6	4	75.2	49
Hillingdon	0.1	1	35.9	48
KCW	46	30	98.2	104
LSL	7.68	25	109.26	168
MSW	1.1	2	107	123
Redbridge & Waltham	0.28	1	63.07	64
Kingston & Richmond	3.1	3	71.7	73
Totals	71.9	80	1208	1437

The creation of the London Initiative Zone allowed FHSAs to make bids for extra funding to provide services for the population they served, with individual authorities receiving varying LIZ allocations. There has been considerable activity using LIZ funding to set up and introduce a variety of mental health initiatives across all HAs. As this funding comes to an end, there is concern about how to evaluate the LIZ programme and ascertain whether outcomes of the projects funded have been satisfactory.

5.8.5 Promising models for delivery of better services

Service development can be considered at two levels: changes which may be achieved within the primary care team and models involving external inputs into the practice.

Within the practice

a. Case registers – This would recognise that for some patients mental illness is a chronic health problem, in much the same way as diabetes and asthma, which in many practices are already managed in chronic disease management clinics based on case registers and a call/recall system (King and Nazareth, 1996). Individuals suffering from long-term mental illness could be readily identified and biannual review of stable problems could be undertaken by the most psychologically minded GP within the practice. This would necessitate initial identification of individuals, by looking at repeat prescribing, discussion with all members of the primary care team, practice computer searches, and checking with all secondary care institutions connected with the practice. Having established a case register, continuing administrative support is essential to operate an efficient call/recall system.

b. Practice protocols – These aim to improve recognition and management of clinical problems. They can be produced in-house, taken from external sources and used as directed or adapted for local use. They endeavour to produce a uniformity of clinical practice which is based on evidence and consensual experience of the best approaches to difficult clinical problems. Guidelines for the management of depression have been produced for use in general practice and disseminated by the Defeat Depression Campaign. The World Health Organisation has developed a primary care version of ICD10 with management guidelines for 22 disorders (Ustun et al, 1995). The difficulty associated with practice protocols is their effective implementation, as the benefits need to outweigh the problems of uptake such as education in how to use them, relevance to general practice and not upsetting the delicate time balance that operates in general practice.

c. Agreed care plans – The development of Case Management and the Care Programme Approach (CPA) has not made much impact on the involvement of general practitioners in the care of their long-term mentally ill patients. Where GPs are invited to CPA meetings, timing usually prevents them from attending. Organising a meeting to suit several different professionals involved in the care of one patient is not always straightforward, but the keyworker should assume responsibility for ensuring that the GP is made aware of the meeting's outcome and any particular actions which are part of his GMS activities. This is especially important concerning physical problems that mentally ill patients suffer (Kendrick et al, 1991), as there is excess morbidity and mortality amongst the mentally ill. The essential component of making agreed care plans is that there is adequate opportunity for effective communication between primary and secondary care.

d. Mental health facilitators – Facilitators have been shown to be effective in assisting GPs managing chronic health conditions (Fullard et al, 1987). The Department of Health recently completed a study based in a London borough, which sent a mental health facilitator to work in six practices (Armstrong, 1996). The facilitator helped practices develop practice protocols for the detection and management of depression and anxiety, enhanced practice knowledge of external support, promoted a programme of educational activities, and advised about the employment of counsellors. This study reports a modest success, improving recognition rates of psychiatric illness, which may encourage further evaluation of this resource to bring about improvements within a practice.

e. Catchment areas – For the most part secondary care facilities define the catchment area for which they assume responsibility. Where general practice surgeries are geographically located on the borders of several defined catchment areas, the GP will have to liaise with different secondary care providers, possibly offering services of different quality, depending on where his patient resides. Where there are already problems in accessing or identifying appropriate secondary services this creates a further burden of administrative difficulty. Catchment areas might more appropriately be defined by a group of general practice surgeries providing GMS services to a set population. Chapter 8 discusses further the conflict which may arise between basing sector boundaries on primary care and on social services boundaries.

External to the practice

a. The 'shifted outpatient' model – The mental health team moves into the primary care setting, holding referral clinics in the surgery (Mitchell, 1985). This aims to reduce stigmatisation for the patient, make access easier for the GP, allow for joint assessment and treatment, and improve inter-professional communication.

b. The 'liaison-attachment team' model – The multidisciplinary mental health team forms a close working relationship with the primary care team (Midgley et al, 1996), with the specific aim of helping the primary care team to develop its skills in the assessment and management of people with mental health problems. When the primary care team is confident with the majority of mental health problems, the mental health team moves on to another practice.

c. The Nunhead 'integrated model' – Joint case registers are developed by primary and secondary service teams (Strathdee, 1993). There is a named liaison nurse, outpatient clinics are held in the surgeries, and practice protocols are developed.

d. Liaison Key-workers – A key-worker on the CMH team – usually a community psychiatric nurse develops close links with (usually) two general practitioners. This key-worker looks after all patients with serious mental illness (SMI); develops 'shared care plans' with the GPs; acts as a facilitator for contacts with other members of the community mental health team as appropriate; provides a familiar face to the two GPs who get to know the key-worker assigned to them; and provides training and support for other members of the primary care team (often primary care nurses and Health Visitors) who are undertaking mental health work in the practice. This enables the CMH team to develop relationships with every general practice in its area: but it involves a very different way of working to the more usual arangements, in which the patients in a key-worker's case-list may come from many different practices. The advantages claimed for this arrangement are that the users, the GPs and the key-workers all prefer this way of working, and it allows the key-workers a more varied case-load, which in turn probably accounts for their better job-satisfaction (Goldberg et al, 1996a).

5.8.6 Shortcomings of existing services

The provision of mental health services in primary care in London is by no means universally poor. There are examples of good practice where individual practices have developed effective in-house services and good links with external services. However, these are the exception rather than the rule, and of the remainder there is still considerable variation in services available. Some of the variation can be explained by inadequate human resources. Practice nurses directly and indirectly by freeing GP time can perform a useful role. The provision of counsellors to practices is inequitable, and this may be due to inadequate practice premises unable to provide space for visiting professionals.

Even where sufficient personnel are available, a fundamental question is whether staff have adequate skills and knowledge for detection and management of mental health problems. This is true of all core members of the primary care; less than fifty percent of GPs undertook a hospital psychiatry post as part of their training (Styles, 1991), and there is little specific training for the management of psychological problems encountered in general practice. Practice nurses are unlikely to have ever received appropriate training in the management of mental health problems, may be responsible for administering antipsychotyic depot medication, and are often seen as more approachable by patients with psychological distress.

That use of case registers and practice protocols is not widespread further reduces the effectiveness of the primary care team. The time and manpower costs in establishing these need to weighed against more structured and efficient practice. The problems associated with accessing secondary services often centre on the knowledge of catchment areas, especially for practices that have to refer to a number of sectorized service providers. This can be further complicated by individual secondary service providers not offering a full range of services and necessitating referral across providers for certain categories of patients. There are no dedicated link workers to liaise between primary and secondary care teams to facilitate knowledge of existing services and offer more effective communication.

Alongside the statutory services there is a wealth of voluntary and charitable institutions undertaking valuable and supportive work with people suffering from mental illness. Who they are, where they are, and what they offer are questions not readily answerable in the local practice context. An adequately maintained resource directory available in each GPs practice would facilitate information giving to patients and carers.

5.8.7 Proposed solutions

Given the complexity of providing adequate mental health services, it is not surprising that there are deficiencies in several areas of service provision. Likewise, interventions to improve service provision in primary care should operate at several levels. These can be considered at the primary care, secondary care and health authority levels. Some of these are clearly important to primary care nationally whilst others are particular to service provision in London.

a. Primary care

Training of primary care staff is a priority. This should focus mainly on general practitioners and practice nurses to improve their detection and mangement skills. The WHO has developed a simplified version of the mental disorders chapter of the 10th revision of the International Classification of Disease which is suitable for use in primary care (ICD10-PHC). The classification is unusual in that it gives detailed advice on management, and is both brief and user-friendly. For each of the 22 disorders there is advice on information for the patient and family, specific counselling for the patient, indication (if any) for medication, and indications for specialist referral (Unstun et al, 1995). The classification has been field tested with British GPs, and found to improve both their confidence and their skills (Goldberg et al, 1996b). Training materials aimed at improving the mental health skills of staff inprimary care are currently being developed by the authors in conjunction with ICD10-PHC. There are several other training packages already available (listed in Appendix).

Central to effective implementation of an education programme are the availability of motivated and trained tutors and protected time from clinical practice for educational activities. Protected time is expensive but increases the likelihood of practitioner attendance and rightly accords importance to continuing education which must be more than added on to a busy working day.

The newly established **RCGP Unit for Mental Health Education in Primary Care** based at the Institute of Psychiatry under the directorship of Dr André Tylee is seeking to improve the Continuing Medical Education (CME) infrastructure by setting up a teacher training course for GP CME tutors and their nearest nurse facilitator/trainers. Suitable pairs of trainers are being recruited for this course in South Thames Region as well as South and West and Northwest Regions. Regions and Health Authorities are currently being asked to fund suitable participants who as a result of the one year course will then be able to provide learner centred, multiprofessional, experiential, skills based, practice-based training using existing training packages. It is hoped that North Thames as well as South Thames based London Health Authorities will see the longer term benefit of sending pairs of tutors on this course.

There should be a **more equitable distribution of counsellors and psychologists** to general practice surgeries. These are probably best administered externally from the practice, using professionals with appropriate qualifications. This would allow good referral policies to be put in place, autonomy for the therapists, and adequate supervision within a professional context.

The development of **case registers** should be adopted as good practice and more promoted by the Royal College of General Practitioners. Practice protocols based on best available evidence or consensus, developed internally or borrowed would help to foster a more systematic approach to clinical problems.

b. Secondary care

Secondary care services would serve primary care in London better if **catchment areas** were aligned to general practice populations instead of operating from a potentially distant hospital site. In connection with this, a community based mental health team could provide a liaison worker attached to a number of GPs.

Community mental health teams should continue to concentrate on **ways of better integrating** mental health services: including dedicated key-workers; clinics by psychologists or psychiatrists and psychiatrists in larger centres; and collaboration between the teams in up-dating shared care registers. The community mental health team has an important function in **enabling** staff in primary care to undertake mental health tasks in primary care: they will do this by assisting in training days, by supervision sessions, and by offering consultation services with difficult patients.

c. Health Authority

A new responsibility here might be to provide primary care teams with an updated **resource directory** of locally based statutory and non-statutory service providers. This has already been done in some places, but the practice now needs to be generalised. Nor can it be thought of as a 'one-off' task: the directories need to be regularly up-dated.

Appendix

Training packages for General Practitioners

Depression – Recognition to management. Videotape with booklet, available from Defeat Depression Campaign, Royal College of Psychiatrists.

Counselling depression in primary care. Videotape with booklet, available from Defeat Depression Campaign, Royal College of Psychiatrists.

Management of depression. Videotape with booklet, available from Defeat Depression Campaign, Royal College of Psychiatrists.

Schizophrenia disease management pack. Ring file containing printed information, acetates for overhead projection and slides, for use by a tutor in a group context. Available from Mental Health Education Fellowship at the Institute of Psychiatry.

Focus on alcohol abuse. Videotape with booklet, available from the Postgraduate Department, University of Manchester.

Suicide. Available from the Samaritans.

Problem solving videotape. Available from Dr Lawrence Mynors Wallace, Warneford Hospital, Oxford.

Depression audit package. Available from Dr Lloyd, Department of General Practice, Exeter University.

Psychological Audit Package. Available from Dr Frank Smith, Department of General Practice, St. George's Hospital Medical School.

Reattribution videotape (somatization). Available from Routledge Educational Videotapes

Primary health care team mental health training package. Contact the Royal Institute of Public Health and Hygiene.

Chapter 5.9

London's ethnic minorities and the provision of mental health services

Kamaldeep Bhui

Summary

- London is characterised by great ethnic diversity, with 45% of all people from ethnic minorities living in the capital, compared with 10% of all White British people. Members of ethnic minorities tend to experience high levels of social adversity, with high unemployment and poor housing, and these factors are likely to increase their mental health needs. Most of the UK's refugees live in London, and levels of unmet mental health needs among this group are likely to be high. How to provide effective, acceptable and appropriate care for members of ethnic minorities is therefore one of the central issues for purchasers, planners and providers of London's services.
- Current statutory services do not seem to be effective in detecting mental health problems across all ethnic groups, in engaging members of these groups in treatment, or in gaining the confidence of Black communities in general. A striking manifestation of this is the marked tendency for Black Caribbeans to reach psychiatric services via the criminal justice system or compulsory admission.
- Professionals in the statutory services currently have generally limited understanding of how to adapt their ways of working so that they can come to a full understanding of the needs and problems of people who do not share their cultural background. Time constraints in a highly pressurised service work against achieving this goal, but professionals are also often unaware of the limitations of the service they can provide.
- Research on the mental health of ethnic minorities has not addressed the concern of these communities that they do not receive services which they see as acceptable and relevant to their needs.
- Some apparently successful models of good practice have been established in the voluntary sector, but tend to be insecurely funded and to have very limited links with statutory services.

Ways of addressing the problems currently encountered include:
- Widespread consultation should take place both with users from ethnic minorities and with other members of their communities on how to make generic services more accessible and appropriate for them.
- In-patient wards could be made more acceptable environments by provision of bilingual workers who could understand the cultural context of patients' experiences, female-only areas or wards, accessible places of worship with closer liaison with those offering spiritual guidance, and integration with non-medical and social models of caregiving.
- Training in culturally sensitive practice should be part of the core professional and continuing education training for all professionals across all statutory and non-statutory providers of mental health care.
- The expertise of voluntary and statutory providers needs to be integrated both centrally and locally, and more effective ways of working jointly need to be developed.
- The workings of the Mental Health Act in relation to ethnic minorities need to be examined, with introduction of advocates or legal representatives at an earlier stage.

A note on terminology

The term black in this paper is taken to mean all non-white ethnic minorities: this is to clarify policy thinking rather than to convey that all issues pertaining to black people can be similarly conceptualised or resolved. The term ethnic minorities is used synonymously, and although it does not have the same political history as the term black, it does convey something more of the diversity within black communities in Britain. Data pertaining to specific groups will be described in accord with the ethnic category classification employed by the researchers in reporting their findings.

5.9.1 Introduction

The current position

The last two decades have seen little increase in the effectiveness of mental health services provided for Britain's black communities despite intense debate about the cause of inequity of service provision. Epidemiological data indicate an excess of schizophrenia amongst Afro-Caribbeans and possibly amongst all minorities, an increased use of the Mental Health Act and medication, an excess of suicides amongst Asian women and possibly young black men. Patients continue to voice intense dissatisfaction with psychiatric services and professionals. Suspicions of racism and oppressive practices have resulted in increased funding of research into the amount of mental illness amongst ethnic minorities; the voluntary sector has emerged as a provider in response to the inflexibility of statutory services and has been charged with the responsibility of developing better services but usually on a short term funding basis and in the mean time the statutory sector remains not only unattractive but aversive to black users. Attention to injustices within existing practice is focused by tragedies such as the death of Jonathan Zito by the actions of Christopher Clunis, a black man with schizophrenia; a black man whose pattern of contact with services was a catalogue of missed opportunities, poor communication and disastrous care provision in terms of service structures, individual professionals and society. The pattern of care received by Clunis has been identified as typical of care received by black communities in Britain (Francis, 1994). So decades of persuasive research findings, tragedies, working parties, committees, enquiries, 'political first aid' and health service restructuring, all designed to deliver effective care to all people, have failed black people. Whilst these facts are well known, the barriers to progress remain diverse, institutionalised and manifest through contradictory ideologies and theoretical frameworks for conceptualising a solution.

The agenda

Cries of racism within health service public institutions have not been limited to mental health care. However, it is surprising that a speciality which demands effective communications and seeks to understand extremes of behaviour has failed to deal effectively with the greatest 'breakdown' of all: that is communication with black communities who mistrust the mental health care system (Wilson, 1993; NHS Task Force, 1994). This persistent and extreme mistrust reflects the inertia of statutory sectors, who have thus far failed to engage actively in spirit as well as on paper with the central issues underlying the rage felt within the black communities: these issues continue to be relegated in favour of more immediate 'merry go round' priorities in a rapidly evolving mental health care system (Hadley et al, 1996).

This document sets out to describe the evidence for inequity of service provision to black communities in London, to isolate responsible factors, to identify significant barriers and to propose solutions. Data about social inequality, special problems amongst London's ethnic minorities, and the particular limitations of London's mental health services will be presented. Barriers to change are discussed with a broad focus on service based issues and the ethos of mental health care including professional attitudes, research ideology, competing priorities and the politics of racism and anti-racism in mental health care. The inclusion of racism in a document focused on the delivery of care is not intended to send the reader into a defensive withdrawal or a guilt trip, nor is it to restrict the debate to black people alone. Injustice is the responsibility of society as a whole and all members of that society have valuable contributions to a resolution. By drawing attention to what for black people is a daily source of distress and concern, a normally very private experience, something personal to black people is shared with the reader – black people's perspective on why the existing services are inadequate and what of their experience is denied by an institutionally determined approach to mental health care delivery in the UK. The intention is to truly involve people of all backgrounds in a task which simply seeks a just system of health care; this common aim is often forgotten in the emotive exchanges when black mental health care is discussed.

5.9.2 London and Britain's black communities

The census and ethnic minorities in Britain

Where do minority ethnic people live?
Examining England and Wales as a whole, just under 60% of the African Caribbean population live in Inner London; a third of the Bangladeshi population are in Inner London; almost a third of the Indian community live in Outer London. Greater London contains 44.8% of all people from ethnic minorities and only 10% of the White UK population (Owen, 1996). London has the highest proportions of ethnic minority populations in the country (Balarajan & Raleigh, 1992). For example, 45% of Brent and 42% of Newham residents are identified as non-white by the census categories.

Problems of measuring the population size and distribution
Census data have increasingly become a means for estimating the distribution and needs of the population, and are heavily utilised for planning purposes. However, under-enumeration is believed to have been very significant for a variety of Black and Asian ethnic groups in the 1991 Census. Census data also conceal the important variations existing within census defined ethnic groups (Bulmer, 1996; Peach, 1996). Specific groups arrived in the UK at different times and during a diverse range of economic and political climates; age distributions, patterns of fertility, morbidity and mortality may vary widely even between populations defined by the Census as belonging to a single group. Thus to speak of black people and ethnic minorities is insufficiently specific when comprehensively considering needs.

Making sense of the 'other': hidden morbidity?
The 1991 census does not contain a category for people of mixed ethnic origin, who are instead included in one of the three 'other' groups. Yet, 12% of ethnic minorities in Britain were estimated to be of mixed origin; over three quarters are UK born and a half

under the age of fifteen (Berrington, 1994). The 'other' category contained 290000 people in total outnumbering the Black African, Bangladeshi and Chinese ethnic groups; Greater London accounts for 5.2% of the 'other' category nationally, 57.1% of the 'Other-Asian' and 41.7% of the 'Other-Other' group. Who comprises otherness? Owen (1996) cites that North-Africans, Arabs and Iranians cannot be distinguished within the Other-Other group of which they collectively form 22.5%. So the existing ethnic categorisation overlooks a significant proportion of people who would require specialist services.

5.9.3 London's mental health services

High risk services

According to the authors of the MILMIS reports (Chapter 6), 'high hospital admission thresholds and few beds concentrate severely ill people on acute units, creating a culture of violence and sexual harassment'. It is not surprising that many patients refuse to accept the intolerable living conditions currently encountered in London's hospitals and are compulsorily detained. With severe bed shortages 'there will be times when suicidal or dangerous patients abscond while waiting for admission' (Lelliot et al, 1995). A recent enquiry has demonstrated that those detained patients who commit suicide after absconding do so usually within a few days (Banerjee et al, 1994). London's services are therefore high risk services to encounter; and they are services which a disproportionate number of ethnic minorities *will* encounter, making their 'high risk' nature an issue of specific importance for individuals from ethnic minority backgrounds.

Community care and ethnic minorities

Ethnic minorities have historically been given consideration only as an afterthought in changing service structures in the NHS, and there is little indication that this is changing as the implementation of community care policies continues (Bhui et al, 1995b; Ahmad & Atkin, 1996). What is likely but unhelpful is that a further series of community care changes will be implemented as part of unevaluated policy fuelled by a new political ideology (Hadley et al, 1996). Examining community service use, Doyle et al (1994, 1995) demonstrated that the amount of care received by disabled, low income people was extremely variable and much of the resources were devoted to providing care for a small percentage of those eligible and in need of care; furthermore the most disabled appeared to obtain care through informal carers. Over half of this group received no formal care at home. Already lagging in terms of equitable service provision in a resource hungry health care system, it is likely that unless the mental health needs of ethnic minorities are given consistent and progressive consideration from the inception of any new ideology, they will continue to receive a crisis only service at the behest of legal powers designed to maintain public order and safety. There are very few studies examining the equity of community care distribution and efficacy across ethnic groups.

5.9.4 Social adversity among ethnic minorities: a double jeopardy

Ethnic minorities living in London are disproportionately exposed to the social problems of living in inner cites as well to services which are themselves in crisis. Unemployment affects under 10% of the white group, over 30% of the Bangladeshi and Pakistani group, over 20% of the Black other and Black African group, between 10 and 15% of the Irish, Indian and Other Asians and nearly 20% of the Other-other and Black Caribbean group (Peach, 1996; Figure 1).

Figure 1 Unemployment amongst black people in inner cities

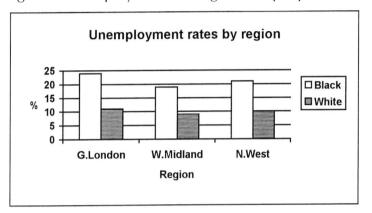

Source: Black and betrayed: a TUC report of black workers experience of unemployment: Data based on labour Force Survey (TUC, 1995a)

The use of local authority housing, the quality of housing, marital status and household constitution also vary by ethnic group with minorities consistently faring badly and the Black African, Bangladeshi, Chinese, Pakistani and Black other groups always having the worst experience (Peach, 1996).

Atri et al (1996), amongst GP registered patients in Tower Hamlets, confirmed that ethnic minorities were five times more likely to be living in overcrowded conditions, less likely to own their own homes (11% vs 36%), twice as likely to be in social classes 4 or 5 and were less likely to be employed (46% vs 20%). Furnham & Shiekh (1993) interviewed 100 Asian immigrants in Greater London. Morbidity correlated significantly with employment, children living at home, being female, and experience of racial abuse/prejudice; having parents living in Britain was a protective factor. Pilgrim et al (1993) confirm that racial prejudice remains a major stressor. There are no systematic studies of the Chinese population in London. Inferences can be drawn from Furnham & Li (1993) who examined how values, social support and expectations across generations influenced mental health in a Chinese community sample in Manchester, Edinburgh and the West Midlands. 44.2% of first generation and 22.2% of second generation had significant morbidity and reported psychological symptoms. Amongst the second generation, the less proficient an individual was in English the more likely it was for him or her to report psychological symptoms. There are also few data on London's Vietnamese communities, though a recent study in Nottingham (Nguyen-Van-Tam et al, 1996a, 1996b) supports the impression in London (Tang & Cuninghame, 1994) that there is considerable difficulty in using English as a second language to secure effective health care. There was low uptake of preventive programmes, and high levels of disadvantage including traumatic experiences.

Thus the social disadvantage, unemployment and poor housing which members of ethnic minorities in London are disproportionately likely to experience are likely to be pivotal factors in their mental health needs. These require attention as part of any overall plan to address their mental health needs (Health Advisory Service, 1994). Targeted mental health care has been demonstrated not to improve patient outcomes in isolation from critical social interventions (Conway et al, 1994). Community care policy is therefore always likely to be less efficacious amongst ethnic minorities, yet no account has been taken of this by policy makers or providers.

5.9.5 Refugees and asylum seekers

The United Nations High Commission for Refugees estimates that there are 20 million refugees world-wide yet less than five percent of them come to Europe (Medical foundation for the care of Victims of torture 1994). Home Office figures suggest that in 1994, 32800 asylum seekers entered the UK and made applications; this was 10,000 greater than in 1993 (Home Office Statistical Bulletin, 1995/96). London is the favoured destination for refugees arriving in the UK and most will live in inner city areas; estimates from studies in North London indicate that 116 000 refugees live in London (Karmi, 1992a, 1992b).

Refugees are especially vulnerable to psychiatric disorders including depression, suicidality and post traumatic stress disorder (Ramsay et al, 1993; Medical Foundation for the care of Victims of torture, 1994; Gorst-Unsworth, 1992). Gammel et al demonstrated that one third of refugees in Newham were depressed, 44% were women. Depression was associated with having spent little time in the UK (36% of recent arrivals), and with not speaking English (37% of those with no English compared with 25% of those who could speak some English). 62% reported constant worrying and about a half reported other symptoms consistent with a diagnosis of post traumatic stress disorder. Their needs for health care are therefore significant. King et al (1994) when measuring the incidence of psychosis amongst ethnic groups in North London found that 11% of their hospital or community contact patients were refugees compared with only 5% of the population of the catchment area, further supporting the evidence that refugees are over represented amongst psychiatric populations.

Children either as victims, or passive observers of violence are often neglected as a focus of therapeutic attention, and this neglect can result in post traumatic stress disorders, depressive reactions, somatic symptoms and what Richman (1993) refers to as the existential dilemma of distrust in others and facing an uncertain future.

Refugees and health, social and legal agencies

70% of the Newham's (Gammel et al, 1993) depressed refugees wished to talk to a counsellor or professional in their own language. Most refugees were registered but often had difficulty registering with GPs who in some instances did not wish to have refugees on their list. Over a third of the refugees who were depressed felt they needed to talk to someone in their own language compared to 10% of those who were not depressed.

The Refugee Arrivals Project annual report (1994) shows great difficulty in meeting housing and basic needs of refugees, with statutory organisations not recognising the special needs of this population. In general, the rules and regulations of social benefits agencies appear to disproportionately deprive ethnic minorities of benefits due to them (TUC, 1995b). Negotiation of such institutional barriers must be considered by any multi-agency service addressing the mental health needs of ethnic minorities in general and refugees in particular (Atkin & Rollings, 1993).

Traumatic experience needs to be conceptualised in terms of a dynamic, two way interaction between the victimised individual and the surrounding society, and not as a relatively static, circumscribed entity to be located and addressed within the individual psychology of those affected (Summerfield, 1995). Health care professionals focus on their limited brief of treating disorders without attending to its social context . The undermining effects of insecurity over deportation, extreme poverty, poor housing, and racism are underestimated and should be distinguished from what is generally meant by the stresses of acculturation (Summerfield, 1995). Refugees are rarely included in the any ethnic monitoring exercise so little attempt is made to plan for their potential needs.

5.9.6 Black people and psychiatric services

a. Cultural competencies of the professionals
In all statutory services time constraints determine the level of attention and degree to which a professional comes to really know the characteristics of any patient. Where a patient presents their distress in a manner which is unfamiliar to the health care professional , more time and attention to detail are required if the level of knowing that patient is to be comparable to that in a patient who shares (with the professional) the same language, social class, culture and world view about health, illness and help seeking (Bhugra & Bhui, 1996). Not only is such time not usually available but professionals are often unaware of the limitations of their own assessment. This is especially a problem in emergency situations where decisions are often made in a hurry, within the constraints of legal and peer group precedents.

Somatisation of depression among non-western communities is a concept of particular significance for the manner in which professionals assess patients from minority backgrounds. Much has been written about this (Bal, 1984; Burke, 1986; Leff, 1988) even though somatisation is common among white British patients also and can occur in any age, social class and intellectual level (Helman, 1990). The absence of shared meanings, lexicon, concept of self and world view contribute to the emphasis on physical symptoms which are more directly amenable to undistorted translation. Somatisation as a term is often applied when, due to premature closure of assessments or of 'cultural distance', there is a poor shared understanding of the therapeutic encounter (Bhui, 1994). Such a scenario has more recently been demonstrated to be associated with non recognition of psychiatric disorder in primary care (Jacob et al 1996). Wilson & MacCarthy (1994) demonstrated that even when patients presented with psychiatric complaints, Asians were more likely to be diagnosed as suffering from physical illness; where physical complaints were presented, more of the white group were identified to have psychiatric problems than the Asian group. Jacob et al (1996) confirmed that a sample of West London GPs correctly diagnosed less than a fifth of those identified by a questionnaire to be ill.

5.9.7 Existing services

Utilisation of London's mental health services

a. General psychiatric inpatient services

Afro-Caribbeans have three to thirteen times the admission rates of white patients. This is for schizophrenia and affective psychoses (Bebbington et al, 1981; King et al, 1994; Moodley & Perkins, 1991; van Os, 1996). Admission rates under a section of the mental health act are also higher for Afro-Caribbeans (Wessley, 1991; Bebbington, 1981; Moodley & Perkins, 1991; Bagley, 1971; King et al, 1994; Davies et al, 1996; Callan, 1996). The magnitude of the excess varies in different parts of London and is likely to be a function of not only the population but the configuration of the local service (Bebbington,1981). Fewer black inpatients are diagnosed as having depression or a neurotic illness (Lloyd & Moodley, 1992; Bebbington, 1981; Cochrane et al, 1977, Cochrane et al 1989; Dean et al, 1981). Diagnostic (schizophrenia) excess and challenging behaviour amongst black patients have been cited as the cause of this finding (Sheehan, 1995; Lloyd & Moodley, 1992). Asians have lower admission rates than white patients, fewer re-admissions, and spend less time in hospital than a comparable sample of white patients (Gupta, 1991). Recently, Callan (1996) reported that Afro-Caribbeans also had shorter re-admissions than a British born white control group; a milder course was hypothesised to exist among Afro-Caribbeans. Black patients more often receive depot medication and physical treatments (Lloyd & Moodley, 1992; Littlewood & Cross, 1980) and along with white immigrants received a poor service as out-patients.

b. Forensic services

Afro Caribbeans are over represented amongst patients admitted to secure units (Jones & Berry, 1986; Maden, 1996, section 4.6 of this report). Among sentenced prisoners the prevalence of mental illness amongst Afro-Caribbeans is 6% compared to a prevalence of 2% amongst the white population (Maden, 1996). Amongst a random sample of remanded mentally disordered offenders diagnosed as having schizophrenia, 17.6% were white, 68.8% were Black Caribbean, 43.8% were black African, 58.3% were black British and 42.1% fell within another non-white ethnic group (Bhui et al, 1996). Black men are more often received by hospitals on forensic sections of the mental health act than are white prisoners (Banerjee et al, 1995; Bhui et al, 1996; Davies et al, 1996). Three quarters of black defendants coming into contact with psychiatric services have had previous contact with psychiatric services whereas a half of the white group have had previous contact with a psychiatric service (NACRO, 1990) suggesting that more of the black group have fallen out of care. Black people comprised 47% of those appearing before courts and in need of psychiatric assessment whereas they represented only 24% of those detained within police stations indicating again that there is a failure to effectively divert black mentally disordered offenders at the pre-court stage (Robertson et al, 1996).

c. Primary care

Consultation Rates
There has been little uniformity in the findings of research on ethnic variations in patterns of consultation in primary care. In an analysis of GP attendees, patients of Indian, Pakistani and Bangladeshi origin consulted the most, but after adjustment for

confounders this finding held for women only (Carr Hill et al, 1996). In the London Borough of Brent male Asians had substantially higher consultation ratios (Gillam, 1989). Consultations for anxiety and depression though were reduced in all immigrant groups (72%-76% of white group rate). British patients more often left the surgery with a repeat appointment, prescription or certificate. Higher consultation rates amongst Black patients have been reported in Brixton (Kiev, 1965). Research in practices in Tower Hamlets (Li et al, 1994) suggests an over representation of White and Black Caribbean patients and an under representation of Bangladeshis, Chinese, Black Africans, and Black Other.

Detecting Psychiatric Morbidity
Amongst Lloyd & St Louis's (1996) sample of Black women primary care attendees, black African women had higher levels of morbidity than a white control group, yet GPs noted psychiatric problems in 26% of black patients and 34% of white women. Jacob et al (1996) examined Asian primary care attendees in West London and found that 42.4% of them presented with non-specific complaints; only 6% reported psychological problems. GPs recognised only a fifth of cases. Significantly, not telling the GP about their complaints was associated with psychiatric morbidity as was dissatisfaction with the GP's treatment and contact with an alternative practitioner. Li et al (1994) report that in Tower Hamlets detection of morbidity for the Vietnamese was almost a quarter of that for the white population. Black African and Bangladeshi patients had nearly a half the detection rates of conspicuous morbidity. In a study of the causes of low rates of detection of depression among elderly members of ethnic minorities, inaccurate translation and embarrassment were problems reported by both Asian and White GPs (Pharoah, 1992). Over 60% of London GPs said it would be helpful to have more staff to provide education and information services.

Studying reasons for difficulty obtaining appropriate services in primary care, Nguyen-Van-Tam & Madeley (1996b) cite evidence from Nottingham that more than half of their sample of Vietnamese had *not* gone to their doctor because of language problems. Lloyd & St Louis (1996) reported that black women less often knew what they wanted from their GP (25% of white rate) and they were less likely to make multiple requests of their GP (23% of white rate). Black patients were less satisfied than white patents and this was especially so for black African women who also were the most distressed and attended the least often. Amongst the Vietnamese in London and Nottingham, there were difficulties in consultations with GPs. 35% reported using children to interpret (Nguyen-Van-Tam et al, 1996a; Tang & Cuninghame, 1994). The NHS Taskforce (1994) reported that of the Chinese community in the Oxford region, nearly half did not know how to obtain a doctor in an emergency. Furthermore 43% of those surveyed report that they prefer western medicine and 50% a combination of western and Chinese medicine.

It is clear that different ethnic groups remain dissatisfied with their GP and this is reflected in differential utilisation of GPs across ethnic groups (Health Education Authority, 1994); longer waiting times than white patients, distance from the surgery, the absence of same sex GPs, GPs less often calling in black patients for health checks and information not being available in the patient's own language all contribute. Loneliness, racist attacks and financial difficulties are also factors which add to morbidity (Pilgrim et al, 1993).

d. Community Studies

Doyle (1995) examined disability and users' views about care received. Despite mental health not explicitly being excluded, there were no psychiatric diagnoses seen but general inferences about care preferences can be made. Amongst young adults with physical disabilities, of whom 43.1% were from various ethnic backgrounds in London, it appeared that those with greater need were not necessarily supported more. Indeed people were actually losing contact with agencies, especially social services (Doyle et al, 1994). Access to respite and social events was very limited. Ethnic minorities were less optimistic about their future and feared that poverty, disability and their ethnic origin would isolate them. Most coped with the aid of family and mothers were the main carers. White GPs tend to emphasise the existence of family support, an explanation which has attracted much criticism for ignoring large populations on the basis of a stereotype (Ahmad, 1996). Yee (1996) argues that support for black carers must become a mainstream service issue, raised at senior management level, describing the three major myths which must be dispelled: that black families look after their own, that a colour blind approach is inherently not racist as carers' (and patients') needs are dismissed as not fitting the needs which are accepted to warrant recognition and that black carers continue to be seen as immigrants rendering their whole claim to better care as an unreasonable demand from a generous state.

e. The Voluntary Sector

A large number of voluntary organisations now deliver social and health care for members of ethnic minorities ; at least a half of those listed by SHARE are located in London. However, there is still a lack of information about the activities and client groups of voluntary sector organisations and about the effectiveness of models used. An overall strategy is urgently required to ensure that provision of specific services meets the care needs of local populations in a systematic way.

Webb-Johnson (1991, 1993) presents a clear account of how the public's perception of services can influence the development of good practice guidelines; it is clear that the voluntary organisations then have a major role to play in such a process. Jamdagni (1996) examined special projects and highlighted many areas of improved quality in comparison to mainstream services. In Camden (Jamdagni, 1996) nearly half of the community workers had come across people who chose not to use statutory services suggesting that services were not acceptable in their current form. Interesting insights into black carers' views about the system of service provision were also gleaned. 28% of carers in Camden did not want to be put in touch with social services or a mainstream voluntary organisation because of previous bad experiences and language barriers. English was not the first language in almost two thirds of carers and 80% of users. 62% of carers had not had a break in the last year.

Special medical problems

Alcohol use

McKeigue & Karmi (1993) reviewed data on alcohol consumption amongst ethnic minorities. Consumption was lower than the British mean in Afro-Caribbean men and women. Among South Asians average alcohol consumption is also lower than native British but within certain sub-populations alcohol related morbidity rates are higher. Thus amongst Sikhs heavy spirit drinking is especially high. They have higher rates of morbidity compared with Hindu and Muslim men and the alcohol related admission rates are increasing amongst South Asians. Although Cochrane et al (1996) indicate that the second generation have moderated their drinking patterns, there remained a tendency amongst the Sikhs and Hindus to drink so as to forget their problems.

Suicide

Mortality statistics indicate that suicide amongst ethnic minorities is on the increase especially amongst Asians and specifically Indian women from India and East Africa; rates of suicide have recently been reported to be between two and two and a half times the all England and Wales rate respectively (MHF, 1995b). Bhugra et al (1996a) recently reported on findings in West London; South Asian women showed crude rates of attempted suicides that were 1.6 times that of white and black women and 2.3 times that of South Asian men. Age specific rates confirm that amongst the 16-24 age group, South Asian women have rates which are 2.6 times that of white women and seven and half times that of South Asian men in the same age band. Balarajan (1996) reports that rates are elevated amongst Indians, Irish and Africans; the suicide rate amongst Caribbeans is reported to be the same as that of the British population. Pakistani and Bangladeshi rates are lower than those of the British population. Methods of suicide vary according to locally available methods and ascertainment may be a problem, hence an assessment of open verdicts is also essential for a full evaluation. For example, self immolation has been shown to be the chosen method amongst many Indian women. but was not found in West London (Bhugra et al, 1996a). Precipitating factors include interpersonal difficulties within families often to do with the second generation's desire to adopt western styles of intimate relationship, but also where conflicts arise from the perceived threat to much cherished values and traditional roles for women. Such values and social roles which normally provide certainty and are a source of strength become rigid and inflexible in the face of adversity. Alcohol use and financial worries also have been invoked as potential explanations (Bhugra et al, 1996b).

5.9.8 Barriers to delivery of effective interventions

Lack of understanding of different explanatory models of distress
Patients' unique explanations of misfortune, including illness, linked with characteristic help seeking behaviours, have been defined by Kleinman (1980) as explanatory models. Such models influence help seeking and hence the nature of treatment received. High levels of morbidity may go undetected if an individual's appraisal of their symptoms involves an explanatory model out of keeping with that expected by GPs and psychiatrists. Thus Beliappa (1991) reported an interpersonal social interpretation of depression by Bangladeshi people in East London, and Krause (1991) in an ethnographic study demonstrated that Punjabis in Bedford could communicate their distress by the use of idioms of a sinking heart (literally translated). MacCarthy & Craissatti (1989) interviewed Bangladeshis in East London and confirmed significant degrees of hidden morbidity and that the impact of life events could not readily be translated across cultures. The GP was seen as a village elder and was often approached for a multitude of difficulties and so detecting illness was just one of many issues presented to GPs. In some instances explanatory models direct patients to other sources of help, for example, prayer or increased attendance at a temple. The specific sources of help will be unique to each culture and are likely to involve traditional healers, complementary medicine practitioners (Bhopal, 1986; Wilson, 1993) as well as GPs. For

example, Balabil & Dolan (1992) report that British Asians attendees of two London GP surgeries had lower expectations of counselling and that this may explain their hesitancy in seeking this form of intervention. Yet, Littlewood & Cross (1980) illustrate that it is not just the patient who determines what help is offered. Black psychiatric outpatients in this study received more physical treatments (major tranquillisers and ECT). Black and white immigrants received intra-muscular injections more often and their pattern of outpatient attendance was characterised by self referrals, missed appointments and being booked in to see the most junior member of the team. The expectations of health professionals therefore appear to be as important.

Pathways into care
Most psychiatric morbidity in the UK presents to the GP, who is thus the focus of delivering community based health care (Goldberg and Huxley, 1980). The low detection rates found despite high consultation rates in primary care contrast with the findings that, as discussed above, black people are over-represented in psychiatric hospitals and forensic units and are more often identified to be in need of psychiatric help through crisis services and by the use of the mental health act (see sections on forensic and general psychiatric services). For example, Bhugra et al (1996c) in a study examining the incidence and outcome of schizophrenia found that only one of thirty six African Caribbean patients with schizophrenia presented through their GPs. Bhui et al (1993) demonstrated that despite 54% of Asian psychiatric hospital admissions having an Asian GP, only 24% were admitted at the behest of their GP. Thus the current structure and functioning of services fails to deliver early interventions for black patients.

Alternative services and sources of help
Black people who were born in other countries have also to negotiate generational changes of attitude to success, work and family commitments; sources of dignity and pride will be under threat. Traditional sources of support may disappear and the statutory sector may attempt to replace them with health and social service funded alternatives which are likely to be unreliable (short term funding) and less culture specific. Traditional remedies and culturally consistent healing strategies may not be within the realms of accepted medical practice especially when there is such a focus on evidence based medicine (Huka, 1995). Yet, the popularity of these approaches bears witness to the failure of statutory services to effectively manage the totality of an individual's distress.

Collaboration between sectors and agencies
Jamdagni (1996) scrutinised the barriers and opportunities for improving service delivery to black populations. The work highlighted three instrumental factors: the political will of the purchaser, access to and relationship with local black communities and a relationship between purchaser and provider which is based on a shared understanding and a degree of trust. An outreach approach and partnership with a community health council are described as mechanisms to improve communication and generate better working relationships between the various players (Hendessi, 1994).

Health service research and black communities

Conflicting research methodology and ideology

Black communities are currently highly suspicious of the intentions of cross-cultural research and see it as a further pathologisation of being Black. The unique position of psychiatry as a discipline of judgement yet entertaining extensive legal powers generates a 'very potent brew of racial suspicion and distrust' (Cochrane & Sashidharan, 1996). Health service research as a discipline is itself evolving. An accepted publication bias was attended to by Donnan (1996) who advocates a need for new broader based but rigorous techniques to test hypotheses and that such an approach should be the foundation of progressive health service research rather than just descriptive studies. Yet here is the paradox, much of the work which is cited by the minority communities themselves to come closer to their experience of mental health services is indeed qualitative and takes account of context rather more than diagnosis (Littlewood, 1990; Fernando, 1988). The methodologies for these approaches have developed largely from the discipline of anthropology. Yet anthropology and epidemiology as approaches have always had an uncomfortable relationship (Inhorn, 1995; Janes et al, 1986) but one which must now be harmonised in order for high quality cross cultural health service research to develop (Smaje, 1996). For example the medical literature on compliance with treatment has entirely failed to encompass the concept of compliance as a medical ideology far removed from the realities of a patient's life and their perception of risk (Trostle, 1988; Bhui, 1996a). Although epidemiology is suited as a methodology in many medical specialities, in the realms of mental health it encounters major limitations in terms of assumptions and inferential validity (Cochrane & Sashidharan, 1996), and even within academic circles consensual and consistent views have not emerged on appropriate methodologies for health services research for culturally distinct communities. The combination of this fragmentation and persisting beliefs in a purist method is evident in a paralysis of service and policy development, where a more pragmatic approach might enable important changes in services to be made even within existing resources (Bhui et al, 1995b). There needs to be a social research agenda concentrating on black people's perceptions and perspectives on health care delivery that are not concerned with fundamental biological and aetiological truths but with making the system fit the needs of the population (Ahmad, 1993). Notable exceptions to this absence of culturised research using integrative methods on mental health are studies by Abas et al (1996) and Lloyd et al (1996) in London and Patel et al (1995) in Harare.

Racism and the anti-racist movement in mental health

Fernando (1992) criticises the historical foundation and contemporary practices within psychiatric establishments as racist and specifically draws attention to the perpetuation of this state by racist ideology in research. Such a notion is supported by the racist categories of violent Caribbean male youths and hysterical South Asian girls as a focus of research (Black health workers and patients group, 1983) and by the clearly documented historical accounts of social sanctions and research that we today would consider blatantly racist (Fernando, 1988, Littlewood & Lipsedge, 1989). Stuart (1996) proposes that there are limits on what ethnic minorities can blame on the inequities of white supremacy; he argues that the term institutional racism has been used in a reductive manner to imply that racist processes are the only primary cause of all the unequal outcomes and exclusions that black people experience … there are two sides to the black experience of subordination, that which is inflicted from without and the response to this from within. Yet ethnic minorities seek no more than an equal opportunity of access in health and social care provision. One must beware that although crude racist conclusions are no longer apparent in transcultural psychiatry research, implicit or subtle racism still pervades the discipline (Cochrane & Sashidharan, 1996). Perhaps what Stuart (1996) alludes to is an unacceptable inertia in the national debate about how to prioritise. A debate which is beset with powerful emotions transmitted through generations of oppressive experiences which, although to some seem redundant in contemporary service developments, may serve to generate mistrust between British people as citizens, patients, carers and providers. This inherent tension affects clinical service developments, the research agenda and ultimately patient care.

An example: a confusion of tongues

An example: Studies do convincingly demonstrate the existence of an excess of diagnosed schizophrenia amongst young Afro-Caribbean men (Wessley, et al 1991; Glover, 1989, Bebbington et al, 1994) A further hypothesis is that Blacks may have relative immunity to minor disorders and vulnerability to major disorders related to denial of mental illness. A search then ensues for why this might be. Such data have not been welcomed by ethnic minorities. It is not the data but the inferential limitations and the potential impact on the public that have escaped researchers' awareness. The difficulty is that the findings are too readily interpreted in the context of favored aetiological hypotheses and conclusions are drawn that the data do not support. This intellectual leap to causal attribution results in the reification of the favored hypotheses.

The flu hypothesis, one example of this process was advanced to explain this effect for Black men born in the 1950s and 1960s. Yet at no point is there any consideration of whether these hypotheses are likely to be welcomed and considered by the Black community as being of public health interest or of direct therapeutic relevance. Consequently what in scientific circles can be considered as a tentative hypothesis worthy of exploration is to the community a far fetched attempt to further exoticise Black mental health with little attempt to explain or interpret the findings to those whom the findings should most affect, that is patients.

An interesting hypothesis based on routine data and with potentially unresolvable residual confounding is identified by the Black media as further evidence of at least disrespectful regard, if not an insidious form of racism. Nonetheless, it was these hypotheses which led to much perplexed disbelief amongst the Black communities where conference speakers were heard to say 'so not only do we have more schizophrenia but they now want us to believe that we get it because our mothers caught the flu'.

The development of this hypothesis is an example of how inferences of public health importance based on a lore of rational scientific principles can neglect the actual impact of this revered scientific rationality on public perceptions. The implementation of public health measures and the pursuit of quality research in this field requires a much greater collaboration at the planning stage taking account of ethical considerations, interpretation and presentation of the findings. Representation on ethics committee could be one useful approach, although ethical committees have been demonstrated to draw inconsistent and questionable conclusions (Alberti, 1995; Hotopf et al, 1995). Greater collaboration or seeking consultation with existing voluntary agencies or a sample of the public or perhaps even the study populations would lead to more creative and fruitful solutions, even though establishing such a process would require much mutual effort especially around issues of ownership and disagreements between parties. Inevitably this would introduce another component to what is often an already complicated process. Many commentators suspicious of the 'schizophrenia epidemic' suggest that the findings summarised above reflect the racism or ethnocentrism of British Psychiatry (Smaje, 1995). The word racism, however, is imprecise and can do violence to the distinctions between injustice based on ignorance, error or omission and injustice that arises from a vindictive prejudicial attitude. Of course the consequences of either may be identical and if one defines racism by the outcome of action rather than the intentions of individuals and organisations then such blunt application is valid; however, conflating these two attitudes will not encourage dialogue or collaboration.

Thus a new research agenda is needed which is closer to clinical practice and which is part of a co-ordinated strategy to addresses the many important gaps in our current knowledge. For example, the Chinese and Vietnamese communities have received far less funding or research than some other communities. Refugees have received relatively little attention despite their growing number and the their burden of morbidity (Mental Health Foundation, 1995a). Service development should be based on reliable data so as to ensure that resources are best spent; however, in view of the dynamic nature of population demographics as well as culture, it appears that whichever model of delivery is adopted it must retain the capacity to change the profile and quantity of interventions provided as well as retain expertise within teams and not rely on single individual to become representatives of whole cultures.

5.9.9 The Voluntary sector and partnerships

Emergence of the voluntary sector

The voluntary black organisations have been identified as the only source of culturally sensitive practice (Gray, 1996). Their freedom from institutional legislation and a professional body of esoteric knowledge are their strength; such procedures although essential as a safeguard do bureaucratise any effort to change existing patterns of service provision. The black mental health dedicated voluntary sector has become the guardian of good practice and the convenient solution for the colour and culture blind approach of the statutory sector. Figure 2 describes some of the London services which may be seen as examples of good practice developed in the voluntary sector.

Joint working: is it happening?
A recent survey of voluntary organisations indicated that 53% had past contact with mental health services (La Granade & Bhugra, 1996). Only one organisation recalled positive experiences from the statutory sector. 26% admitted negative perceptions and 47% acknowledged negative experiences. These included eurocentric practice, slow response to crisis, lack of preventive measures, lack of respite services, racist treatment, bureaucracy, poor support, lack of cultural and religious sensitivities and an inflexible approach. 52% of agencies said that they did network. 33% of agencies wanted more information from the statutory sector on mental illness and on local services. Information available on a 24 hour basis was deemed essential, training of voluntary organisation workers and joint working was regarded as important perhaps again reflecting that the statutory sector may not be receptive.

Figure 2 Examples of good practice in the voluntary sector

- The Brixton Circle project provides to the black community what the community care act suggests should be provided to all patients. Attention is given to accommodation, education, counselling, employment and even involving the users after a period of stability and training in service provision (Brixton Circle Project Annual Report, 1991/2).

- The Chinese Mental Health Association is one of the few Chinese organisations providing alternative models of engagement and therapeutic work for members of the Chinese community. They avoid the label mental illness as this is heavily stigmatised and people would be unlikely to attend. Counselling, advocacy, befriending and support are provided but as with very many voluntary sector organisations, funding is an ongoing issue. The organisation actively works with the statutory sector, from which it received over a third of its referrals last year. A quarter of referrals have depression and a fifth have schizophrenia. In over 40% of cases further services are offered and accepted (Chinese Mental Health Association , 1995).

- The Afro-Caribbean Mental Health Association, Brixton, epitomises the response of the black community to poor statutory sector services and created an alternative to hospital based care whilst using a multidisciplinary approach. Housing, counselling and legal advice as well as therapeutic alternatives were all available.

- Nafsiyat in North London is a well established source of intercultural therapy; the founders of the organisation and those who work in an intercultural context have been successful at providing counselling in a friendly and culture sensitive manner, adopting existing models as required (Acharyya et al, 1989). For example, an empowering adaptation is the right of clients to express an opinion on the ethnic origin of their future therapist; not all want an ethnically matched therapist. Furthermore clients can bring a friend, relative or confidant with them during therapy sessions which allays much anxiety about communication and trust. Robins (1992) reports that 90% of patients reported a 'good outcome'. Referrals included rape and sexual abuse amongst women (25%), psychoses (15%), 46% had depressive syndromes and only 12 of 52 had pre-treatment GHQ scores that were less than 12 and 38 had post-treatment score of less than 12.

- The Manchester action committee for action on health care for ethnic minorities. This appears to be the first city wide, independent multi-ethnic umbrella body dedicated to health and community care. Thus direct access to decision makers is made possible for all black groups. This scheme is in the process of being replicated in Camden and Islington (Camden Health and Race Group et al, 1992).

A study in the North West Thames region (NW Thames RHA, 1994) confirmed that both the voluntary and statutory sectors lacked an understanding of each others' sector; specifically there was a low level of mutual knowledge between commissioners and voluntary providers about the structure, policies, planning, ethos and management processes of each other's sector. There were few examples of commissioning from the voluntary sector. One specific recommendation was that the voluntary sector infrastructure needs improvement and information standards that yield comparable voluntary sector cost and performance data should be developed. There is a lack of evaluative criteria which are agreed by voluntary provider and purchaser and which provide clear evidence about the usefulness of innovative services. It is essential that those voluntary sector services which are clearly valuable should be assured of longer term secure funding.

The voluntary sector has now been raised to a level of responsibility to resolve the difficulties faced by the statutory sector, but is often obliged to provide services on a short term basis with limited funding (Jamdagni, 1996). These groups often face severe marginalisation as a result of their campaigning role or race focus which can set them at odds with conventional services. A lack of information and of a supportive infrastructure and under-resourcing further limit their impact (Jennings, 1996). Such organisations are set the double task of being providers of services and evaluating them according to unspecified criteria that would have to satisfy both the statutory services and the purchasers, all within the budget designed to provide a service (Ahmad & Atkin, 1996). It is conspicuous that there is very little research evidence about the effectiveness of voluntary organisations, yet it is clear that such organisations bridge a gap in service provision and provide high quality culturally sensitive care. Even when monitoring and evaluation data are available they receive scant attention from service providers and purchasers (Watters, 1996).

What responsibilities should the statutory sector retain?
Having established that the voluntary sector providers can deliver quality care, where does this leave the responsibilities of the statutory sector who are charged by their professional bodies with clinical and ethical responsibilities and by the public (through the law) with civil and potentially criminal responsibilities to provide care and to protect the public and the patient. The majority of the black severely mentally ill are still cared for by the statutory sector. Can hospitals and consultants divest themselves of responsibilities in all these arenas? Is the voluntary sector prepared to adopt a professional code of ethics and to take legal responsibilities which any government of the day will not readily welcome? All these dilemmas arise if one conceptualises the two sectors as separate in ideology, geography and funding. Separatist services fiercely retain their autonomy and have an important advocacy role to play for those who are most dissatisfied with and alienated from health services (Mental Health Foundation, 1995a). However, if the psychiatric professions simply delegate all responsibility for the care of ethnic minorities to specialist services in the independent sector, they will betray their responsibility to care for the whole community and not just those who piously adapt to the ideology of free NHS care at the cost of personal choice. Joint working between statutory and voluntary sectors with an equal share of clinical and legal responsibilities working harmoniously in the best interests of the patient is an achievable. In some instances smaller independent providers would fear a loss of autonomy or an unwelcome alteration of their service ideology and working practice so

as to be consistent with that of the more powerful statutory partner (Atkin, 1996). Where there are high risk decisions the parties and individuals regarding themselves as having legal and ethical responsibility will try and override the opinions and suggestions of other team members. So even if black organisations were to become accepted as team members, the scope for their work to be compromised is significant. Psychiatrists like all professions are members of a political system whose ideologies and institutional structures shape the conditions of knowledge applied to such work (Kleinman, 1988). If the voluntary sector were also to 'professionalise' in this way would they be able to retain their closeness to the perspective of black service users? All of these crucial questions remain unanswered.

Psychiatric service models

There is no consistent view about the best mainstream model of delivering mental health care to ethnic minorities. Some advocate a separate statutory service for black people as a speciality, and such a service may be necessary where the statutory sector blatantly neglects the mental health needs of black people and influential local people and organisations lack the will and the capacity to develop integrated services which are suitable for all. Although such services have generated much expertise (for example, Lynfield Mount Unit in Bradford) the problem of collaboration is displaced to that of defining roles and responsibilities in relation to general adult psychiatric services. Furthermore, such a service is then likely to be referred all patients that the general services experience as 'beyond their expertise' and the general services then no longer feel they have to acquire expertise. Fully integrated multicultural services remain elusive, but have the strengths of built in funding, the possibility of developing long term strategies, and the development of expertise in cross cultural psychiatry in generic psychiatric services. There are no published British evaluations comparing patient satisfaction for these two styles of service; while this debate has remained unresolved black patients continue to receive care from existing statutory services when in crisis. What happens in between crises and whether community interventions are effective across cultural and ethnic groups is untested. The general crisis of mental health services has distracted all from the plight of black patients as if their interests were subsidiary. The home treatment movement was hoped to be a more humane and satisfactory solution (Sashidaran, 1994) but again has not been evaluated across cultures. It may be that a lack of resources, lack of managerial skills, the weight of institutional inertia and the external imposition of other priorities continue to frustrate attempts to create better and more responsive services (Cochrane & Sashidharan, 1996).

Training and education

Health sector professionals

There have been numerous publications, books and an annual calendar of conferences on cross cultural psychiatry, the ineffectiveness of existing services and the need to develop new models of working. In all these arenas, the need for further training for health and social care providers has been emphasised. Aims of such training include sharpening the professionals' ability to define states of distress across cultures so as to know which states can appropriately be identified as manifestations of illness within existing psychiatric nosology. The institutions that supervise the main professional groups in mental health care do not appear to be addressing the issue of race and culture to a significant extent, possible because they are inherently conservative bodies (Fernando, 1996). Furthermore in view of the recent critical changes in the provision of health care, the list of professionals requiring additional training has lengthened: managers, purchasers, tribunal representatives, police officers and indeed anyone that may come into contact with the mentally ill have now been deemed to be in need of additional training. This is often tactically presented as part of continuing education or as exhibiting anti-racist measures. Yet therein lies the dilemma. The whole process is not seen as an essential part of core professional training. Although psychologists and social workers do now have some race and culture training modules, psychiatrists have been slow to take up the challenge. Continuing medical education is one vehicle of intervention, but may be too little too late for the development of the full awareness and sensitivity required. The undergraduate medical curriculum, although now grasping communication and interview styles as being of importance, has not delved into race or cultural awareness training and where it has done so the focus remains on numbers rather than meanings; although inequalities in health are raised in terms of indices of deprivation, ethnic minorities remain an index of deprivation rather than acquiring attention for comprising a group with specific needs and therefore requiring modification of the skills, competencies and knowledge components of medical education. The BMA survey of multi-cultural education demonstrated that 44% of undergraduates, 25% of postgraduates and 59% of GPs reported the inclusion of health and culture in medical education programmes (BMA, 1995). Only 9% of house officers reported that health and culture in relation to the local population was included in their induction. For those institutions without courses, 58% of undergraduates, 42% of postgraduates and 50% of GPs thought there was no need for a course. Although this refers to all medical specialities the psychiatric post-graduate curriculum is similarly unimpressive. Consideration of existing psychiatric concepts in relation to black people appears under Social Sciences in the Basic Sciences and Clinical Curricula for the MRCPsych. Thus 'prejudice and stigma', 'ethnic minorities and mental health' and 'social anthropological' methodology are on the curriculum but are not an essential or necessarily examined part of the examination. The report of the working party to review psychiatric practice and training in a multi-ethnic society suggests rather non-specifically that convenors of approval visits might determine whether Transcultural Psychiatry is incorporated into MRCPsych courses (Royal College of Psychiatrists, 1996). There is no mention in the ethical or legal section of the MRCPsych curricula about black minorities' mental health. Such a position is untenable in light of the significant mistrust between the black communities and the profession. The assertion that most psychiatrists will work in rural areas where there are few black people, and therefore a just component of the training curriculum cannot be devoted to black and ethnic issues, is flawed. It firstly assumes that black people can only expect an equitable service if they live in an area with a high proportion of black people. Secondly it assumes that white people in the UK are the same all over the country, as if all white people are either devoid of culture or have a culture which does not warrant attention in mental health settings. On the basis of the rapidity with which the user movement is gaining momentum in Britain, perhaps psychiatrists have miscalculated. There has been concern that ant-racist training, or even training in cross cultural psychiatry was somehow a political activity not befitting a profession with the highest ethical standards and those who have undergone an arduous and clearly scientific career choice. Yet in every country psychiatry as a profession is enshrined in a social and political system and a recognition of that is essential in all branches of psychiatry but more so where cross cultural issues are concerned (Kleinman, 1988).

Voluntary and independent sector professionals

The training received by voluntary and independent sectors is often similar to that of the statutory sector in that fully qualified former NHS and social service employees may transfer to this way of working, seeing it as more effective and less oppressive for black people. People usually avail themselves of courses and conference attendance but there are no studies which indicate the levels of expertise or indeed the deficits. Sections of the voluntary and independent sectors have indicated a need for mental health training and more liaison with psychiatric services. The training requirements and support with supervision is usually built into the provider function but again these needs remain ill defined other than where there are examples of projects not being able to function (see Jamdagni, 1996). The expertise within the black independent sector is certainly not recognised by mainstream providers as a resource. A mutual exchange of expertise could be fruitful, but the task of providing and focusing on training with limited budgets and little desire within psychiatric service provider units to develop joint training has compounded a breach in joint working.

5.9.10 Creating sensitivities and solutions

'The primary functions of racial prejudice are psychological and cultural.

The primary functions of racism are economic and political'

(Lago & Thompson, 1996)

Progress will be achieved not just through formal contracting processes but also because key staff in purchaser and provider organisations care about the outcomes (Chandra, 1996). For many of the problems discussed there are no obvious immediate solutions. Indeed the pattern of immediate short term solutions to allay political pressures is counterproductive. Each of the problem areas mentioned below could in themselves be the focus of working parties, committees, literature reviews, special projects and more searching. Yet, what is required for each is an ongoing commitment to the issue, an annual plan of action, ongoing generation of expertise, co-ordination and evaluation as well as financial investments. Britain's multi-cultural society is not temporary or static, and requires a flexible, consistent and evolving mental health service strategy. There are *key priorities* that require urgent action, and it should be possible to implement such changes in practice with few additional resources. ***Longer-term priorities*** are areas where action is necessary but likely to require substantial extra resources. If they are not met in the medium to long term other efforts will be undermined. Any strategy must include a plan of action incorporating the full range of remedial interventions comprehensively integrated with service and training innovations.

5.9.11 Key Priorities

Mental health services: can't change or won't change?

Hospital and community based services all need to recognise that patients or users of services are dissatisfied not only with personal interactions of staff but also with the locations, hotelling aspects, decor and information about services. Inpatient wards can be very disturbing places to be and this has become increasingly so since many wards took on a psychosis only function in view of bed shortages. London has been especially hard hit by bed closures. Specific changes include: bilingual workers who understand the cultural context of a patients biographical experiences, female only areas or wards, accessible places of worship, closer liaison with those offering spiritual guidance (therapists, religious leaders) and an integration with social models of care giving. All of these serve to holistically address distress experiences and not to deny aspects of the patient which do not conveniently fit into the accepted range of recognised problems and interventions.

- **The culture of ward and community treatment environments must change so as to re-capture the purpose of caring for the distressed; nowhere is this disparity more detrimental to patients than when the patient's cultural norms differ from those of the decision makers and providers.**

- **The involvement of families, religious leaders and advocates in consultation and treatments is essential if trust is to be restored and if we are to begin to offer equitable care. Attention to the detail of the environment in which we meet with patients engenders a first stage of respecting our patients' distress.**

- **Purchasers should ensure that quality standards are met and for those standards regarded as essential there should be financial penalties attached to complacency. In a market economy only issues with financial incentives seem to be prioritised.**

- **Nationally agreed standards of care need to be established by examining in detail the process of contact with health and social care agencies in terms of environment, decision making and degree of culture working in relation to all procedures and practices. Purchasers should have quality criteria which must be adhered to** (Bhui, 1996b; HEA, 1996; NAHAT, 1996; Gunaratnam, 1994).

Professions or pretenders?

Health services and especially primary care facilities have, since the introduction of the marker economy, changed in many aspects but there is no convincing evidence that a more just system of mental health care for black people is even on the agenda of individual practices, provider units and commissioners. Black patients may require more time, differ in their styles of communicating distress, and indeed English may be their second language. None of this is reflected in any systematic way either in vocational training or in the undergraduate curriculum (Huby et al, 1989. Not in any other arena of medical practice would such a professional 'limitation of competence' cause any difficulty for clinicians to appreciate the ethical dimensions; expertise and information would be sought. Race, culture and mental health issues appear to frighten, threaten and confuse our ethical sensitivities. Hence the subject remains taboo and is left to the individual's and the profession's delicate sense of self esteem rather than being determined by ethical debate or by patients' preferences.

- **If any of the professional bodies wish to seriously tackle the issues set out in this document then training in race, ethnicity and mental health is essential.**

- **The General Medical Council, the Royal Colleges and provider units must make such training a part of the core professional and continuing education training. This should be for *all* professionals and not only for white professionals.**

- **Providers and purchaser could also be influential in organising training events and indeed could make such a process integral to personal career development.**

- **Collaboration between organisations involved in training is needed so that cross-cultural training curricula become available to all professions, grades and organisations. Development of training packages and establishment of regular courses might act as one measure of the motivation to develop skills and competencies** (Huby et al, 1989).

Generating and retaining of expertise

All provider units within the statutory sector and the voluntary sector are familiar with situations in which special expertise is required. Yet, there continues to be little attempt to integrate the expertise of the voluntary and statutory providers.

- **Purchasers and providers must ensure that a local system of expertise and mutual consultation is readily accessible for all clinicians, independent and voluntary sector practitioners, service planner, managers and those with expertise in the implementation of policy.**

- **Joint planning of services, joint training and joint conferences can add to mutual confidence which takes time but need not be more expensive.**

Specific communities previously neglected

Balarajan & Raleigh (1992) advocate that ethnic monitoring of health service staff be actively linked to ensuring adequate representation of the communities which they serve; a process which has not been realised by any of the Royal Colleges or providers on a formal basis. The Chinese and Vietnamese communities have so far been largely neglected in term of health service research. Thus there are special groups for whom specific services may be necessary. Women generally and women from ethnic minorities specifically are likely to have different treatment and professional preferences (Ismail, 1996; Mills, 1996).

- **Little work has attended to consumer preferences in these groups or to special circumstances which shape the therapeutic choices available to them, choices which will be different from those offered. For example, single sex wards, regular contact of the ward with religious bodies and access to places of worship.**

Longer-term priorities

Community psychiatry & the voluntary sector

A diversity of global models of dealing with suffering exist. There has been much difficulty within the statutory and voluntary sectors regarding joint working. There is no critical evaluation of potential models of joint working or in which circumstances it should be adopted.

- **This whole area needs much greater scrutiny regarding existing practice, organisational management models which could be adopted for joint working and which of these methods are generalisable.**

- **Clear accounts of when joint working is not acceptable are also required if a credible level of care is to be offered to all patients regardless of whether they happen to live in an area of best practice.**

The Mental Health Act

The Mental Health Act needs evaluation, particularly with regard to potential prejudicial interpretations. 'Law does not exist in a vacuum. The interpretation and application of the law will vary in accordance with those in influential positions. Successful health promotion requires legal equality ... not all of our actions are governed by law but many are governed by tradition, convention or even informal agreement' (Bhopal & White, 1993). The Mental Health Act is already under close scrutiny by the public, government and the Royal College of Psychiatrists. Not only is community care bringing new clinical situations requiring greater clarity and/or amendments to the legislation but there is a developing view that the existing legislation, although effective is unjust and does not adequately protect civil liberties (Bradley et al 1995; Pelosi et al, 1995). 'The law must protect human rights as its fundamental purpose. If it does not it will become oppressive' (Juss, 1995).

- **The Mental Health Act and its use requires closer examination in terms of potential biases against minority groups and viable amendments which would ensure a just system of care. Leaving treatment decisions to the judgment of clinicians conveys an impartiality in the process that is not borne out by the data. Legal representation at sectioning, alternative models of mental heath legislation, prompt advice on admission and legal advice for clinicians also is essential.**

- **This issue requires some urgency. Relegation to resource starved working parties and committees is unlikely to yield results. Contact with lawyers and the judiciary should be formalised as well as examining alternative legal systems of mental health care in other countries. The mental health act and all its suppositions must be examined in detail and decision making around ethnicity scrutinised.**

Academic Departments

Responsible research in conjunction with black communities is essential. Patients and relatives want research on better ways to live with their ill-health, and some will declare that clinical trials based on a narrow medical model of disease have neglected their prime concerns (Fox, 1996). The training of undergraduates, postgraduate and offering professional courses has for too long been a haphazard process.

- **Academic departments should form links alongside provide units with the independent and voluntary sector and should act in closer harmony with black** communities, perhaps the very ones whom they wish to involve in research. There is a great need for the development of appropriate training materials and for local and national courses rather than purely scientific conferences as these have a difference purpose. The exact content of training will of course depend on the target trainees. A core of anti-racist and equal opportunities training is presumed to be an essential foundation and should of course be applied across disciplines.

- New models of academic, voluntary sector, public and statutory sector working need to be developed for training, research and service provision. The academic component as with the others should be multi-professional and representative ethnically and culturally of the target locality.

Service provision

Service provision, clinical care and communicating dissatisfaction as well as generating solutions to problems in the true spirit of a culture of diversity has progressed at a haphazard pace and in a poorly coordinated way. Although this diversity of solutions is heralded as the pinnacle of owning local solutions to local problems, undoubtedly there is a learning curve; there are inevitably some solutions which are counter-productive. Short term funding for projects followed by no proper evaluation is a waste of money and ideas, and serves only to defer a proper solution with long term planning.

- The major funding bodies and charities as well as government bodies must have a coordinated strategy of action for the country retaining enough flexibility such that more effective local solutions can be implemented and owned by local people at the same time ensuring that there is an overall minimum standard of care for all patients.

- There should be a forum for ongoing dialogue and representation of the ideologies of each of the organisations (including voluntary and patient groups). One of the roles of such an umbrella organisation could be to examines new projects and research proposals for their viability and value to patients as well as their research quality rather than the applying criteria of research quality suited only to conventional treatments (Ernst, 1995; Vincent & Lewith, 1995).

- All new and existing models of service delivery require thorough evaluation, with attention also given to the limitations of existing health services research methodologies. Thus care management and court diversion are currently being heralded as solutions without due attention to the efficacy for different ethnic groups, whilst no attempts are made to consider the effectiveness of other potential interventions which may be more acceptable to some groups (Complementary treatments and traditional healing strategies).

Chapter 6

Mental health services in London: evidence from research and routine data

Sonia Johnson & Paul Lelliott

Summary

A series of previous research studies have reported on aspects of the state of London's mental health services in the 1990s, and some recent information is also available from routinely collected national data. This body of evidence is outlined in this chapter, and suggests the following major conclusions:

- During the 1990s, there has been a growing 'bed crisis' on London's acute wards, with very high bed occupancy levels, admissions for which have increased substantially over the past five years.
- Admission rates are higher in inner London than elsewhere in the country, particularly for young men.
- Patients on wards in London are more likely to have psychotic illnesses, to be compulsorily detained, to have significant social problems and to be aggressive than those elsewhere in the country – this both suggests that the threshold for admission is higher in London and that staff have to contend with a more severely disturbed population than elsewhere.
- A major factor contributing to this 'bed crisis' is likely to be a shortage of alternatives to hospital care, particularly highly staffed residential facilities in the community, and a lack of suitable placements for patients when they are ready to be discharged from hospital.
- The very severe pressure on beds has arisen despite the fact that inner London purchasers spend a high proportion of their health budgets on mental health compared with purchasers elsewhere in the country and provide large numbers of acute beds.
- This pressure on beds is likely to be at least in part a reflection of the extremity of needs for services in London. Despite this, current national capitation formulae mean that the resources available to most inner London purchasers will decline relative to the rest of the country.
- 'Old long stay' patients discharged from the long-term wards of the large hospitals appeared to have fared reasonably well after discharge. In contrast, community and residential provisions for 'new long-term' patients who require high levels of support appear to be very limited.
- Patients who are placed in community residential facilities clearly prefer them to hospital residence. Mechanisms for monitoring such services are weak, but most facilities seem to provide reasonable care and a reasonable environment.
- Placements in community residential care often fail to achieve a good match between level of support and patients' needs.

6.1. Introduction

This section will summarise a number of significant studies carried out in the 1990s which have described aspects of routine service delivery in London. It will also outline some evidence available from routinely collected national statistics, which allows comparison with service use in other areas of the country.

The existence of a number of research centres of excellence in London has meant that as well as the studies of routine service delivery described here, there are various important papers describing and evaluating innovative services set up as part of research studies. These have not been discussed here as they are generally not examples of routine practice in London. However, work such as the descriptions and evaluations of the Daily Living Programme in Camberwell (Muijen et al, 1992a) and the Early Intervention Service at St Mary's (Merson et al, 1992) provides very helpful insight into the feasibility and outcome of the application in inner London of various innovative models of community care.

6.2 London's place in national patterns of service use

This section is based on national, centrally collected data. Recent changes in national patterns of service use are first outlined, and an account is then given of current service use patterns in inner and outer London.

6.2.1 Changes in service use in the UK, 1950s to 1990s: the national picture

a. In-patient care
From a peak in 1954 of 152,000 (Tooth and Brooke, 1961) the number of people occupying psychiatric beds in England fell by 74% to 39,500 in 1993 (House of Commons Health Select Committee, 1994b). The location of psychiatric beds has also changed. As the large, single-specialty hospitals were run down, beds were placed increasingly in small units, often in district general hospitals. This process, however, progressed much more slowly than the development of the policy which drove it (see Chapter 4) and was still in its early stages in 1985. By March 1993 there were still about 20,500 patients in large hospitals, 52% of the national total patient population. 38 of the original 130 'water tower hospitals' had actually closed at this date (Davidge et al, 1993). The proportion of patients in beds in large psychiatric hospitals who were under 65 years (52%) resembles closely the proportion for all NHS psychiatric beds. This, together with the fairly low average length of stay (76 days), suggests that by 1993 the beds in large hospitals were used for similar purposes to those in other settings. Figure 1 shows the declining overall numbers of residents in hospitals over this 40-year period.

Trends in service activity over this period allow some inferences to be made about changes in the make-up (casemix) of the patient population. In spite of the massive bed closures, admission rates have increased. Between 1969 and 1991, a period which saw the number of hospital residents fall by two-thirds, the number of admissions per 100,000 population increased by 8% (from 371 to 399 per 100,000). This was possible largely because of a great reduction in the number of resident patients with protracted lengths of stay. In 1991, 65% of discharged patients had lengths of stay of less than one

Figure 1 Residents in psychiatric hospital in-patient units

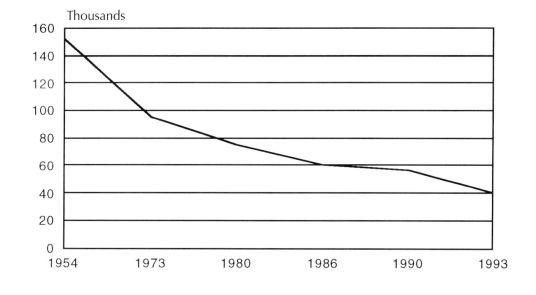

Figure 2 National bed occupancy figures: 1982–1992

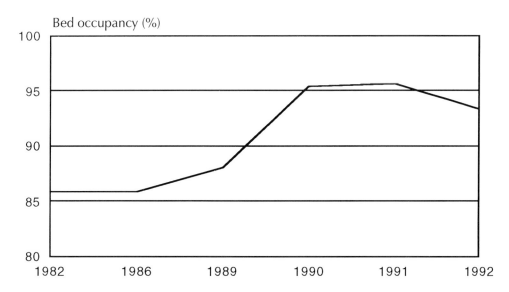

month, and 90% less than three years. There has also been a slight national increase in bed occupancy levels, as shown in Figure 2.

The composition of the in-patient population has also changed over the past decade in terms of age and gender. Between 1982 and 1992, the number of hospital residents aged 15 to 44 actually increased by 7% (from 12,670 to 13,500). For all other age groups, there was a substantial fall; by 50% for those aged 45 to 64 (from 19,050 to 9,600), 51% for those aged 65 to 74 (from 15,570 to 7,600) and 39% for those 75 years and over (from 23,180 to 14,200). During this period, the percentage of younger patients (15 to 44 years) in wards for adults rose from 40% to 58%. Men accounted for a greater proportion of psychiatric episodes in 1992 than in 1982 (46% vs 41%). Much of this change appears to have been accounted for by men aged 20 to 44 who had a 39% increase in episodes over this period compared with a 10% increase for women in the same age range.

After remaining constant since the Mental Health Act was amended in 1983, the absolute number of formal admissions increased by 27% between 1989 and 1993, although this only represents an increase from 7.4% to 8.1% of all admissions.

b. Other residential provision

Only a small proportion of the NHS hospital beds which have been closed have been replaced by residential places provided by other agencies in other settings. At the end of 1969, when about 50,000 hospital beds had closed, there were 1,602 places in 92 local authority homes for mentally ill people in England and Wales and 1,087 places in 51 voluntary and private homes (Department of Health and Social Security and Welsh Office, 1975).

Over the last decade for which there are complete data (1983–1993), 29,330 further NHS psychiatric beds closed, a 43% reduction in provision, and 7,700 new places opened in residential facilities managed by other agencies. This represents replacement of only 26% of the beds lost (House of Commons Health Select Committee, 1994b). More than 80% of these new residential places were provided by the voluntary and private sectors, the remainder by local authorities.

This changing pattern of provision meant that by 1993, 27% of all residential provision (including hospital beds) was managed by agencies other than the NHS, compared with just 9% in 1983. As the balance of provider agency has shifted so has the nature of the residential provision available to the mentally ill. While almost all psychiatric hospital beds have 24-hour cover with nursing staff on duty and awake at night, residential accommodation provided by other agencies is much less likely to have high staffing levels. A recent survey of 35 UK health districts and health boards found that only about half of the non-NHS residential facilities had either high levels of staffing (a ratio of staff: residents of 1:1) or 24-hour cover with staff awake at nights (Faulkner et al, 1992).

c. Day hospitals and day centres

Figure 3 shows changes in the total numbers of places in day hospitals and day centres.

Following a 73% increase during the 1980s, from 12,950 in 1979 to 22,400 in 1989, the number of psychiatric day hospital places has subsequently remained virtually static, with 22,900 provided in 1993 (House of Commons Health Select Committee, 1994b). During this recent period the number of total attendances was unchanged but the number of new attendances increased by 13% (from 56,000 in 1989 to 72,000 in 1994) (Department of Health, 1995h).

Day centre places provided by local authorities for mentally ill people under 65 years increased by 74% (from 8,700 to 15,100) during the decade up to 1992 (House of Commons Health Select Committee, 1994b). A further 14,700 places were purchased from other agencies during 1992.

c. Clinical staff

Figure 4 shows changes in numbers of CPNs and of consultant psychiatrists employed in the NHS.

Figure 3 Trends in day care provision: 1979–1993

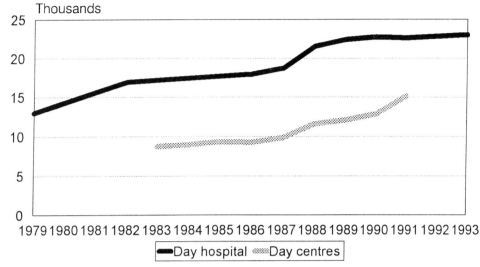

Places in day hospitals and in local authority and mixed day centres

Figure 4 Consultant psychiatrists and Community Psychiatric Nurses: numbers employed by the NHS 1969–1991

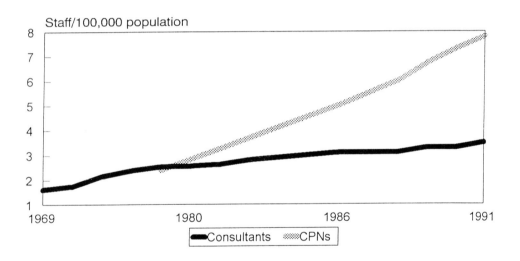

The development of more comprehensive community-based services has been accompanied by a doubling of the number of consultant psychiatrists and by substantial increases in the numbers of psychologists and occupational therapists (Department of Health and Social Security, 1980; Department of Health and Office of Population Censuses and Surveys, 1992). Although the number of community psychiatric nurses (CPNs) trebled between 1979 and 1991, it started from a low baseline. Even by 1991 there were only 3,600, which represents about 7.5 per 100,000 total population.

6.2.2 Current service provision in London in a national context: HES data

The Department of Health statistics division have supplied for this project Hospital Episodes Statistics (HES) data from the year 1994/5, which allows comparison between current service activity in London and that in the rest of the country.

Comparisons have been made between four groups, as shown in Figure 5:

Figure 5 Groupings of local authorities for HES data analyses

1 INNER LONDON
Camden, City of London, Greenwich, Hackney, Hammersmith & Fulham, Islington, Kensington & Chelsea, Lambeth, Lewisham, Southwark, Tower Hamlets, Wandsworth, Westminster

2 OUTER LONDON
Barking & Dagenham, Barnet, Bexley, Brent, Bromley, Croydon, Ealing, Enfield, Haringey, Harrow, Havering, Hillingdon, Hounslow, Kingston, Merton, Newham, Redbridge, Richmond, Sutton, Waltham Forest

3 OTHER LARGE INNER CITIES
Birmingham, Bradford, Gateshead, Leeds, Liverpool, Manchester, Newcastle, North Tyneside, Salford, Sheffield

4 THE REST OF THE COUNTRY
All other local authorities

---

a. Finished Consultant Episodes in 1994/95

Figure 6 shows total psychiatric Finished Consultant Episodes (FCEs) per 100,000 population for each geographical group and Figure 7 FCEs per 100,000 for people aged 16-64. Rates for men and for women are shown separately in each figure.

Overall, inner London had the highest rate of FCEs of any of the four groups and outer London the lowest. For all ages, inner London had 58% more FCEs per 100,000 than outer London, 9% more than other large cities and 37% more than the rest of the country. These differences were more marked for people aged 16–64, where inner London has 83% more FCEs than outer London, 22% more than other large cities and

Figure 6 FCEs per 100,00 – all ages

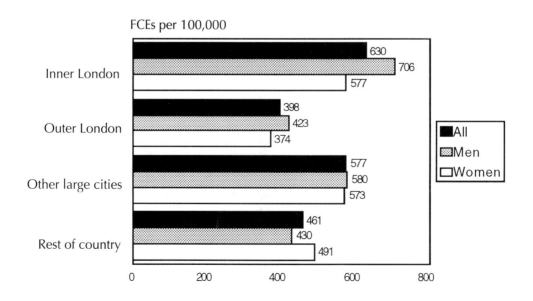

FCEs per 100,000

Figure 7 FCEs per 100,000 – people aged 16 to 64

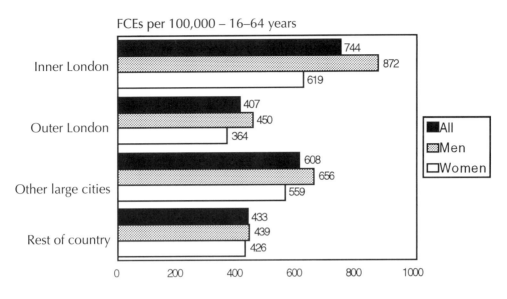

72% more than the rest of the country. For men aged 16–64 only, the differences are still more pronounced, with Inner London having a rate 94% above that of Outer London, 33% above that of other large cities and 99% above the rest of the country.

Figure 8 and Figure 9 show in greater detail profiles of FCE rates for age bands of the population between 16 and 64.

These are the age bands where inner London's rates of FCEs exceed those for the rest of the country: for bands over age 65 the trend reverses, with relatively low rates of FCEs in inner London. Comparing Figures 8 and 9 indicates that these differences between inner London and other large cities for those aged 16–64 are largely accounted for by an increased number of FCEs for men, particularly young men. Overall, men

Figure 8 FCEs per 100,000 by age band – males

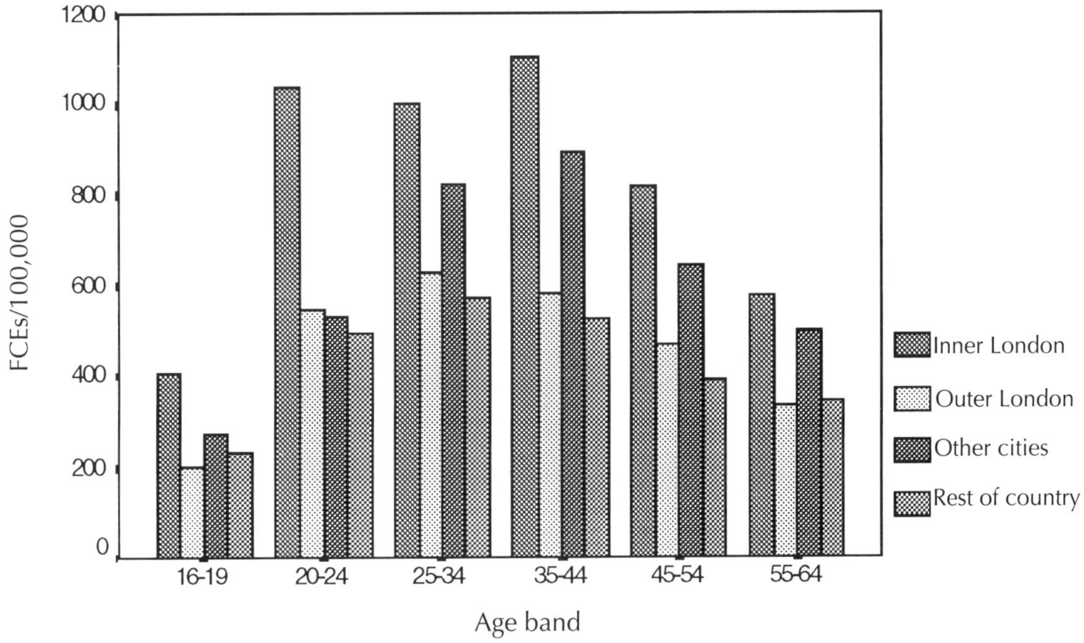

Figure 9 FCEs per 100,000 by ageband – females

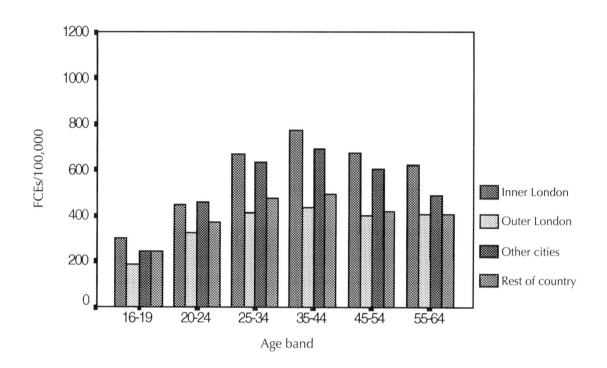

under 34 make up 30% of all FCEs in inner London, whereas in outer London they represent 26%, in other large cities 24% and in the rest of the country 22%.

Trends over time

HES returns have also been obtained and analysed for 1989/90. Table 1 compares FCE rates for 1989/90 with those for 1994/5.

Table 1 FCEs per 100,000 population aged 16–64: Rates in 1989/90 and in 1994/5

Geographical group	Males – FCEs per 100,000 population aged 16–64 yrs			Females – FCEs per 100,000 population aged 16–64 yrs		
	1989/90	**1994/5**	**% change**	**1989/90**	**1994/5**	**% change**
Inner London	723	911	+26%	666	635	–5%
Outer London	420	511	+22%	399	393	–2%
Other cities	551	678	+23%	549	568	+3%
Rest of country	386	456	+18%	431	436	+1%

The most marked change over this five-year period is an increase in the number of FCEs for males. This has occurred in all geographical groups of local authorities, but is slightly greater in inner London (inner London: 26% increase; outer London: 22%; other cities: 23%; rest of country: 18%). The increase is greatest among men aged between 16 and 24 years (31% nationally). By contrast, there has been no increase in numbers of FCEs for women.

Given the already pressurised state of London's services and the predominance of younger people in the city, this rising rate of admissions among young men is likely to have a considerable impact on the city's services. The reasons for the rise remain uncertain. Possibilities include professionals' concerns about risk of violent or other dangerous behaviour, a risk which may be seen as greater for young men, or socio-economic factors such as the effects of unemployment and the increasing social alienation of young men.

Detention under the Mental Health Act

Table 2 shows rates of compulsory admission under the Mental Health Act in the four geographical groups in 1994/5:

Table 2 Compulsory admissions to NHS facilities per 100,000 gender-specific population in 1994/5

	Total	Males	Female
Inner London	164	193	136
Outer London	79	93	67
Other cities	52	58	45
Rest of the country	37	38	37

Compulsory admission rates are one of the characteristics where inner London deviates most markedly from the rest of the country. Inner London has around twice as many compulsory admissions per 100,000 population as outer London, around three times the number in other inner cities, and more than four times the rate for the rest of the country. The compulsory admission rate for men in inner London is 50% higher than that amongst women: in contrast, male and female rates for the 'rest of the country' group are equal, with intermediate findings in the other two geographical groups. These findings strongly suggest that the casemix in London is more severe than in other cities, and that the crisis in acute bed provision discussed below is likely to be due to real differences in needs and demands for services.

Discharge Destinations

About 12% of all people discharged from hospital go to other NHS residential facilities, or to local authority or independent residential care settings. The figure increases to over 20% for people aged over 65 years. Figures 10 and 11 show for men and for women in different age bands the proportions of discharges which are to such NHS, local authority and independent sector residential care settings.

Figure 10 Proportion of males discharged from hospital who went to NHS, local authority or independent residential services, 1994/5

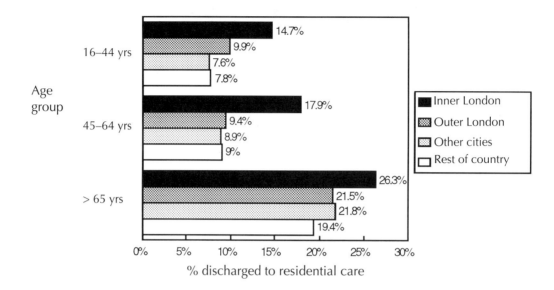

% discharged to residential care

Figure 11 Proportion of females discharged from hospital who went to NHS, local authority or independent residential services, 1994/5

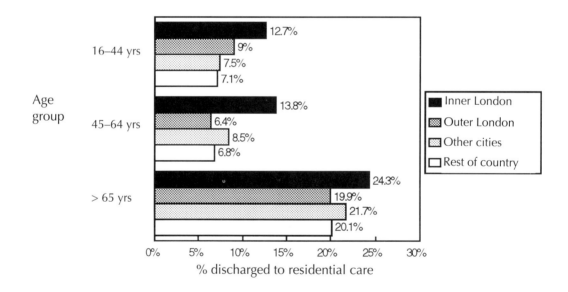

% discharged to residential care

Thus both men and women in each age group in inner London are more likely to be discharged to one of these residential care settings than people in other areas. The difference appears particularly marked for people in the 45 to 64 age group, who in inner London, unlike the other areas, are more likely than younger people to be discharged to a residential setting. These differences may reflect the greater isolation and lower levels of family support experienced by inhabitants of inner London (see Chapter 3).

Marital status
Figure 12 shows the proportion of male and of female FCEs in each area accounted for by people who are single, widowed or divorced.

Figure 12 Proportion of all FCEs which are of people who are single, divorced or widowed

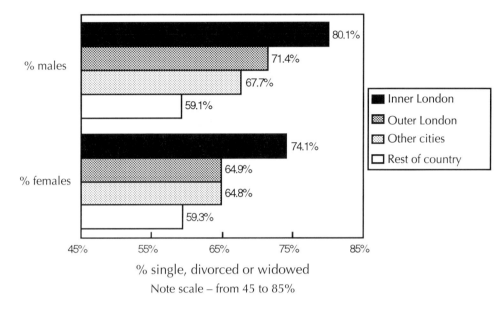

% single, divorced or widowed
Note scale – from 45 to 85%

There are major caveats attached to the HES data on marital status, in that numbers of missing cases are considerably larger than in other categories, some people who are cohabiting will be classified as single and some who are separated as married. However, the differences between London and other areas, with inner London having the greatest proportion of single, divorced or widowed individuals, again suggest that London services may be dealing with a more socially isolated population than exists elsewhere.

Diagnoses

Figure 13 shows proportions of FCEs with a diagnosis of schizophrenic psychosis in each area:

Figure 13 Proportion of FCEs with a diagnosis of schizophrenic psychosis

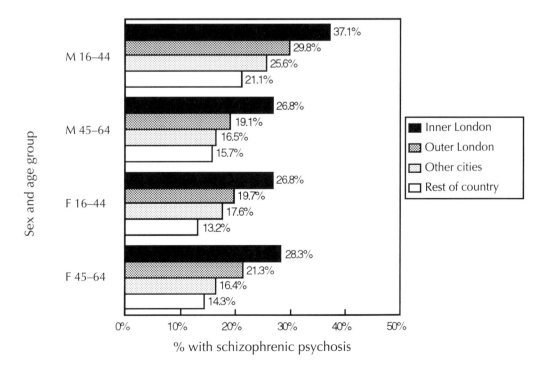

% with schizophrenic psychosis

Thus for this indicator of casemix, inner London is again markedly different from elsewhere, with a higher proportion of finished consultant episodes being for people with a diagnosis of schizophrenia than in the other geographical groups. This applies to both sexes and each age group, but is most marked for men between 16 and 44, for whom in inner London 37.1% of finished consultant episodes carry a diagnosis of schizophrenia, compared with 29.8% in outer London, 25.6% in the other large cities and 21.1% in the rest of the country.

6.3 Monitoring of Inner London's Mental Illness Services (MILMIS)

The Monitoring of Inner London's Mental Illness Services (MILMIS) project group was set up in response to:

- observations that bed occupancy in inner London had become unacceptably high;
- concerns among psychiatrists and others about conditions on wards, with the concentrating effect of bed closures resulting in a high proportion of disturbed young patients detained under the Mental Health Act and frequent violent incidents on psychiatric wards;
- the fact that government data on bed use do not provide a clear picture of bed occupancy or the state of wards, and are not generally published until several years after collection.

So as to set up a mechanism for collecting clear indicators of the state of London's services, psychiatrists from 12 inner London Trusts, including 10 of the 17 most deprived in the country, established the project (MILMIS Project Group, 1995; Lelliott et al, 1995). Data collection is based at the Royal College of Psychiatrists Research Unit. Four censuses have been carried out at six month intervals since June 1994, with the most recent conducted in early 1996. Table 3 shows the results for MILMIS 1 and MILMIS 2: MILMIS 3 and 4, for which results will shortly become available, suggest there has been no substantial subsequent change (Bernard Audini, personal communication).

Thus the bed occupancy rates for inner London short stay beds appear to be very high. When a count was made of the true demand on census days, mean occupancy rates were between 114% and 122% (this excludes those patients on leave whose beds did not need to be kept available). Patients who should have been in London short-stay wards were elsewhere, including in the community, in prison or police cells and in distant psychiatric hospitals. There were about 100 people in the latter category; these were admissions as 'extra-contractual referrals' (ECRs), which are paid for by the local health authority and represent an outflow of funds from inner London to other provider services.

It is also likely that at least some of the over-occupancy found in MILMIS was due to bed-blocking. One third of patients on inner London 'short-stay' wards had been there for more than three months and 12% for more than six months – nearly twice the national average.

The MILMIS data also give indications of the conditions in these overcrowded short stay wards. About one-half of patients were detained on Sections of the Mental Health act on census days and incidents of assault and sexual harassment were frequent.

Table 3 The MILMIS Surveys

		MILMIS 1	MILMIS II
		June 1994	January 1995
1.	Number of services	12	12
2.	Combined population	2.6 million	2.9 million
3.	Total admission beds	1109	1235
4.	Patients in admission beds	1236	1321
5.	% in beds 3-6 months	27%	20%
6.	% in beds 6-12 months	8%	9%
7.	% in beds >12 months	4%	3%
8.	% patients detained	50%	48%
9.	No. in other beds in trust	53	43
10.	No. in medical beds	5	7
11.	No. in NHS ECR beds	42	18
12.	No. in private ECR beds	60	84
13.	No. in home/in community	30	29
14.	No. in prison/police cells	14	8
15.	Admission unit occupancy	111%	107%
16.	"True" bed occupancy[A]	130%	123%
17.	"True" bed occupancy[B]	122%	115%
18.	"Requirement" bed occupancy	140%	N/A
19.	No. 1st degree assaults	67	84
20.	No. 2nd degree assaults	37	43
21.	No. 3rd degree assaults	1	4
22.	Incidents of sexual harassment	53	37
23.	Incidents of sexual assault	8	4

Key

2. Changes in the population figures across the three surveys are due to the changing boundaries of the provider trusts and are higher in MILMIS II because activity was recorded for only part of one service in MILMIS I.

3. **Admission beds** are psychiatric beds allocated routinely for admitting people from the community for short-term care (less than 3 months). Bed numbers are higher in MILMIS II, because: a) a few more have been opened since MILMIS I and b) activity was recorded for only part of one service in MILMIS I.

4. There are more patients than beds because: a) some patients are sent on leave and their beds are filled by other patients, "hot bedding" and b) additional beds are put up at times of bed crisis, "beds in corridors".

5-7. These figures refer to the percentage of patients who have been in admission beds for a long time. Stays of more than 6 months in short-stay beds might be considered inappropriate.

8. Refers to the percentage of people in admission beds who are detained under Sections of the Mental Health Act. These figures are much higher than the national average.

9-14. These are the number of patients who needed to be in admission bed on census day but who could not be admitted because beds were full. ECR ("extra-contractual referral") is the term used by the NHS to describe and admission to a hospital distant from the patients home: here it refers to admissions to other psychiatric hospitals, often many miles away outside of London. These hospitals are either NHS, if beds are available, or private if not.

15-18. There are different ways of considering bed occupancy (see MILMIS project group 1995 article for a fuller explanation). **Admission unit occupancy** relates to the number of people actually on the lists of admission units i.e. who are supposed to have a bed available that day in that unit. **True bed occupancy**[A] takes account of patients who should be in admission beds but are elsewhere because beds are full (9-14). **True bed occupancy**[B] excludes patients who were on leave and who were stable enough not to have needed a bed kept empty on the night of the census – it represents the absolute minimum bed occupancy level for all patients who need to be accommodated.

19-23. Represent the number of these incidents committed by patients on the admission units and reported during a week before or after census day; most such incidents are committed against nurses or other patients, **1st degree assaults** are those that result in no detectable injury; **2nd degree assaults** result in minor physical injuries such as bruising, abrasions or small lacerations; **3rd degree assaults** result in major physical injuries including large lacerations, fracture, loss of consciousness, or any assault requiring subsequent medical investigation or treatment.

The group's reports make a number of comments on the background to the situation they have found:

- They observe that in reducing bed numbers in psychiatric hospitals, an important distinction between short stay and long stay beds has been overlooked. Short stay beds (stay less than 6 months, or preferably less than 3 months) provide short-term treatment, care or respite for people with acute illness, or exacerbations of chronic illness. It remains uncertain how far other services (other accommodation, additional support in the community etc.) are realistic and sustainable alternatives for short stay beds. When planners talk of reducing beds, they need to understand that whilst there is evidence that other community based-services can be substituted for long-stay beds, the evidence that alternative provisions can be substituted for short stay beds is less substantial. Reductions in short-stay beds may thus have taken place without evidence that their replacement is feasible.

- With regard to the substantial numbers of longer stay patients found on London's short-stay wards, this substitution of short-stay beds for longer stay facilities means that patients requiring longer term care and rehabilitation are cared for in an inappropriate environment. It also has an adverse effect on availability of these beds for their intended function, which is short term treatment, care or respite.

- Unlike beds used for short term care of those with acute illness or exacerbations of chronic illness, long-stay hospital beds are inter-changeable with high staffed non-hospital (and often non-NHS) facilities for all but a few. In a survey of 50 English mental health services, Lelliott and Wing (1994) found that 2,000 beds in England were occupied by 'new long stay' patients aged 18 to 64, who remained in hospital despite being 'medically fit' for discharge. About one third of all these patients were resident on short stay wards. Thus many of the substantial numbers with longer stays on London's short stay units are likely to be people who could be cared for in an appropriate non-hospital setting.

- Throughout the history of hospital closures, there has been rhetoric about resources being transferred from hospital beds to community services. However, the massive bed closures which have taken place have not generally resulted in equivalent investment in alternative facilities or staff (Lelliott et al, 1993). Also, for many services there is little further scope for releasing money from closures of long-stay hospital beds – Lelliott and Wing (1994) found that more than 40% of services now have fewer than 15 long-stay beds per 100.000 population. Thus there has been a lack of investment in alternative services for those patients who are 'blocking beds' for longer periods in London's services, and there is no obvious future source of money for provision of the required services.

- The overcrowded, highly aroused atmosphere of London's short-stay wards, with their frequent assaults and high rates of detention, are likely to be an unhelpful and inappropriate environment for the treatment of psychosis. In such an atmosphere, containment rather than therapy, rehabilitation and resettlement is likely to be the priority for staff, and recovery is likely to be further delayed. The environment is a particularly inappropriate one for patients with longer stays.

6.4 London's mental health purchasing: data from the Regional Offices

6.4.1 Introduction

A further data set which allows London's mental health services to be considered in relation to other areas in the country is the assessment of purchasing by Health Authorities (HAs) carried out by NHS Executive Thames Regional Offices in late 1995. These data and comparable information for purchasers in other large cities have been drawn from purchasing information used by the NHS Executive. They allow comparison between areas of London with different demographic characteristics and between inner deprived London and other deprived city areas. Based on a King's Fund classification of the socio-demographic characteristics of purchaser catchment areas, the data are grouped as follows:

Groups of health authorities

1 Inner Deprived London
Kensington, Chelsea & Westminster; East London & the City; Camden & Islington; Lambeth, Southwark and Lewisham

2 Mixed Status London
Brent & Harrow; Ealing, Hammersmith & Hounslow; Redbridge & Waltham Forest; New River; Merton, Sutton & Wandsworth

3 High Status London
Barnet; Hillingdon; Barking & Havering; Bromley; Bexley & Greenwich; Croydon, Kingston & Richmond

4 Inner Deprived – outside London
Sunderland; South of Tyne; Newcastle & North Tyneside; Bradford; Leeds; Sheffield; South Birmingham; Liverpool; Newcastle

---

6.4.2 Needs assessment and strategic planning

Regional offices assessed to what extent Health Authorities (HAs) had carried out a number of tasks important for rational planning of services. Table 4 shows the results.

There are no very striking differences between areas in extent of completion of these essential activities – for most items, most but not all health authorities have carried out the task. Inner Deprived London Health Authorities tend to have relatively high rates of having carried out these tasks.

6.4.3 Care Programme Approach implementation

By June 1996, all HAs in the country reported that the Care Programme Approach had been fully implemented.

Table 4 Activities informing purchasing by health authorities

	1 Inner Deprived London (4 HAs)	2 Mixed Status London (5 HAs)	3 High Status London (7 HAs)	4 Inner Deprived outside London (9 HAs)
HAs which have carried out comprehensive assessment of local needs for mental health services	4 (100%)	3 (60%)	6 (86%)	7 (78%)
Assessment of needs for services for mentally disordered offenders carried out	4 (100%)	3 (60%)	5 (71%)	5 (56%)
HAs which have conducted a review of district's existing mental health services for adults	3 (75%)	4 (80%)	6 (86%)	8 (89%)
Review conducted of child and adolescent services	2 (50%)	3 (60%)	3 (43%)	3 (33%)
Review conducted of elderly mentally ill services	3 (75%)	4 (80%)	6 (86%)	6 (67%)
Review conducted of secure services	3 (75%)	3 (60%)	4 (57%)	4 (44%)
Mental health strategy developed by HA	3 (75%)	3 (60%)	6 (86%)	5 (56%)

6.4.4 Service availability

For each HA, consideration was given to how many of the following 8 services providing 24 hour access to specialist psychiatric care were purchased locally: crisis house; crisis team; 24 hour community mental health team; intensive home support team; telephone helpline; drop in centre; on call community mental health nurses; and on call doctors. The mean number of services from this list of 8 purchased in Inner Deprived London was 4.75 (with a range from 1 to 7), compared with 3.67 average for other Inner Deprived areas, 3.4 for Mixed Status London and 3.3 for Middle Status London. The mean nationally was 2.71. Thus there is limited evidence for greatest development of innovative 24 hour crisis services in inner London, with the other urban areas also having a greater range of crisis services than is average nationally. However, in inner London in particular, purchasing authorities are large and span several catchment areas, so that these findings may be a reflection of different models of crisis service available in different parts of the catchment area, rather than of a wide range being available throughout the catchment area.

Consideration was also given to length of stay and occupancy rates in acute psychiatric services during the period from April to September 1995. Table 5 shows these.

Table 5 The bed state on acute wards

Bed state	Inner Deprived London (4 HAs)	Mixed Status London (5 HAs)	High Status London (7 HAs)	Inner Deprived outside London (9 HAs)
90% + bed occupancy **and** > 20 patients in acute beds for more than 6 months	3/4 (75%)	3/5 (60%)	0	1/9 (11%)
90% bed occupancy **or** >20 patients in acute beds for more than 6 months	1/4 (25%)	2/5 (40%)	7/7 (100%)	5/9 (56%)
bed occupancy below 80%	0	0	0	2/9 (22%)
80–90% bed occupancy **and** less than 20 patients in acute beds for longer than 6 months	0	0	0	1/9 (11%)

These data indicate some geographical variations. No London HAs achieve the most desirable bedstate of 80 to 90% bed occupancy **and** no more than 20 'new long stay' patients, whilst a single Inner Deprived HA outside London does so. The majority of Inner Deprived and Mixed Status London HAs have both very high bed occupancy and an accumulation of new long stay patients, whilst all High Status London HAs and the majority of the Inner Deprived HAs outside London have one of these problems, but not both. Two HAs outside London have bed occupancy below 80%, a situation which is not encountered in London and may suggest the possibility of over-provision of acute beds. Thus there is some evidence here that more deprived areas of London may have particular pressure on their acute beds. However, an important reservation about these data is that they do not take HA population into account – the significance of having accumulated a total of 20 new long stay patients will vary according to the total catchment area population; and they are based on a single period of 6 months in 1995.

6.4.5 Secure services

Table 6 shows mean level of purchasing of medium secure beds in the first and second quarter of 1995/6, adjusted for population size.

The level of medium secure place purchasing per 100,000 during the first six months of the 1995/6 financial year in Inner Deprived London was thus around four times the level of such purchasing in Inner Deprived areas outside London, with more than ten times as much purchasing of such places on an ECR basis. Mixed Status London, although substantially below Inner Deprived London, also considerably exceeded the level of use of this type of provision in deprived areas elsewhere. The cost of such places is high, particularly on an ECR basis (see Chapter 5.6), so that these differences, if sustained, make a very significant impact on demands for expenditure on mental health services in inner areas of London compared with elsewhere. Possible reasons for these striking differences in use include the extreme socio-demographic characteristics of London (see Chapter 3) and/or a shortage of other secure services provision, such as less secure intensive care provision.

Table 6 Levels of purchasing of medium secure beds

Mean places purchased per 100,000 population	Inner Deprived London	Mixed Status London	High Status London	Inner Deprived out of London
Medium secure places/100,000 on an extra-contractual referral (ECR basis) (range)	8.74 (5.99-14.57)	3.67 (0-11.61)	0.36 (0-1.61)	0.73 (0-2.07)
Total medium secure places/ 100,000 population (range)	11.52 (5.99-14.57)	5.33 (2.42-11.61)	1.50 (0-4.37)	2.85 (1.01-7.29)

6.4.6 Service activity

Figure 14 shows mean FCEs per 100,000 reported in each group of HAs.

Figure 14 FCEs per 100,000 population in 1994/5, by area

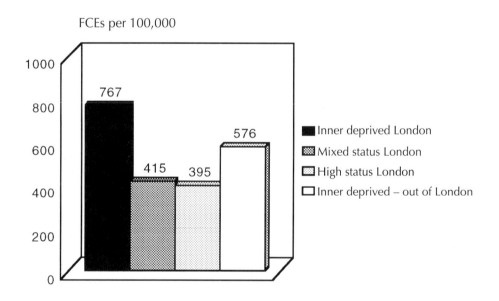

FCEs per 100,000

Again, Inner Deprived London appears to be at an extreme in this aspect of service activity, although here Inner Deprived areas elsewhere are intermediate between Inner Deprived and other areas of London. The Regional Offices were also asked to give details of planned and of forecast numbers of FCEs for 1995/6, the financial year during which data collection took place. In High Status London and Inner Deprived areas outside London, planned and expected activity levels for 1995/6 were each close to 1994/5 levels. In Mixed Status London, planned number of FCEs had increased by around 14% from 1994/5 use, and the mid-year forecast of service activity for the year was close to this planned level. For Inner Deprived London, the mid-year forecast was that actual activity would exceed planned number of FCEs for the year by approximately 10%.

6.4.7 Proportion of budget spent on mental health

Figure 15 shows the average proportion of total HA budget spent on mental health in each geographical group. This indicator is an estimated spend and has a low level of reliability, as there are differences in the interpretation of which elements of expenditure should be involved.

Figure 15 Proportion of total health budget spent on mental health

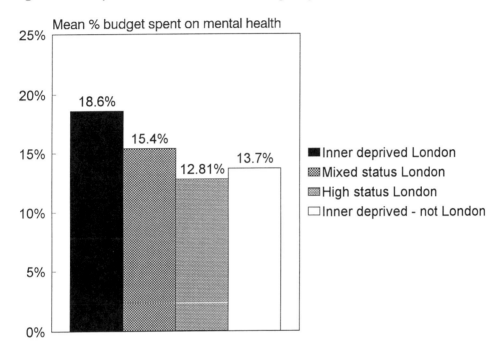

Again there is a clear gradient within London, with proportion of budget spent on mental health decreasing with decreasing social deprivation. Inner Deprived areas outside London again do not resemble the Inner Deprived areas in London – their mean proportional spend on mental health is between those for Mixed and High Status London. However, the range for Inner Deprived areas outside London is particularly wide, from 9.9 to 20.7% of total health budget. In Inner Deprived London the range is from 17.7% to 19.3% of total health budget (with one HA missing), in Mixed Status London from 12.1% to 17.7%, and in High Status London from 9.0% to 18.0%. Thus Inner Deprived London authorities appear to be uniformly high spenders on mental health, whilst within the other groups there is considerable variation.

6.5 The Sainsbury Centre for Mental Health Acute In-patient Study (ACIS)

A view of differences at an individual patient level between London acute services and those elsewhere in the country is provided by the Sainsbury Centre's Acute In-patient Study (Shepherd et al, in press), a large national study of in-patient characteristics and service use. Sampling for this study was carried out on a stratified basis, with social deprivation, as indicated by the Jarman UPA score, as the main variable on which this stratification is based. The study as a whole therefore provides a view of service use across areas with nationally representative range of levels of deprivation.

In-patients in four London Trusts (West Lambeth, North West London, Haringey and Oxleas) were compared with those in three non-London urban Trusts (Aintree in Liverpool, Sheffield and Cardiff). The Jarman indicators of London and non-London districts have not been matched: they are not necessarily drawn from the same stratum and the non-London urban districts are likely to be less severely deprived. The following table compares the demographic, diagnostic and service use characteristics of in-patients on acute wards in London and non-London areas:

Table 7 In-patients in London and in other cities: demographic, diagnostic and service use characteristics

Characteristics	London (n = 353)	Other cities (n = 363)
% of patients who are male	57.3%	47.7%
mean age	37.5	42.2
% who are white	50.9%	93.3%
% who have a diagnosis of psychosis	55.0%	45.3%
% who are detained under MHA	47.6%	27.8%
% who are 'new long stay' patients, defined as patients who have been in hospital for more than 6 months	12.4%	5.5%

All these differences reach statistical significance at least at the conventional $p = 0.05$ level, and most at a very much higher level of statistical significance. The severity of patients' clinical and social problems was rated using the Health of the Nation Outcome Scales (HoNOS), on which a higher score indicates more severe problems (Wing et al, 1996). The variables on which there was a statistically significant difference between the mean score for London in-patients and for those elsewhere are shown in Table 8:

Table 8 HoNOS scores for patients in London and elsewhere

HoNOS variable	Mean for London	Mean for other cities
Aggression	1.27	0.68
Alcohol/ drug problems	0.74	0.49
Housing	1.41	0.87
Activity & employment	1.42	0.75
Memory problems	0.56	0.36
Psychotic symptoms	1.57	1.33
Global rating of severity of impairment of functioning	12.66	9.95

Differences for the other five HoNOS variables did not reach statistical significance. Thus these data confirm the evidence from the HES and MILMIS data that the in-patient population on London wards is significantly different from that in the other cities studied – London patients tend to be younger, and are more often to be male and much more often from an ethnic minority community. They are also more likely to have been compulsorily detained, to be rated by staff as aggressive, to have a diagnosis of psychosis and to have substance abuse problems and difficulties with housing and with activity. This suggests that the threshold for admission to an in-patient unit is likely to be higher in London than elsewhere, with people who are not psychotic and have not been compulsorily detained less likely to gain access to an acute bed. It also suggests that the clinical and social problems with which staff on London in-patient wards have to deal may be more severe than elsewhere, although again it must be remembered that the urban areas outside London were not selected to have equivalent levels of deprivation to the London areas in the study.

6.6 The TAPS Project

The TAPS project has involved a detailed prospective study over the past decade of the outcomes of all those who were long-stay in-patients with functional illness at two large asylums, Friern Barnet and Claybury, when reprovision began in 1985. The very detailed information collected on the social and clinical outcome, costs of care and service use of these groups provides the best London information on the fate of former long-stay psychiatric hospital inpatients. A series of papers have discussed the study design and results including Dayson (1993), Anderson et al (1993) and Leff (1996).

In general the TAPS results support the conclusions of "Better Off in the Community?" (House of Commons Health Select Committee, 1994a), that former long-term in-patients are relatively well provided for. Results indicate that, comparing those who leave with those who stay, discharged patients are happier with their placement, have more opportunities for autonomy and more diverse social networks. The incidence of crime, vagrancy and suicide was very low. Almost all the patients were resettled in some form of supported accommodation, particularly group homes.

Extensive reprovision of "Water Tower Hospitals" [large Psychiatric Hospitals with at least 100 beds (usually substantially more)] has taken place in North and South Thames and is a continuing process. For example in South Thames Region one Water Tower Hospital closed in the 1970s, two in the 1980s and seven in the 1990s so far, with closure of six more planned this century. The process of resettling all the former long-stay patients at these hospitals is likely to be occupying a substantial proportion of the places currently available in residential care in London. (Figures for hospital closures provided by the Department of Health, 1996.)

A number of the residents in the TAPS project did prove relatively difficult to resettle. Seventy-two of the five-hundred and fifty were thought too disturbed to live in standard community homes, and were placed in highly staffed facilities which were usually on hospital sites. This was the group for whom the economic costs were by far the greatest (Leff, 1996). The one major new difficulty which seemed to have arisen following reprovision was with general admission beds. Following the complete closure of one of the hospitals the local district general hospital admission facilities came severely under pressure, partly because of the presence in the community of the former long-stay patients. The admission facilities at the old psychiatric hospital were thought preferable to those in general wards both by patients and by staff.

6.7 Sainsbury Centre Survey of Residential Care Provision

Shepherd et al. (1995) have carried out a survey of a group of residential facilities for the mentally ill selected at random from lists of residential care providers in Greater London. Twenty community homes and five long- stay hospitals wards were studied (one voluntary and one private community home declined to take part). The sample included private homes, local authority hostels, voluntary homes and joint provision by Housing Associations and Health Authorities.

In general, the researchers evaluated the physical environment, staff interactions with residents and resident satisfaction in the community-based homes as fairly good, with no very serious concerns expressed about any of them. The hospital settings, on the other hand, appeared physically and socially impoverished environments.

The residents of the jointly commissioned homes were usually former long-term in-patients with an average age of fifty-five. A younger group was represented in the social services and private sector homes, but the mean age of residents in the voluntary sector homes was also over fifty, reflecting the fact that they had often been set up in response to hospital closures. Some specific points arising about the community-based homes were:

- There seemed to be a tendency, although not a very marked one, for independent sector homes to provide a pleasanter environment.
- There is not necessarily a very good match between levels of support provided and the needs of residents, so that greater attention needs to be paid to this in placing individuals.
- Resident satisfaction is very much influenced by the amount of privacy available to them and by the restrictiveness of the rules imposed at the home.
- Currently there are few quality assurance programmes in place, especially in the voluntary sector, and better monitoring of care provided is needed.

6.8 'The 1994 Crisis in Acute Mental Health Beds' – a report by Hilary Guite and colleagues

This research report was prepared by Guite et al (1995), commissioned jointly by the Task Force on London and local purchasers. It is one of a series of studies which have focused mainly on difficulties in meeting the demand for acute beds in London. It refers primarily to the catchment area of one inner London Health Commission (Lambeth, Southwark and Lewisham), but aims to use this specific information to draw some conclusions about the general situation in inner London.

The report describes the "bed crisis" which began in April 1994 when an overflow developed from local hospital beds into the private sector at the cost of 1 million pounds overspend in the Health Commission on private sector mental health beds. Prior to this date, use of such beds for extra-contractual referrals (ECRs) had been at a low level, but subsequently it remained considerable.

Developments in bed use from the late 1980s onwards are summarised. From 1975 to 1987, bed occupancy had been stable at around 85%. In about 1988 the demand for acute psychiatric beds seems to have begun to rise, so that by 1992 bed occupancy had risen to close to 100%. A further rise in bed occupancy of 5% seems to have occurred in 1993 and then a further increased demand of 5% in April and May 1994 led the acute bed capacity to be finally exceeded, resulting in the overspill in to the private sector. Guite and her colleagues discuss why this increasing demand for bed may have occurred. The major causal factors they identify are:

- Changes in mental health policy, with increasing pressure to identify severely mentally ill people, make discharges safer and improve the quality of life of the severely mentally ill. The authors suggest that the one major event which coincided with the final rise in demand for beds in April 1994 was the introduction of Supervision Registers.
- An increase in homelessness and a lack of development of special needs supported housing, leading to both increased numbers requiring admission and greater difficulties in arranging suitable accommodation on discharge.
- Increased unemployment, which may compromise the community's ability to cope with severely mentally ill people.
- Demands particularly for secure beds created by schemes for diversion of mentally disordered offenders from courts and prisons.

The report also emphasises that the number of acute beds in the hospitals within the Health Commission's catchment area fell by only a total of eight beds between 1989 and 1994, so that it is unlikely that loss of acute beds in itself accounts for the developing bed crisis, at least in this particular inner city area.

6.9 The Inner London Collaborative Audit of Admissions in two Health Districts

The Inner London Collaborative Audit of Admissions in two Health Districts (Flannigan et al 1994a, Bebbington et al 1994, Flannigan et al 1994b) examines the use of acute beds in two inner London Health Districts, Hammersmith and Fulham and South Southwark. The study began in 1990 and involved collection of information on a sample of people who were in-patients in acute wards on a particular census day or were admitted over the three months following the census day.

In both districts the major reasons identified by staff as having led to admissions were self neglect, risk of self harm, poor functioning and poor acceptance of medication. A substantial difference in bed use between the two Districts was noted, with higher bed availability and a greater admission rate in South Southwark. Major differences in patterns of admission between South Southwark and Hammersmith and Fulham where that in South Southwark some patients were admitted with affective disorders, a group hardly represented in Hammersmith and Fulham, and relief of carers or patients' requests for admission were significant reasons for admission in Southwark but not in Hammersmith and Fulham. The authors raise the possibility that very high demand for acute beds may make it difficult to admit people with affective disorders when indicated, and that it may also make it excessively difficult to provide admission because of carer relief or patient request. The authors also comment on the rate of detention under the Mental Health Act, much above the national average in both districts.

Researchers also interviewed keyworkers about whether any alternative might have been found to acute admission. Staff in Hammersmith and Fulham rarely saw an alternative to the admission, but in South Southwark staff thought that around a quarter might have been cared for in the setting of a hostel with 24 hour supervision. No other facilities were considered by staff to be a reasonable alternative to admission for patients on their wards. The authors also note that there appeared to be significant numbers of "revolving door" patients in each District, with almost a quarter of those admitted having been discharged from a hospital inpatient stay within the previous month.

6.10 Powell, Hollander and Tobiansky: a four year survey of London's acute bed state

This study was carried out by Powell and colleagues (1995), in order to make a formal longitudinal assessment of the impression held by many London psychiatrists that at the beginning of the 1990s obtaining access to acute admission bed was becoming increasing difficult. The study procedure was to make enquiries by telephone to all the NHS managed acute psychiatric units in Greater London on each of four census days a year, all on Bank holiday weekends between Easter 1990 and Christmas 1993. The focus of the study was on numbers and occupancy of acute beds. Their main findings were as follows:

- Acute bed provision for inner London Health Districts was about twice that for outer London (0.466 beds per thousand compared with 0.255 beds per thousand).
- The overall number of acute beds declined steadily between Easter 1990 and Christmas 1993, with an overall reduction during this period of 10.3%.
- For inner London the mean bed occupancy over this period was 99.79% with means for individual districts ranging between 91.08% and 104.89%. For outer London the overall mean was 95.1% bed occupancy, with means for districts ranging between 84.29% and 109.28% (this figure of 109% which is considerably out of the range for most outer London Health Districts is for Greenwich, which is a highly deprived area, despite being classified as outer London.) The difference in occupancy between inner and outer London was statistically significant.
- There was a non-statistically significant trend for bed occupancy to increase over the four years of the census.
- Both acute bed provision and bed occupancy had significant associations with Jarman score, with more deprived districts having both greater provision of acute beds and higher bed occupancy levels.

The lower bed occupancies found in this study compared with MILMIS reflect a different definition of bed occupancy: MILMIS takes into account extra-contractual referrals to other hospitals and patients who are awaiting admission or should have been admitted if space were available, whereas the denominator used by Powell et al consists only of patients who are actually on the ward or on leave. The authors note that extra-contractual referrals increased considerably over this period, so that the study data is not likely to give a complete indication of the rise in demand over this period.

The authors conclude that bed occupancy is unacceptably high. They argue that there is a considerable risk that premature discharge will lead to danger for patients and others, and that adequate management of patients admitted many miles from their homes is difficult. The marked rise in extra-contractual referrals resulting from these high demands for beds appeared likely to lead to disinvestment in local services as commissioning agencies have to cut local budgets in order to finance these flows of patients elsewhere. They note that from a financial perspective, 'there is a flow of tens of millions of pounds each year from deprived urban areas to suburban and rural areas and to the private sector'. They also observe that the severe difficulties faced by inner London as deprived districts were likely to be compounded by a new capitation system for resource allocation, which required them to save 11.9% over the following five years.

The authors followed this work with a further census conducted in May 1996 (Hollander et al, 1996). This found that over the two and a half years intervening, a sharp rise in mean bed occupancy had occurred in Greater London, from an overall mean of 101% at the end of 1993 to 113% in 1996.

6.11 Cochrane, Conroy and Lewis: A Profile of London's Mental Health Services

This report on the state of London's Mental Health Services in the Financial Year 1993-1994 was produced by Cochrane and colleagues at Conrane Consulting for the Mental Health Task Force on London. Their procedure was to ask for completion of a detailed questionnaire and then to carry out visits in each of the Commissioning Authorities within the London Implementation Group (LIG) area. The report includes information on local populations' current service utilisation, forensic and challenging behaviour services and expenditure. The report both summarises the current status of services in the London Implementation Zone as a whole and provides an individual description of each of the twelve Commissions' catchment areas. Important observations made include:

- The mean admission rate across London is 4.55 finished consultant episode per year per thousand population under sixty-five. The range was wide (2.21 to 8.58 per thousand). Overall bed use ranged from 0.26 to 0.78 beds per thousand population aged under sixty-five. The range outside London in a comparable survey was between 0.2 to 0.5 per thousand, and five of the twelve districts had acute bed use above 0.5 per thousand, thus placing them above the top end of the range for the country as a whole.

- Pressure on acute beds, indicated by occupancy and turnover, was "undoubtedly high" in some districts. The authors comment that there seemed to be considerable variation in this degree of pressure, and their view is that this is not readily explained in terms of bed provision or the characteristics of the area. As was also noted by Powell et al (1995), some areas with high levels of acute bed provision also appear to have high occupancy. A suggested explanation is that a common characteristic of areas where there is such pressure for beds is that there is a high concentration of patients with relatively long stays on in-patient wards. This suggests that access may be restricted by beds becoming "silted-up" with longer stay cases, whom it may only be possible to discharge when other residential or secure facilities become available.

- Compared with figures for the rest of the country, the spend on mental health in London is high. The mean for London Commissions was for mental health to represent 16.35% of total expenditure on health, compared with a national mean of 11%. The range within London was very wide: between 10-22% of the overall health spend. The average sum spent was 6.5 million pounds per 100,000 population, with again a wide range from 3.5 to 12 million per hundred thousand. Social Services expenditure seemed relatively low, representing around 11% of the combined NHS and Social Services spend on mental health. Again the range was broad, from 7% to 24% (including the Mental Illness Specific Grant). The proportion of total mental health spend devoted to community services appeared to be low and was on average 19%, with in-patient provision accounting for the rest. Again the range was wide, with between 54% and 95% of the total budget spent on in-patient services. The authors suggest that those districts that are planning a service which appears well balanced between hospital and community are anticipating spending around 60–70% of their budgets on in-patient services. Generally the low community costs appeared partly to reflect the fact that there were very few community services operating out of hours.

- Comparing findings in London with their work elsewhere in the country, the authors suggest that in London services for the long-term highly dependent mentally ill are under-developed, with little specialist intensive community support available and limited "rehabilitation" facilities.

- Staffing is also examined and London appears to have high proportions of qualified and higher grade mental health staff in most professions. The report suggests that the London workforce should be reviewed, and that this expensive workforce cannot necessarily be justified. However, subsequent evidence of considerable recruitment difficulties for mental health staff in London (Lelliott et al, 1996) suggests that the down-grading of London's mental health workforce may not be helpful.

- Overall the authors suggest that the "silting-up" of acute beds by patients with a longer length of stay is preventing money being diverted to provision of community services. Proposed strategies for relieving this include the provision of community services which can provide more intensive support, of residential rehabilitation facilities and of an increased number of medium secure beds.

6.12 The Thames Bed Census

A further source of information on acute bed provision in London is the Thames Bed Census, carried out in June 1994 and reported by the NHS Executive in their recent briefing paper on 'Mental Health in London' (NHS Executive, 1996b). A survey of all acute and low level secure beds for adults and of acute assessment beds for the elderly mentally ill in the NHS and the private sector was carried out on a single census day in London, Hertfordshire, Kent, Surrey, Sussex and Essex. The main conclusions, as summarised in the NHS Executive's report, were as follows:

- Of the 3,710 adult acute patients covered, 23% (843) appeared no longer to require acute beds.
- 45% of these inappropriately placed patients (n = 380) could have been discharged to the community if there had been professional staff available to support them at home (72%), a place to live or more suitable housing (61%), or more day care (29%).
- 52% (437) could have been discharged or transferred to long-stay residential care, such as a group home, staffed housing or in-patient rehabilitation.
- Bed occupancy rates were very high, even by the relatively conservative definition adopted in this study – rates of up to 98% were found in inner and outer London, despite the exclusion of people on long term leave.
- The conclusion is drawn that a more effective and wider range of community services is required to lessen the need for so many acute beds.

Acknowledgement
We are very grateful for the help of Ms Sylvia Kingaby, statistician at the Department of Health Statistics Division, who analysed the Hospital Episode Statistics data.

Chapter 7

Levels of in-patient and residential provision throughout London

Rosalind Ramsay, Graham Thornicroft, Sonia Johnson, Liz Brooks and Gyles Glover

Summary

This chapter reports on a detailed survey of in-patient and residential mental health services in each London Borough, conducted in the first half of 1996. Information was collected from Local Authorities and from NHS provider Trusts on levels of provision for the catchment area's population. We compare the figures with the expected levels of service produced by expert consensus. Regarding the collection of these data, our main findings are that:

- data are extremely difficult to collect as no agreed national categories of service exist
- many Boroughs and provider Trusts have incomplete data about what they provide
- Trust boundaries which are not co-terminous with local authorities and which are susceptible to change make reconciliation of data from different sources difficult.

In relation to the levels of provision in Inner London, we have found:

- a wide variation in numbers of acute beds per 100,000 population (32–66)
- 10 fold variation in the numbers of intensive care beds
- 6 fold differences in the use of medium secure beds
- 5 fold difference between the number of 24-hour staffed residential care places in the most compared with the least well provided Boroughs
- 10 fold differences in the numbers of places in lower staffed residential care

Outer London:

- provides or purchases about three-quarters of the average level of acute bed provision for Inner London, but the *range* of acute bed use in the Outer London Boroughs is almost the same as Inner London
- uses about half as many intensive care bed as Inner London
- consumes less than a fifth of the Regional Secure Unit beds
- uses 70% of the Inner London levels of 24 hour staffed residential care places
- has about 75% of the Inner city level of lesser staffed specialist housing

In terms of the expected number of places needed in each category, we have shown that the ranges of provision most widely cited, upon which the present version of the MINI (mental illness needs index) computer programme bases its estimates of facilities required, substantially underestimates need in inner London. They suggest that less provision is required than is actually in place in respect of acute, intensive care and medium secure beds, 24-hour staffed housing and lower supported accommodation. This contradicts all the other evidence in this report, and the repeated strong impressions of clinical staff.

We conclude therefore that the MINI estimates are inadequate for current needs in London. Since many districts lie near the top of the range of MINI scores, this indicates that the top end of the ranges are set too low. On the basis of this evidence a revised set of ranges has been developed, and a new version of the MINI software programme has been produced incorporating these. Estimates from this appears more commensurate with other evidence on mental health services in London.

7.1 Levels of in-patient and residential service provision throughout London

This section describes the results of a major survey conducted at PRiSM of levels of in-patient and residential service provision across health, local authority and voluntary sectors in all London boroughs. The survey was confined to these aspects of provision not because community and day services were seen as unimportant, but because previous experience has indicated that it is extremely difficult to obtain an accurate view of service provision, particularly outside the statutory sector, and that the difficulties are often greatest for non-residential services. Given the short timescale for this study, it was therefore necessary to limit the aspects of service provision to be quantified – in-patient and residential care seemed an appropriate focus as these are the aspects of London's services about which debate has recently been most intense and which currently carry the greatest costs. Chapter 8 provides some information about the availability of day, community and work services.

We first describe the methods used and the difficulties encountered. The obstacles we faced in trying to obtain an overview of current London provision are significant in that they indicate how difficult it remains to obtain information of a quality adequate for the rational planning of local services. We will then outline the levels of provision to be found throughout the city, and will explore how far variations in level of provision appear to be related to some major socio-demographic indicators.

As well as describing these actual levels and their variation, we wished to compare them with estimates of how much provision one would expect to be required in each area of London. Until recently, there has been little available technology for determining on the basis of local area characteristics how much provision is needed. Improved understanding of the relationships between socio-demographic factors and service utilisation has allowed the development in the past five years of quantitative indices of need based on demographic attributes of areas. One of these, the MINI (mental illness needs index), has been operationalised as a computer programme (Glover, 1996). This estimates the likely level of facilities required for a geographical areas by calculating where the area lies within the range of need levels for districts within England and applying this to published estimates of the range of necessary provision of various sorts of facility. These methods remain very much in their infancy, but the MINI (mental illness needs index) is based on substantial development work, has taken into account both epidemiological work on need and data on actual service utilisation and is widely used. It therefore appeared appropriate use this in a comparison of actual and expected levels of service provision throughout London. The results of this are described in the final section of the chapter. The need levels estimated by the MINI software programme appeared a relatively poor reflection of service provision in London, so that further work was undertaken to develop a new version compatible with evidence on service use in London. This development work and its results are described in sections 7.5 and 7.6 of the chapter.

The data discussed in this chapter have also formed the basis for cost analyses by the Centre for the Economics of Mental Health. This chapter should be read in conjunction with Chapter 11, which describes this health economic work.

7.2 Method and obstacles encountered

7.2.1 Data collection

A brief questionnaire was designed, based on the categories of in-patient and residential care included in the MINI software programme. The definitions used for each category are shown in Figure 1:

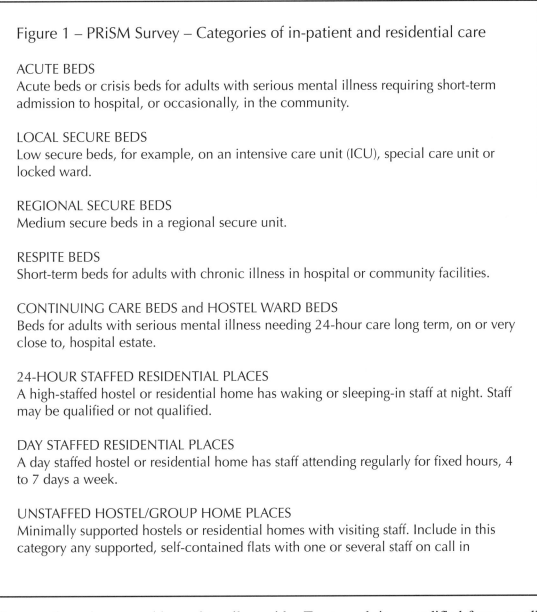

Figure 1 – PRiSM Survey – Categories of in-patient and residential care

ACUTE BEDS
Acute beds or crisis beds for adults with serious mental illness requiring short-term admission to hospital, or occasionally, in the community.

LOCAL SECURE BEDS
Low secure beds, for example, on an intensive care unit (ICU), special care unit or locked ward.

REGIONAL SECURE BEDS
Medium secure beds in a regional secure unit.

RESPITE BEDS
Short-term beds for adults with chronic illness in hospital or community facilities.

CONTINUING CARE BEDS and HOSTEL WARD BEDS
Beds for adults with serious mental illness needing 24-hour care long term, on or very close to, hospital estate.

24-HOUR STAFFED RESIDENTIAL PLACES
A high-staffed hostel or residential home has waking or sleeping-in staff at night. Staff may be qualified or not qualified.

DAY STAFFED RESIDENTIAL PLACES
A day staffed hostel or residential home has staff attending regularly for fixed hours, 4 to 7 days a week.

UNSTAFFED HOSTEL/GROUP HOME PLACES
Minimally supported hostels or residential homes with visiting staff. Include in this category any supported, self-contained flats with one or several staff on call in

The questionnaire was addressed to all provider Trusts and, in a modified form, to all Local Authority Social Services. In the Trusts, the Clinical Director was generally contacted in the first instance, although the questionnaire often seemed to have been passed around the department, with a variety of members of staff often involved in its completion, including Business Managers, Directors of Operations, Directors of Mental Health and General Mangers of Mental Health Services. In Local Authorities, considerable research time was often required to locate the person most likely to be in a position to respond to the questionnaire. The most frequently occurring titles for respondents were Principal Officer for Mental Health, Commissioning Officer or Assistant Director of Community Care, and Policy Development Manager.

A 'snapshot' of numbers of clients aged 15 to 65 currently placed was requested, in preference to annual client figures or data on the numbers of places 'available'. In a situation where an unused bed or place is likely to be sold on to another borough or Trust, a record of places available by geographical location would be misleading, and annual client figures would produce distortions for the short-term types of accommodation. The 'snapshot' method based on numbers of clients placed is the only way to obtain an impression of how many **places** are being provided for residents of a particular Borough. Obtaining such a picture was necessary for the data to be comparable with MINI estimates for cross-sectional numbers of places available in each category.

Social Services Departments were asked for a 'snapshot' of the number of residents of their Borough who were currently in places provided, commissioned or purchased by the Borough, including places funded by other agencies, and places both in and out of Borough. Trusts were asked for a 'snapshot' of the number of residents of the Trust's catchment area (for Acute Mental Health services) who were currently in places managed or funded by or through the Trust, including Acute ECRs and patients in Regional Secure Units (this latter being the only category which included forensic services).

In some cases funding for RSUs and private acute ECRs had not devolved to the Trust, but remained with the Health Authority. Where possible, Health Authorities were asked for supplementary information – this however remains incomplete, and more comprehensive information about RSU provision is given in Chapter 5. Purchasers were also asked for the numbers of adults in "Section 28A" funded places (reprovided for clients of old psychiatric hospitals). These places are funded directly through the Health Authority and will not be recorded by Trusts or by Social Services Departments. It was ultimately decided to exclude this category from our survey, as both funding and (often) the residential place itself are client-specific and expire with the client.

Besides figures on the numbers of clients being placed, the location of the placement was recorded (in or out of Borough/catchment area), along with the management and the main funder/s. The questionnaires were sent out between February and March 1996. Because of difficulties in obtaining a response from some Trusts and Local Authorities data-gathering continued into July 1996.

7.2.2 Data analysis

In order to compare actual provision with MINI estimates of need based on both the Wing (1992) and the Strathdee and Thornicroft (1992) ranges, data from Trusts and Local Authorities were brought together and divided up by Borough. In cases where a Mental Health Trust had boundaries coterminous with a Borough, this was relatively straightforward. However, in some instances, Trusts' contracted catchment areas straddled two or more Boroughs or parts of Boroughs, and in some cases, Trust boundaries were not coterminous with electoral wards. In these cases the proportion of the Trust's catchment population living in each Borough was calculated and the number of beds 'available' to each estimated by applying these proportions to the total number of places used. The resulting figures, rounded to one decimal place, were then added to the Local Authority figures and, where appropriate, Health Authority figures to produce a total number of all kinds of residential provision being currently used by residents of each Borough. For this reason, Trust-provided places are frequently given to one decimal place.

In general, the Trust would record only Health Service funded places, while the Local Authority would record both these and local authority funded places. As a rule of thumb, if the stated funding source of places was the same, the places were assumed to be duplicates, and if it was different, they were assumed to be distinct. In the case where information on provision came from two different sources, and was in conflict, the agency funding the residential care was assumed to have the more accurate account.

Respondents were asked to code the data given with an information quality code:

1 = good/accurate
2 = approximate
3 = possible omission/overestimation
4 = guess
5 = information not available

A further assessment of information quality was made at data entry stage, using the following criteria. All bed numbers which resulted from dividing Trust figures by Borough percentages were given the Information Quality coding 3, which represents possible omissions or overestimations. All bed numbers which resulted from summing such "derived" Borough figures with "non-derived" figures were also given Quality Code 3, no matter how reliable the data with which they were summed. Inspection of these data quality codes indicated that the number of '3' codes was regrettably large.

7.2.3 Limits to the accuracy of the data

- Often no single individual person within the Trust or Local Authority would have access to an overview of services provision and the questionnaires would need to be passed to several different respondents.

- Our way of classifying provision was seldom compatible with classifications used by the agencies concerned, both for their own internal requirements and for public information purposes, neither was there consistency between the way agencies in different areas classify services. This meant that provision had to be re-audited according to our categories, which might be time-consuming for respondents, particularly in services undergoing major changes. The March date of the survey also coincided with the busiest time of the year for many departments – one of our general recommendations is that it is unwise to undertake surveys of service provision in the last three months of the financial year.

- Where complete data was not obtained until June or July, a considerable time lag developed between information given by different agencies in the same area, so that the information was not a true 'snapshot.'

- Local Authorities, in particular, often lacked an overview of the specialist mental health housing used by Borough residents. Two thirds of Local Authorities gave details of schemes funded or part-funded by Local Authority, Health Authority or

DoH monies, but only 1/3 included private or voluntary sector schemes *without* such funding, paid for out of D.S.S. benefits. Unregistered homes were unlikely to be included, yet some of these may offer quite high levels of personal care (as long as they do not also offer board, they are not required to register).

• Two kinds of residential provision were found which did not fit neatly into our categories: family placement schemes and supported, self-contained flats. It was generally decided to exclude the former from the survey and reclass the latter in the 'unstaffed home' category. However, since supported tenancies were not explicitly enquired about in all areas and seemed to be viewed in some places as a category distinct from those we enquired about, there may be some omissions here.

• The 'respite' category, as seen in the Strathdee and Thornicroft tables is in practice hard to do justice to in a 'snapshot' survey. A return marked "0 respite beds" could mean any of three things: respite care is never provided as such; there are respite beds but they were not being used at the time of the survey; there are no beds designated (set aside) for respite use, but it is bought in when required.

• The method of dividing up Trust catchment areas by Borough brought down the overall quality of the information as presented by Borough, and will in some cases lead to unrepresentative results, particularly where a Trust straddles an under-privileged and a privileged Borough, such as Oxleas NHS Trust which covers the London Boroughs of Bexley and Greenwich. In such cases, it may be more helpful to view the results by Health Authority (see Chapter 11).

• Data were gathered for the 16–65 age group only. However, a difficulty arising from this was that many services do not have a very clear age cut off point for 'graduates' of the services (individuals who have entered services as adults, and continued in them after passing the age of 65). In 10 Local Authorities and 5 Trusts there was at least one residential service in which data was only available for adults plus "graduates" (those who had entered services as adults and continued in them after passing the age of 65). In this case, the optimal Information Quality Code for the category of residential care in question, was 2 = approximate). In 9 Local Authorities and 3 Trusts it occurred that, for at least one of the residential service, figures were only available for 'adults + elderly' and in this case the optimal Information Quality Code is 3 (= omissions/overestimation).

7.3 Levels of provision in London Boroughs

Tables 1 and 2 summarise the information obtained on current service provision for inner and outer London. As the above caveats about data quality should make plain, the information about individual Boroughs should not be used as the basis for planning without checking its accuracy. However, the information is probably of sufficient quality to give an indication of overall patterns in service provision in London.

Table 1 'Snapshot' of levels of service provision per 100,000 in inner London Boroughs

Borough	Acute beds per 100,000 population (i)	Local secure/ intensive care places per 100,000	Regional Secure Units (Incomplete – see also chapter 5.6) per 100,000	24 hour staffed non-acute places per 100,000 (including hostel wards, continuing care beds, community beds with 24 hour staffing)	Day staffed/lower staffed supported accommodation per 100,000 Including supported tenancies and respite beds
Camden	38	4.2	not given	not given	NG
City of London	53	14.5	21.8	273	48
Greenwich	35	1.5	3.6	57	117
Hackney	59	16.2	23.2	51	37
Hammersmith & Fulham (ii)	58	8.1	not given	73	10
Islington	38	4.2	not given	143	26
Kensington & Chelsea (ii)	66	5.4	not given	78	78
Lambeth	43	9.3	13.1	126	90
Lewisham	33	3.4	8	55	40
Southwark	43	8.5	9.4	90	74
Tower Hamlets	56	3.7	not given	64	42
Wandsworth	32	2.1	8.4	59	18
Westminster (ii)	41	8.7	not given	146	50
Range in levels of provision /100,000 for Inner London	32-66	1.5-16.2	3.6-23.2	51-273	10-117
Overall provision/100,000 for Inner London Boroughs	44	6.2	10.6	85	55

(i) Excludes ECRs
(ii) There was incomplete medium secure bed, respite bed and residential place information for these Boroughs because each is partly served by Riverside Trust, which did not give data for these categories

Table 2 'Snapshot' of levels of service provision per 100,000 in Outer London Boroughs

Borough	Acute beds per 100,000 population (i)	Local secure/ intensive care places per 100,000	Regional Secure Units (Incomplete – see also chapter 5.6) per 100,000	24 hour staffed non-acute places per 100,000 (including hostel wards, continuing care beds, community beds with 24 hour staffing)	Day staffed/lower staffed supported accommodation per 100,000 Including supported tenancies and respite beds
Barking	21	1.3	2.7	57	22
Barnet	35	6.8	1.4	63	19
Bexley	35	1.5	3.5	63	8
Brent	36	4.9	4.9	88	87
Bromley	19	0	2.6	43	19
Croydon	23	3.2	0	61	11
Ealing	36	8.7	10.2	70	35
Enfield	29	1.4	8.9	56	12
Haringey	49	8.0	not given	103	34
Harrow	23	0	0	58	30
Havering	21	1.4	2.7	41	7
Hillingdon	22	0	0	40	33
Hounslow	30	0	2.1	24	11
Kingston	24	5.7	4.1	120	25
Merton	34	2.8	not given	58	66
Newham	25	2.4	8.5	114	6
Redbridge	36	4.4	0.9	66	28
Richmond	27	0	0	41	26
Sutton	21	8.9	0	37	64
Waltham	28	4.7	0	41	32
Outer London range	**19-49**	**0-8.9**	**0-11.3**	**24-120**	**6-87**
Overall provision per 100,000 for Outer London	**29**	**3.3**	**3.4**	**62**	**28**

(i) Excludes ECRs

Even taking into account the likely variation due to error discussed above, the heterogeneity in these results is striking – for most forms of provision some Boroughs have several times as much provision per 100,000 as others. In each category, the mean provision per 100,000 for London Boroughs is greater for Inner London than for Outer London, though there is substantial overlap in the ranges.

For acute beds, levels of Outer London provision in most cases cluster within a fairly narrow band between around 20 and around 35 per 100,000. In Inner London, the spread appears rather wider, but most fall somewhere between 30 and 65 places per 100,000.

For both local secure/intensive care beds and medium secure ones, the spread is very wide – in Inner London some Boroughs appear to be using around 10 times as much secure provision as others, and in Outer London the spread is also wide and includes a number of Boroughs not using any such provision at the time of the survey. In both Inner and, by a small margin, Outer London, mean level of use of medium secure is greater than lower secure provision. This raises questions about the relative availability of these types of provision, as, if both were freely available, one would predict that more people would be appropriately managed at the lower level of security. This may thus indicate a shortage of local secure/intensive care beds.

For non-acute residential care, the spread again seems very wide in both Inner and Outer London (though in Inner London, the highest rate for staffed residential care, seen in the City, should probably be considered with caution because of the City's very small size and its geographic and service links with some exceptionally deprived parts of the adjacent boroughs). Local substitution effects cannot account for this as a wide spread in provision is still seen if the categories of 24-hour staffed and day staffed and lower support accommodation are combined.

7.4 Levels of provision and demographic variables

One potential explanation of the considerable heterogeneity in levels of provision around the city is that it may reflect different socio-demographic characteristics producing different levels of need. Jarman's UPA score is a composite indicators of deprivation derived, on the basis of a large survey of the views of general practitioners, to predict levels of pressure on primary care services. It has been shown also to be related to mental health service use (see Chapter 4). Glover's Mental Illness Needs Index (MINI) is also based on socio-demographic characteristics and was derived specifically to try to quantify patterns of need for secondary level mental health care. It was based on studies of the pattern of in-patient mental health care in the North East Thames Region. Figure 1 shows acute bed provision per 100,000 for each Borough plotted against Jarman score and Figure 2 acute bed use plotted against MINI score. Both scores are derived from 1991 Census data.

Figure 1 Jarman UPA scores and acute bed provision/100,000 – London Boroughs

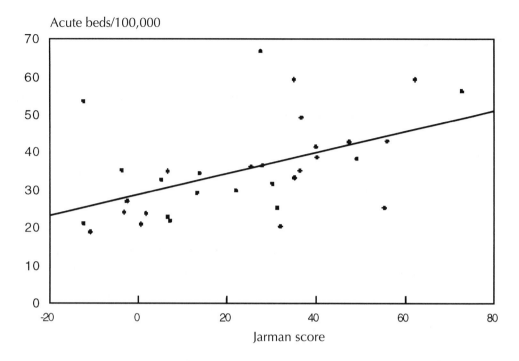

Figure 2 MINI score and acute bed provision/100,000 – London Boroughs

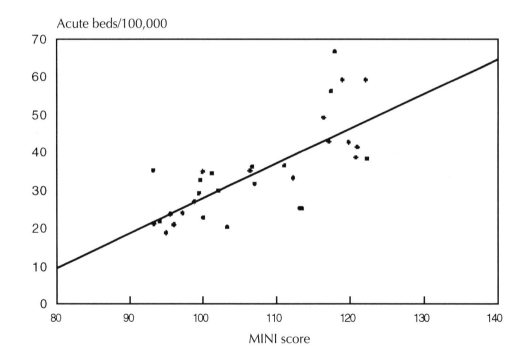

As indicated by the regression line plotted on the graph, there is some relationship between both Jarman and MINI scores and acute bed use – analysis indicates that there is a statistically significant, moderately high correlation of 0.64, with 38% of the variation in bed use explained by variations in Jarman scores.[1] Corresponding results for MINI scores are a correlation of 0.75 and 56% of the variance explained. Inspection

---

[1] All analyses for this section were carried out using SPSS 6 for Windows. Where associations are referred to as 'statistically significant', this indicates that they reach at least the conventional level of significance at p=0.05. Statements about 'variation explained' refer to the adjusted R squared when each

of the graph indicates that there are still some substantial differences in bed use between Boroughs with similar scores on these composite socio-demographic indicators, but generally the association between level of deprivation and acute bed use appears close.

As discussed in Chapter 3, other area characteristics which might be expected to be associated with variations in need for psychiatric services are levels of homelessness, the representation in the local population of ethnic minorities in general and Black Caribbeans and Black Africans in particular, and the unemployment rate. These were each plotted against acute bed provision, and corresponding statistical analyses carried out. Each is significantly correlated with acute bed use, but to a slightly lower degree than the Jarman or MINI scores. Unemployment rate is the most strongly related to acute bed use of these indicators, with a correlation of 0.61 and 35% of the variation in acute bed explained. Homelessness has a correlation with acute bed use of 0.45, with 19% of variation in acute bed provision explained), whilst the correlation with acute bed use for proportion of Black Caribbeans and Black Africans in the local population is 0.51, with 23% of variation explained. We also related bed use to overall proportion of the population belonging to any ethnic minority group, but the resulting association was less strong than that for Black Caribbean or African ethnicity, explaining less than 10% of variation in bed use. These demographic indicators are all highly correlated with one another and with the composite indicators of deprivation, so that it may be more appropriate to consider them all as markers of a general relationship between poor social conditions and bed use, rather than as each having a more specific relationship with service use. When all these variables are entered into a stepwise regression model, MINI score emerges as the only significant predictor of acute bed use, confirming that the contributions of these various demographic variables to explaining bed use are not clearly distinct from one another.

The relationship of other types of provision with socio-demographic variables may be explored in a similar way. Figure 3 shows 24-hour staffed bed provision plotted against MINI score. Here the correlation is 0.60, which again is statistically highly significant. 33% of the variation in use of 24 hour staffed non-acute beds explained by MINI score. Again the other variables examined are positively correlated with service use, but at lower levels: the correlations are 0.43 for Jarman score, 0.42 for unemployment, 0.41 for proportion of the population who are Black Caribbean or Black African, and 0.28 for rates of homelessness. Looking at the plot indicates a substantial number of instances of Boroughs with similar MINI scores having very different levels of provision from one another.

We also examined the association between these demographic indicators and level of provision of all non-acute residential places, including 24 hour staffed, day staffed and lower support care. Again, the association with MINI score was strongest, with a correlation of 0.61 and 35% of the variation explained. Figure 4 shows this relationship.

---

demographic variable is entered into a linear regression with place provision as the dependent variable. The 'best predictor' in each instance was confirmed by entering all the demographic variables as independent variables into stepwise multiple regression model. The City has been excluded from these analyses, as its scores on some variables are extreme and given that its population is below 5,000 people, the validity of including these outliers seems low.

Figure 3 MINI scores and levels of 24-hour staffed bed provision – all London boroughs

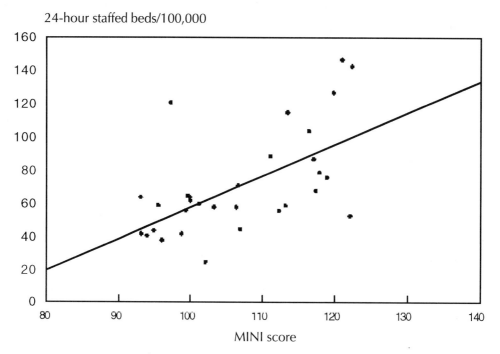

Figure 4 MINI scores and non-acute residential provision (24 hour staffed, day staffed and lower support accommodation)

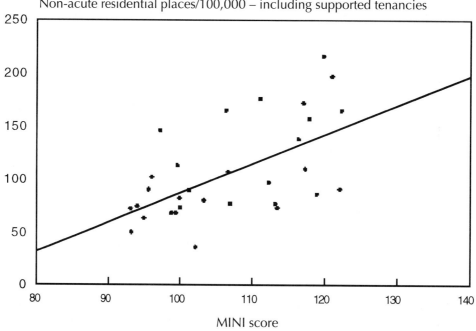

Correlations for provision of supported residential care with other demographic variables were 0.43 for Jarman score, 0.42 for unemployment rate, 0.50 for the proportion of the population who are Black African or Black Caribbean and 0.24 for rates of homelessness: al but the last of these reach statistical significance. For both 24 hour staffed residential care and all supported residential care, MINI score emerged as the only significant predictor when all the demographic variables were entered into a regression model.

Finally levels of intensive care bed provision were also examined. This had highly significant positive correlations with both MINI score (0.58) and Jarman score (0.47), as well as with rates of homelessness (0.58), unemployment rate (0.50) and proportion of the local population who are Black African and Black Caribbean. For this service type, proportion who are Black Caribbean or Black African appears the best predictor, explaining 35% of the variation in intensive care bed provision and emerging as the only significant predictor when all the demographic variables are entered into a regression model. This may be a reflection of the tendency discussed in Chapters 5.7 and 5.10 of this book for Black people to come into contact with the mental health services. However, it must be noted that the association of this variable with intensive care bed use is not much stronger than those for the other demographic variables, and it may be functioning here more as a general indicator of social deprivation than as a marker of a specific association between ethnicity and intensive care service use. Figure 5 shows the relationship between proportion of the population who are Black Caribbean or Black African and use of intensive care places:

Figure 5 Intensive care provision and proportion of population who are Black Caribbean or Black African

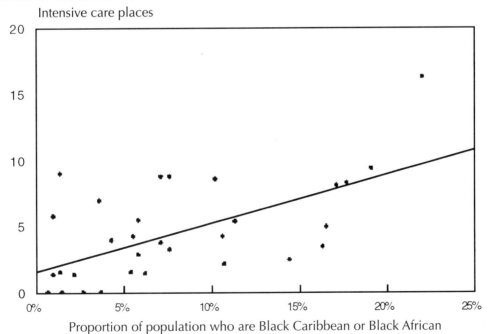

Proportion of population who are Black Caribbean or Black African

The relationships between levels of each types of provision were also explored – levels of each type of place were positively correlated with each other type, indicating that places where there is a high level of one type of care tend also to have large amounts of the other types. This is likely to be at least in part a reflection of the association between level of each type of care and social deprivation. However, it does suggest that no very clear-cut or large scale substitution of any one type of bed for any other is taking place.

Thus socio-demographic variables make a considerable contribution to understanding the large variations which exist across London in service use, with greater social deprivation strongly associated with higher rates of use of all categories of in-patient and residential service use. However, inspection of Figures 1 to 5 indicates that some substantial differences remain between areas which are demographically apparently similar in how much of the various categories of in-patient and residential care are provided. Factors which might explain some of the remaining variation in service use include bottle-necks in local systems preventing movement out of certain types of care, traditions and individual ways of practising among local professionals which influence how patients are managed and where they are placed, and the extent of development of non-residential services, such as community mental health team and local crisis services. It may also be that there are high levels of unmet need in those areas which have relatively low levels of service provision relative to their levels of social deprivation. As discussed earlier in this chapter, the likely limitations to the accuracy of our data must also be borne in mind.

7.5 Mental Illness Needs Index

Staff at the PRiSM team collaborated with Dr. Gyles Glover to compare the actual data for service provision (given above) with three estimates of levels of service provision which could reasonably be expected to be provided in each Borough. There are no official figures or broad consensus available on how much service should be provided in any given area of Britain, so our approach has been to use the best available estimates, to explain the rationale for these estimates, and to show the differences between actual and expected levels of service provision. We have adopted the approach of a sensitivity analysis: that is, we have made three sets of assumptions and calculated for each the consequences in terms of the expected number of places for seven categories of service. This therefore consists of three 'what if' exercises. This section sets out the assumptions behind each of the three estimates, the detailed process of calculating the estimates using the MINI computer programme devised by Dr. Glover, the results, a discussion of the strengths and weaknesses of this procedure, and our interpretations of the findings.

The computer programme which is supplied to calculate the MINI (Glover, 1996) applies the score for any chosen area to the ranges of provision for district health authorities suggested in 1992 by Wing and by Strathdee and Thornicroft. On the basis of where the chosen area's MINI score lies between that of the least and the most needy health districts, it suggests required levels for a number of types of facility. The purpose of this is to assist health authority planners in assigning resources for mental health care and to assist managers and clinicians at provider unit level seeking to make sense of observed variations in rates of service use between geographical sectors.

The MINI computer programme was used to derive 'Wing-based' and 'Strathdee/Thornicroft-based' estimates of local requirements for each London Boroughs. These were compared with the observed levels described above. An outline of the derivation of the MINI needs index and the process of calculating local service levels using it is given as an appendix to this chapter.

Wing's (1992) estimates (column B in Table 3) are derived from his extensive expert review of the literature and are described in detail in his chapter in Stevens and Raftery's 'Health Care Needs Assessment' (Wing, 1994). Wing's figures include services for general adult patients and assessment and treatment for adults aged over 65 with non-organic mental illnesses. The Strathdee and Thornicroft (1992) estimates were made after a national Delphi exercise in which 30 experts in the field were asked (i) to give the categories of in-patient and residential care that should be provided in each local area, and (ii) estimate the mean number of places that should be provided for an average local area, and the range given that requirements are likely to vary with social deprivation. The values given Column C of Table 3 are the composite values established by this process. These figures relate only to services for general adult patients aged 16–65. Tables 4 and 5 show the gaps between actual figures and estimates derived from Wing's work for each Borough in Inner and in Outer London, whilst Tables 6 and 7 show the gaps between the actual figures and the expected figures derived from Strathdee and Thornicroft.

In this work for the London Commission it became clear that the figures obtained by comparing Wing's and, to a lesser degree, Strathdee and Thornicroft's estimates of expected service provision with actual provision were widely at variance with all the other evidence gathered in the other sections of this mental heath service report in that, based upon assumptions of service needs at the national level, they predicted some overprovision in services that by all other accounts were operating beyond their capacity. In other words, the actual figures for service provision (given in Column E of Table 3) alongside the evidence of how London's mental health services are operating strongly suggest that the level of need in the most morbid parts of the capital exceeds even our highest previous estimates.

We therefore produced in 1996 a third set of estimates at PRiSM (column D in Table 3). These figures have been produced using the following assumptions derived from data reported elsewhere in this book. For acute beds, we have assumed that about 20% of current acute bed occupancy is inappropriate use by new long term patients who could be better accommodated in 24-hour staffed (nursed or non-nursed) residential care, that our actual acute beds figures (which do not include private or NHS ECRs) should be increased by about 10% to take account of current in-patient activity in ECR beds, and that a desirable level of bed occupancy is 85%. For Medium Secure beds, and for local secure beds (intensive care units) we have taken 1992 estimates and increased the upper end of the range to reflect actual provision. For 24-hour nursed staffed residential care we have based our figures on the 1996 NHS Executive report on 24-hour nursed staffed accommodation required per 250,000 population (Department of Health, 1996c). For other 24-hour staffed accommodation, and for 'lower staffed accommodation' our estimates reflect the views of many clinicians and managers contacted by the staff of the four teams commissioned to undertake the mental health services report, that there is very considerable underprovision of these categories in many areas. The day staffed hostels category reduces previous estimates to reflect the actual levels of provision, and the lower priority attached to them by many of those interviewed for this study. Tables 8 to 10 show the requirements for each borough estimated from these ranges by the MINI programme, and compare them with actual levels of service provision in each London Borough.

Table 3 Estimated Need and Actual Provision General Adult Mental Health Services (aged 15–64 only), (In-patient and Residential Care), Places per 250,000 population (ii)

A. Category of service	B. Wing 1992 (iii) Range	C. Strathdee Thornicroft 1992 Range	D. PRiSM 1996 (i) Range	E. Actual level of provision per 250,000 Outer London (overall)	Inner London (overall)	Range in London
1 Medium Secure Unit	1-10	1-10	5-30	8	27	0-58
2 Intensive Care Unit / local secure unit	5-15	5-10	5-20	8	16	0-41
3 Acute ward	50-150	50-150	5-175	73 (iv)	110 (iv)	48-165
4 24 hr nurse staffed units/ hostel wards/staff awake at night	25-75	40-150 for these 2 categories	12-50	55	35	0-164
5 24 hour non-nurse staffed hostels/ night staff sleep-in	40-110		50-300	99	162	28-330
6 Day staffed hostels	25-75	30-120	15-60	17	43	14-292 for these 2 categories
7 Lower support accommodation (v)	n/a	48-100	30-120	55	95	

NB   i) PRiSM 1996 estimated need levels based upon: London actual values, and an assumed 4 fold variation of need from least to most deprived parts of England, for most categories of service, with a far greater variation in medium secure beds, and Department of Health (1996c) guidance for an average of 25 places in 24-hour nursed staffed accommodation per 250,000

(ii) all estimates given assume that each category of service exists in the given appropriate range of volume

(iii) the Wing 1992 estimates include old age assessment places, & the Strathdee and Thornicroft figures apply only to general adult services for those aged 16–65

(iv) actuals exclude ECRs

(v) includes respite beds and supported self-contained flats. As not all agencies gave information on these categories, these estimates should be regarded as conservative

Table 4 Difference between actual and predicted levels of service provision in Inner London – Wing version of MINI

Borough (ii)	Difference between actual and predicted for **acute and crisis care** (i)	Difference between actual and predicted for **intensive care unit**	Difference between actual and predicted for **medium secure beds**	Difference between actual and predicted for **hostel staffed wards & highly staffed (24-hr) residential care**	Difference between actual and expected for **day staffed hostels and visited group homes**
Camden	+1.9	**-3.5**	**not known**	**not known**	**not known**
City of London	+1.0	+0.4	+ 0.8	+8.8	+0.3
Greenwich	+22.4	**-5.2**	+ 3.8	+12.9	**-36.8**
Hackney	+42.9	+18.8	+ 35.3	**-38.0**	**-27.0**
Hammersmith & Fulham (iii)	+32.0	+3.0	**not known**	**-4.2**	**-67.7**
Islington	+0.5	**-3.5**	**not known**	+106.4	**-63.6**
Kensington & Chelsea (iii)	+40.8	**-1.0**	**not known**	+2.8	+33.3
Lambeth	+14.9	+7.8	+ 22.9	+124.1	+76.8
Lewisham	+7.3	**-3.7**	+12.6	**-15.4**	**-11.5**
Southwark	+21.4	+6.6	+ 13.7	+47.5	**-28.8**
Tower Hamlets	+40.2	**-2.3**	**not known**	+1.1	**-15.2**
Wandsworth	**-2.1**	**-8.3**	+ 13.9	**-22.7**	**-76.5**
Westminster (iii)	+5.4	+4.3	**not known**	+119.6	**-29.3**
Net difference between actual and expected in inner London	**+228.7**	**+13.4**	**+ 103 (incomplete data)**	**+342.9 (incomplete data)**	**-246 (incomplete data)**

Positive figures indicate that actual provision is greater than predicted by MINI, negative ones that MINI suggests a deficit. All apparent deficits appear in bold.

(I) Excludes ECRs

(ii) To compensate for the Census undercount, all Wing estimates have been increased by 1.04 for Inner London Boroughs. (see Table 7, 1991 Census user guide 58, " Undercoverage in Great Britain".)

(iii) There was incomplete medium secure bed, respite bed and residential place information for these Boroughs because each is partly served by Riverside Trust, which did not give data for these categories.

Table 5 Difference between actual and predicted levels of service provision in Outer London – Wing 1992 version of MINI

Borough (ii)	Difference between actual and predicted for acute beds (i)	Difference between actual and predicted for intensive care beds	Difference between actual and predicted for medium secure beds	Difference between actual and predicted for 24-hour staffed beds – including hostel wards and continuing care wards	Difference between actual and expected for day staffed, respite and lower staffed beds (unlike Tables 1 & 2, does not include supported tenancies for which no estimates in MINI)
Barking	-0.4	-3.2	+1.9	+17.1	-13.9
Barnet	+43.0	+10.2	+0.6	+60.3	-35.8
Bexley	+41.3	-2.4	+6.1	+62.9	-33.3
Brent	+18.8	+0.5	+6.4	+69.7	+108.1
Bromley	+5.6	-8.1	+5.2	+21.6	-18.3
Croydon	+6.0	-0.8	-3.8	+53.7	-64.6
Ealing	+28.6	+12.3	+22.9	+45.6	-23.6
Enfield	+24.0	-5.1	+20.1	+35.1	-55.6
Haringey	+31.3	+5.0	not known	+69.5	-33.1
Harrow	+12.1	-5.8	-1.7	+41.7	-13.3
Havering	+12.6	-2.8	+4.6	+18.8	-35.3
Hillingdon	+11.6	-6.4	-1.8	+10.9	-5.5
Hounslow	+14.9	-7.6	+1.3	-46.6	-45.0
Kingston	+7.0	+3.5	not known	+107.2	-4.4
Merton	+20.7	-1.4	+16.7	+21.1	+55.9
Newham	-8.1	-5.2	+12.6	+115.1	-82.9
Redbridge	+34.8	+2.5	-0.5	+52.7	-5.1
Richmond	+10.6	-5.4	-1.8	-3.4	-23.8
Sutton	+5.5	+10.1	-1.5	-0.9	+64.5
Waltham	+5.5	+0.9	-3.8	-23.7	-11.8
Net difference between actual and expected for outer London	+325.4	-9.2	+ 88.6 (incomplete data)	+728.8	277.6

(i) excludes ECRs

(ii) To compensate for the Census undercount, all Wing 'estimates have been increased by 1.02 for Outer London Boroughs. (See Table 7, 1991 Census user guide 58, 'Undercoverage in Great Britain'.

Table 6 Difference between actual and predicted levels of service provision in Inner London – Strathdee and Thornicroft 1992 version of MINI

Borough **(ii)**	Difference between actual and predicted for **acute beds** (i)	Difference between actual and predicted for **intensive care beds**	Difference between actual and predicted for **medium secure beds**	Difference between actual and predicted for **24-hour staffed places (including hostel wards)**	Difference between actual and expected for **day staffed, respite and lower staffed beds** (unlike Tables 1 & 2, does not include supported tenancies for which no estimates in MINI)
Camden	**- 36.3**	**- 0.1**	**not known**	**not known**	**not known**
City of London	+ 0.3	+ 0.4	+ 0.8	+ 9.5	**- 0.9**
Greenwich	**- 7.9**	**- 3.3**	+ 3.8	+ 40.9	**- 80.2**
Hackney	+ 2.4	+ 22.2	+ 35.3	**- 11.9**	**- 88.0**
Hammersmith & Fulham (iii)	+ 1	+ 5.8	**not known**	+ 19.5	**- 118.8**
Islington	**- 37.0**	**- 0.1**	**not known**	+ 131.5	**- 110.2**
Kensington & Chelsea (iii)	+ 10.2	+ 1.6	**not known**	+ 25.4	**- 16.0**
Lambeth	**- 38.8**	+ 12.5	+ 22.9	+ 161.9	+ 1.4
Lewisham	**- 34.1**	**- 0.6**	+12.6	+ 18.4	**- 74.3**
Southwark	**- 21.6**	+10.1	+ 13.7	+ 79.8	**- 88**
Tower Hamlets	+ 10.2	+ 0.2	**not known**	+ 23.3	**- 63.5**
Wandsworth	**- 51.2**	**- 4.5**	+ 13.9	+ 16.8	**- 154.0**
Westminster (iii)	**- 34.5**	+ 7.8	**not known**	+ 147.3	**- 89.5**
Net difference between actual and expected in inner London	**-239.3**	+ 52	+ 103 (data incomplete)	+ 662.4 (data incomplete)	**-882** (data incomplete)

Positive figures indicate that actual provision is greater than predicted by MINI, negative ones that MINI suggests a deficit. All apparent deficits appear in bold.

(i)   excludes ECRs

(ii)   To compensate for the Census undercount, all Strathdee and Thornicroft estimates have been increased by 1.04 for Inner London Boroughs. (See Table 7, 1991 Census user guide 58, 'Undercoverage in Great Britain'.)

(iii)   There was incomplete medium secure bed, respite bed and residential place information for these Boroughs because each is partly served by Riverside Trust, which did not give data for these categories.

Table 7 Difference between actual & predicted levels of service provision in Outer London – Strathdee and Thornicroft 1992 Version of MINI

Borough (ii)	Difference between actual and predicted for **acute beds** (i) (iii)	Difference between actual and predicted for **intensive care beds**	Difference between actual and predicted for **medium secure beds**	Difference between actual and predicted for **24-hour staffed places – including hostel wards and continuing care wards**	Difference between actual and expected for **day staffed, respite and lower staffed places** (unlike Tables 1 & 2, does not include supported tenancies for which no estimates in MINI)
Barking	- 19.8	- 2.2	+ 1.9	+ 35.2	- 43.4
Barnet	+ 5.6	+ 11.9	+ 0.6	+ 97.8	- 95.8
Bexley	+ 19.7	- 1.9	+ 6.1	+ 87.9	- 69.4
Brent	- 25.1	+ 3.4	+ 6.4	+ 105.1	+ 42.7
Bromley	- 25.2	- 7.2	+ 5.2	+ 56.2	- 69.1
Croydon	- 35.1	+ 1.0	- 3.8	+ 95.0	- 130.7
Ealing	- 16.0	+ 15.0	+ 22.9	+ 84.6	- 90.9
Enfield	- 8.5	- 3.6	+ 20.1	+ 68	- 98.0
Haringey	- 11.4	+ 8.3	not known	+ 100.1	- 96.4
Harrow	- 10.0	- 5.1	- 1.7	+ 66.0	- 27.2
Havering	- 10.0	- 2.3	+ 4.6	+ 45.1	- 74.1
Hillingdon	- 12.8	- 5.7	- 1.8	+ 38.6	- 39.8
Hounslow	- 14.0	- 6.1	+ 1.3	- 19.0	- 90.7
Kingston	- 8.7	+ 4.1	not known	+ 123.9	- 29.2
Merton	- 2.6	- 0.3	+ 16.7	+ 43.7	+ 20.3
Newham	- 46.8	- 2.4	+ 12.6	+ 144.6	- 142.2
Redbridge	+7.7	+ 3.6	- 0.5	+ 80.2	- 48.8
Richmond	- 9.9	- 4.5	- 1.8	+ 17.6	- 57.0
Sutton	- 13.3	+ 10.7	- 1.5	+ 19.6	+ 33.4
Waltham	- 26.7	+ 2.9	- 3.8	+ 4	- 60.7
Net difference between actual and expected for outer London	**- 262.7**	**+ 19.6**	**+ 83.5** (data incomplete)	**+ 1294.2**	**- 1167.0**

(i) excludes ECRs

(ii) To compensate for the Census undercount, all Strathdee and Thornicroft estimates have been increased by 1.02 for Outer London Boroughs. (See Table 7, 1991 Census user guide 58, 'Undercoverage in Great Britain'.)

Table 8 Difference between actual and predicted levels of service provision in Inner and Outer London – PRiSM 1996 version of MINI (Service Categories 1-3)

Inner London Boroughs	Category 1) Medium Secure Unit			Category 2) Intensive Care Unit/local Secure Unit			Category 3) Acute Ward (iii)		
	Actual	Expected	Difference	Actual	Expected	Difference	Actual	Expected (iii)	Difference
CAMDEN	NG	19.9	NK	7.1	13.5	-6.4	65.2	119.0	-53.8
CITY	0.9	0.3	0.6	0.6	0.2	0.4	2.2	2.1	0.1
GREENWICH	7.4	12.7	-5.3	3.2	9.7	-6.5	72.5	89.5	-17.0
HACKNEY	42.1	20.8	21.3	29.4	14.0	15.4	106.8	122.9	-16.1
HAMMERSMITH (i)	NG	16.8	NK	12.1	11.6	0.5	86.8	102.5	-15.7
ISLINGTON	NG	20	NK	6.9	13.4	-6.5	62.8	117.6	-54.8
KENSINGTON (i)	NG	15.3	NK	7.5	10.7	-3.2	91.6	94.5	-2.9
LAMBETH	32	27.7	4.3	22.7	19.0	3.7	104.1	167.2	-63.1
LEWISHAM	18.5	19.2	-0.7	7.8	14.0	-6.2	76	125.7	-49.7
SOUTHWARK	20.5	21.3	-0.8	18.5	14.9	3.6	92.9	132.7	-39.8
TOWER HAMLETS	NG	15.0	NK	6	10.4	-4.4	90	92.6	-2.6
WANDSWORTH	21	23.1	-2.1	5.3	16.6	-11.3	79.4	149.4	-70.0
WESTMINSTER (i)	NG	20.7	NK	15.3	14.1	1.2	71.5	124.2	-52.7
TOTALS (iv)	**142.4**	**125.1**	**17.3**	**142.4**	**162.1**	**-19.7**	**1001.8**	**1439.8**	**-438.0**

Outer London Boroughs	Category 1) Medium Secure Unit			Category 2) Intensive Care Unit/local Secure Unit			Category 3) Acute Ward		
	Actual	Expected	Difference	Actual	Expected	Difference	Actual	Expected (iii)	Difference
BARKING	3.9	7.4	-3.5	1.9	5.9	-4.0	30.1	54.8	-24.7
BARNET	4	13.4	-9.4	20	11.1	8.9	102	104.2	-2.2
BEXLEY	7.6	6.6	1.0	3.3	6.0	-2.7	75.5	58.1	17.4
BRENT	12	19.2	-7.2	12	14.2	-2.2	88	128.2	-40.2
BROMLEY	7.5	9.7	-2.2	0	8.6	-8.6	54	83.0	-29.0
CROYDON	0	14.8	-14.8	10	12.2	-2.2	71	114.7	-43.7
EALING	28	18.2	9.8	24	14.0	10.0	99	128.3	-29.3
ENFIELD (ii)	23	11.6	11.4	3.5	9.6	-6.1	75.4	90.5	-15.1
HARINGEY	NG	20.4	NK	16.2	14.3	1.9	98.6	127.3	-28.7
HARROW	0	7.2	-7.2	0	6.3	-6.3	47	60.2	-13.2
HAVERING	6.2	6.8	-0.6	3.1	6.2	-3.1	48.1	60.3	-12.2
HILLINGDON	0	7.6	-7.6	0	6.8	-6.8	50	65.7	-15.7
HOUNSLOW	4.2	10.8	-6.6	0	8.7	-8.7	60.4	81.3	-20.9
KINGSTON	NG	5.3	NK	7.6	4.5	3.1	31.7	43.0	-11.3
MERTON	19	8.6	10.4	4.7	7.0	-2.3	57.4	65.3	-7.9
NEWHAM	18	17.7	0.3	5	12.7	-7.7	53	114.3	-61.3
REDBRIDGE	2	9.6	-7.6	9.6	8.0	1.6	77.7	75.5	2.2
RICHMOND	0	7.2	-7.2	0	6.1	-6.1	43.1	57.1	-14.0
SUTTON	0	6.1	-6.1	15	5.3	9.7	35	51.0	-16.0
WALTHAM	0	13.3	-13.3	9.4	10.2	-0.8	56.3	92.9	-36.6
TOTALS (iv)	**135.4**	**196.1**	**-48.7**	**145.3**	**177.8**	**-32.5**	**1253.3**	**1655.6**	**-402.3**

(i) Hammersmith and Fulham, Kensington and Chelsea and Westminster are each partially served by Riverside Trust, which did not provide data for medium secure beds, respite beds or (Trust funded) residential places. Other categories of data for Riverside Trust were derived from the MILMIS data. (ii) Enfield is partially served by Haringey Healthcare Trust, which gave no data for medium secure places, so the figure given must be seen as incomplete. (iii) actuals exclude ECRs. (iv) All expected values for Boroughs where actuals are not known were excluded from calculations of totals.

Table 9 Difference between actual and predicted levels of service provision in Inner and Outer London – PRiSM 1996 version of MINI (Service Categories 4-6)

	Category 4) 24 hour nurse staffed units			Category 5) 24 hour non-nurse staffed units			Category 6) Day staffed accommodation		
Inner London Boroughs	Actual	Expected	Difference	Actual	Expected	Difference	Actual	Expected	Difference
CAMDEN	NG	33.7	NK	NG	198.8	NG	NG	40.5	NG
CITY	0.3	0.6	-0.3	11	2.9	8.1	2	0.7	1.3
GREENWICH	69	24.0	45.0	49	126.6	-77.6	17	29.2	-12.2
HACKNEY	16.6	34.9	-18.3	77	207.6	-130.6	0	42.0	-42.0
HAMMERSMITH	37	28.9	8.1	72	168.3	-96.3	13	34.8	-21.8
ISLINGTON	21.6	33.5	-11.9	213	199.7	13.3	19	40.2	-21.2
KENSINGTON	37.9	26.5	11.4	70	153.0	-83.0	44	32.0	12.0
LAMBETH	26.7	47.3	-20.6	281.4	277.3	4.1	58	56.9	1.1
LEWISHAM	18.5	34.6	-16.1	109	192.4	-83.4	49.6	41.9	7.7
SOUTHWARK	12.8	37.1	-24.3	182.6	213.0	-30.4	76.4	44.8	31.6
TOWER HAMLETS	10	25.9	-15.9	94	149.6	-55.6	40	31.3	8.7
WANDSWORTH	43.9	41.3	2.6	102.7	230.8	-128.1	21.1	49.9	-28.8
WESTMINSTER	25	35.2	-10.2	231	207.2	23.8	22	42.3	-20.3
TOTALS	**319.3**	**369.8**	**-50.5**	**1492.7**	**2128.2**	**-635.5**	**362.1**	**445.9**	**-83.8**
Outer London Boroughs	Category 4) 24 hour nurse staffed units			Category 5) 24 hour non-nurse staffed units			Category 6) Day staffed accommodation		
	Actual	Expected	Difference	Actual	Expected	Difference	Actual	Expected	Difference
BARKING	33	14.5	18.5	48.3	74.4	-26.1	6	17.7	-11.7
BARNET	90	27.1	62.9	95	134.3	-39.3	0	33.3	-33.3
BEXLEY	72	14.5	57.5	64	66.1	-2.1	0	18.0	-18.0
BRENT	157	35.1	121.9	57	191.9	-134.9	8	42.5	-34.5
BROMLEY	22	20.9	1.1	103	96.9	6.1	17	25.9	-8.9
CROYDON	25	29.9	-4.9	166	147.6	18.4	22	36.6	-14.6
EALING	34	34.5	-0.5	159	182.4	-23.4	26	42.0	-16.0
ENFIELD	16.9	23.5	-6.6	126.9	115.8	11.1	0	28.9	-28.9
HARINGEY	34	35.6	-1.6	174.9	203.6	-28.7	48	42.9	5.1
HARROW	75	15.3	59.7	41	71.9	-30.9	21	18.9	2.1
HAVERING	68.8	15.0	53.8	26.1	68.1	-42.0	0	18.6	-18.6
HILLINGDON	18	16.5	1.5	75	76.1	-1.1	0	20.4	-20.4
HOUNSLOW	15.3	21.4	-6.1	34	108.3	-74.3	3	26.2	-23.2
KINGSTON	87	11.0	76.0	72.8	52.8	20.0	0	13.6	-13.6
MERTON	35	17.2	17.8	63.5	86.2	-22.7	30.9	21.0	9.9
NEWHAM	94	31.6	62.4	148	177.3	-29.3	0	38.2	-38.2
REDBRIDGE	59	19.6	39.4	84.4	96.5	-12.1	16	24.1	-8.1
RICHMOND	13.7	14.8	-1.1	51.6	72.5	-20.9	0	18.2	-18.2
SUTTON	12	13.0	-1.0	50	61.0	-11.0	92	16.0	76.0
WALTHAM	0	25.1	-25.1	82.6	133.3	-50.7	0	30.5	-30.5
TOTALS	**961.7**	**436.2**	**525.5**	**1723.1**	**2217.1**	**-494.0**	**289.9**	**533.4**	**-243.5**

Table 10 Difference between actual and predicted levels of service provision in Inner and Outer London – PRiSM 1996 version of MINI (Service Category 7)

Inner London Boroughs	*Category 7) Lower support (actuals)*			Category 7 Lower support accommodation		
	Unstaffed	*S&T Respite*	*Supported S-C Flats*	Actuals	Expected	Difference
CAMDEN	NG	11.2	18.0	29.2	81.1	-51.9
CITY	0	0	NK	0	1.3	-1.3
GREENWICH	20	6	200.0	226	58.5	167.5
HACKNEY	67	1	NK	68	84.0	-16.0
HAMMERSMITH	0	2	0.0	2	69.5	-67.5
ISLINGTON	9	13.9	0.0	22.9	80.5	-57.6
KENSINGTON	64	0	NK	64	63.9	0.1
LAMBETH	150	11	0.0	161	113.7	47.3
LEWISHAM	40	4	NK	44	83.8	-39.8
SOUTHWARK	0	10	75.0	85	89.5	-4.5
TOWER HAMLETS	18	0	9.0	27	62.6	-35.6
WANDSWORTH	22.3	1.6	NK	23.9	99.9	-76.0
WESTMINSTER	46	4	15.0	65	84.6	-19.6
TOTALS				**818**	**972.8**	**-154.8**
Outer London Boroughs	*Category 7) Lower support (actuals)*			Category 7 Lower support accommodation		
	Unstaffed	*S&T Respite*	*Supported S-C Flats*	Actuals	Expected	Difference
BARKING	25	1	NK	26	35.5	-9.5
BARNET	51	0	4.0	55	66.6	-11.6
BEXLEY	17	1	0.0	18	36.0	-18.0
BRENT	202	2	0.0	204	85.0	119.0
BROMLEY	36	1	NK	37	51.7	-14.7
CROYDON	9	0	2.0	11	73.3	-62.3
EALING	54	2	15.0	71	84.0	-13.0
ENFIELD	20	10	0.0	30	57.7	-27.7
HARINGEY	18	2	NK	20	85.8	-65.8
HARROW	17	23	NK	40	37.7	2.3
HAVERING	17	0	0.0	17	37.3	-20.3
HILLINGDON	51	7	19.0	77	40.9	36.1
HOUNSLOW	19	0	NK	19	52.4	-33.4
KINGSTON	32	1	0.0	33	27.2	5.8
MERTON	79	1.4	0.0	80.4	42.0	38.4
NEWHAM	7	0	5.0	12	76.5	-64.5
REDBRIDGE	42	0	2.0	44	48.1	-4.1
RICHMOND	24	0	18.0	42	36.3	5.7
SUTTON	16	0	NK	16	32.0	-16.0
WALTHAM	63	1	NK	64	60.9	3.1
TOTALS				**916.4**	**1066.8**	**-150.4**

The Strengths and Weaknesses of this Approach

The procedures described in sections 7.5 and 7.6 offer one view of how far London's mental health services meet expected need. The advantage of this view is that it is explicit, it is based upon reasonable assumptions of the expected capacity which should be provided in each Borough on the basis of local social characteristics, it relates (for the 1996 estimates) to actual provision and known occupancy rates, and it allows costing to be based upon these figures. These figures, however, are best estimates and should be viewed cautiously. They provide predictions for the provision of in-patient and residential care services only. We do consider it likely that intensive extended hours or 24 hour home treatment services can, for example, substitute for some of the requirement for in-patient beds, but as yet the evidence for how far such an offsetting effect will operate in routine urban clinical practice (as opposed to operating in small select patient groups under optimal experimental conditions) is weak, and indicates a pressing need for such cost-effectiveness research. Second, a key issue in considering the substitutability of services for in-patient beds is the displacement of new long term patients from acute beds to 24 hour staffed (especially nurse staffed) residential places. The current substantial under-provision of such places leaves clinicians deciding between over-provision (patients remaining in acute beds) or under-provision (patients being discharged to low support accommodation), and being likely to undergo early readmission to hospital.

Interpreting the Results

Three sets of estimates have been presented in this section as illustrations of how many services could be expected in the London Boroughs under three sets of conditions. It is our view that the Wing (1992) and Strathdee & Thornicroft (1992) versions substantially underestimate the requirements for services in that they indicate overprovision in some categories of service, which the evidence from the other sections of this mental health report consistently show to be operating well beyond their reasonable capacity. Our own interpretation of these findings, therefore, is that the PRiSM 1996 data offer the closest correspondence to the quantitative and qualitative information presented in other chapters here.

The first model, that of Wing, suggests that most Boroughs currently have an excess of most types of provision (details are presented in Appendix 16.6). The only exception is in the category of day-staffed and unstaffed accommodation, where both models strongly suggest a deficit. These findings based on Wing's model are highly problematic, in that they are seem to fly in the face of the ample evidence presented elsewhere in this report that London's services are under great pressure. The tension between this version of the model and the evidence we currently have about reality is sufficiently great that the model does not at present seem to offer a useful framework for considering services in most parts of London. The only way in which one might envisage London's mental health services functioning adequately with the very much lower levels of in-patient, 24-hour staffed and secure beds predicted by the Wing version of the MINI would be if community services became able to offer very much more intensive home support than at present. This might allow community support to be substituted on a large scale for in-patient and residential. However, as yet we do not have good evidence that such a substitution is possible, and indeed there is some

London-based work which has suggested that more intensive community care may result in an increased demand for beds, resulting from better identification of people needing care (Tyrer et al., 1995; Conway et al., 1994).

The second model, based on the ranges proposed by Strathdee and Thornicroft, (1992) suggested that across nearly all of Inner and Outer London, the current provision of 24-hour staffed accommodation is excessive and while there is a shortfall in day and lower support provision. In Outer London the apparent surplus of 24 hour staffed places is close in extent to the apparent deficit at lower levels of support, whilst in Inner London the apparent shortfall of lower support places is about one and half times the apparent excess of 24 hour staffed accommodation.

The finding in this model of an apparent excess of 24-hour supported beds is one which may cause some bewilderment, as it fits neither with the evidence discussed in Chapters 6 and 8 that access to this form of provision is sometimes problematic, nor with recent central policy statements encouraging the development of more highly supported accommodation. The apparent discrepancy means that this finding requires scrutiny with a particularly critical eye. There are a number of possible explanations. First, this category includes remaining continuing care beds in hospitals and hostel wards, and it may be that these still largely contain an old long stay population awaiting resettlement, rather than being accessible to or appropriate for a newer generation of patients. Second, some of this accommodation may qualify as '24-hour staffed', but night-time support may in fact be of a fairly minimal variety, with a sometimes unqualified member of staff sleeping on the premises overnight. Most registered nursing homes and registered care homes will qualify as 24 hour staffed, but the level of support really available at night, and in particular, the capacity of staff for coping with very disturbed behaviour may in reality be very limited. Thus it may be appropriate to regard much of this accommodation as in practice having a lower level of support – this would lead to an overall better fit between this model and reality. Third, as discussed in more detail in Chapter 10, many older established 24 hour staffed houses may in fact be largely occupied by older, very long term residents, whose long-term homes they have become, regardless of whether they still require this intensity of support. Thus places in some of these establishments may very rarely become available, the atmosphere and conditions may not be acceptable to younger people who have not experienced long-term institutionalisation, and staff may not be equipped to deal with a high through-put of young, acutely disturbed individuals. Finally, it is also possible that this apparent surplus is directly related to the apparent deficit in lower staffed provision – some patients may be placed in 24 hour staffed accommodation when more appropriate lower support accommodation is unavailable.

In the third model, that by PRiSM 1996, as would be expected from the previous examination of information about provision per 100,000, there is considerable variation, with some Boroughs having considerably less than the expected levels of some types of provision, others considerably more. However, some overall patterns may be identified. Acute beds are one of the categories where variation appears greatest between areas, but overall, both Inner and Outer London emerge as having substantially fewer acute beds than the model predicts. This fits with the evidence discussed in Chapters 6 and 8, which suggests great pressure on acute beds in London.

The overall picture from model 3 is that services in all categories (with the exception of Medium Secure beds in Inner London) are insufficiently provided throughout the capital. The excess in some Boroughs of Medium Secure over Intensive Care beds raises a question about whether the current balance between these two types of provision is correct. The apparent shortage of acute beds might contribute to this apparent excess provision. However, a more likely explanation may be that the need for this most extreme element of mental health care shows an even sharper concentration in some inner city areas than does the need for more general specialist mental health services. If this is the case, a new needs index will be required for this type of provision. Inspection of the data on provision per 100,000 in Tables 1 and 2 seems to suggests this. Most of the most deprived inner city areas, are using high levels of secure provision regardless of local level of acute bed use, whereas some of the more affluent areas are using none, or only minimal quantities of this provision.

In interpreting the calculations based on all three models, several points should be emphasised. First, this exercise provides estimates for each category assuming that the other categories of service are present in sufficient quantity. If some types of service, for example, are entirely absent, patients requiring them are likely to be inappropriately placed, and either receive to high or too low a level of support. Second, these are estimates based on the overall social indicators for each area (based upon a combination of the values of the constituent electoral wards) and cannot take into account specific local factors beyond the general social-demographic characteristics, such as levels of homelessness or refugees. These can therefore be seen as baseline figures which will need to be modified in the light of detailed local information. Third, the categories should not necessarily be taken literally. The apparent shortfall for acute in-patient beds, for example, may lead local purchasers to commission more beds, or to invest in alternatives to such beds, which might include home treatment teams, acute day hospitals, crisis houses or other forms of short term and intensive support. Fourth, the estimates in Table 3, Column D are somewhat conservative, and do not substantially exceed the what is already actually provided in some parts of the capital. Fifth, the cost calculations in Chapter 11 use these actual and expected data alongside London unit costs for each category of service to explore the financial implications of these models.

Acknowledgement
We are very grateful to Dave Shiress, Special Needs Housing, London Borough of Southwark, and to Lyn J. Hampton, Housing Liaison Officer, Lewisham and Guys Mental Health NHS Trust for very helpful guidance regarding the data collection for our survey.

Appendix Using the MINI to estimating a district's needs

The Mental Illness Needs Index (MINI) is a score indicating how great an areas requirement for specialist mental health services is likely to be. The computer programme which calculates it produces a predicted one year period prevalence of admission (persons likely to spend at least some time in hospital within a year) based on data from the North East Thames Region for 1991. For district health authorities in England (1991 boundaries) this figure ranges from 140.8 (Huntingdon) to 467.9 (Bloomsbury and Islington) persons per 100k population. Published estimates of need suggest district ranges. e.g. Wing suggests a district will need between 50 and 150 beds per 250k total population. The calculation for each facility type and for each chosen area thus rests on three assumptions:

1 The district with the lowest predicted prevalence should require the lower end of the range and that with the highest, the upper end.
2 If a district had a predicted prevalence of zero, it should require zero places (i.e. the plot of places required against predicted prevalence should pass through the origin).
3 The gradation should be smooth.

The range in numbers of places recommended has proportionately greater variation for some types of facility than for others. For acute beds, both sets authors concluded that the highest need was three times the lowest. However for regional secure beds, Strathdee and Thornicroft found consensus that there was a tenfold range in need. In order to satisfy all these requirements an equation was constructed using the concepts of a 'base rate' (b), the number of places which would be required if the admission prevalence (ap) was 100 people per 100k population aged 15-64, and an 'elasticity factor' (ef). The requirement per unit population was calculated as:

$$\text{requirement} = b \times (ap^e)$$

Base rates and elasticity factors were derived for each type of facility to meet the range conditions set out by a process of iteration. Within the relevant range of predicted admission prevalence for districts this gave only very slightly curved distributions.

Chapter 8

The structure and functioning of London's mental health services

Sonia Johnson, Liz Brooks, Rosalind Ramsay and Graham Thornicroft

Summary

A survey of mental health service organisation, functioning and availability in all London provider Trust catchment areas was carried out in early 1996. Its findings are reported in detail in this chapter, and give rise to the following major conclusions:

- London's general adult mental health services are in transition towards a community- based model. Elements in community services which require no major initial expenditure, such as sectorisation and the creation of multidisciplinary teams, have largely taken place, but in many areas community based premises such as community mental health centres are not yet available.
- In most areas, services are not as yet able to deliver sufficiently intensive acute community-based treatment for such services to be a realistic alternative to admission to an acute ward.
- For most major components of comprehensive community services, there are significant shortages in many areas of London, so that few areas seem likely to be able to deliver reliably the 'spectrum of care' advocated in recent policy guidance. Services such as employment schemes and carer support are reported to be entirely unavailable in some areas.
- There are very large variations in service availability, both between Trusts and within Trust catchment areas. It appears that residents of a few areas have most major services available without serious delays or shortages, whilst the population of neighbouring Trusts or even neighbouring sectors are experiencing significant gaps in the provision of essential services.

8.1 Introduction to the PRiSM Study of the Structure and Functioning of London's Mental Health Services

Many of the empirical studies of London's mental health services, in common with the PRiSM study reported in chapter 7 of this book, have focused primarily on provision of in-patient and residential places. The second element in PRiSM's London-wide data collection broadens this focus, and yields information on various important aspects of the structure and functioning of the mental health service system in each Trust. There are two particular focuses. First, the models of service organisation adopted have been surveyed, with an emphasis on studying how far Trusts have moved towards the community-based multidisciplinary teams advocated in a series of recent reports, such as 'Building Bridges' (Department of Health, 1995a), 'Finding a Place' (Audit Commission, 1994a)and the Mental Health Task Force Report on London (Department of Health, 1994a). Second, we have elicited from Trusts ratings of the local availability of a range of forms of care which make up part of the spectrum required for local provision of comprehensive mental health services (Department of Health, 1996a).

A brief questionnaire was developed, examining the extent of sectorisation, the development of multidisciplinary Community Mental Health Teams, the availability of home interventions, emergency assessment practices, service user involvement in planning, and availability and delays experienced in accessing a range of hospital and community services. The questionnaire was briefly piloted by circulating it to the members of the group preparing this report and asking them to attempt to apply it to services with which they were familiar: no more extensive piloting was feasible within the limited time available. The questionnaire is available on request from the authors.

The questionnaire was sent by post to all NHS Trusts in Greater London who are contracted to provide services for mentally ill adults (18–65). The boundaries of these Trusts are shown in Map 1. Trusts were first contacted to attempt to identify appropriate respondents: usually the questionnaire was directed in the first place to the Manager of the Community Directorate. Respondents involved in completing the questionnaires included consultant psychiatrists, business managers, general mangers of mental health services, locality managers, directors of operations and directors of mental health. In most cases, the questionnaire seemed to have been passed around several individuals in the local services before all or most of it could be completed. In the case of the Trusts involved in MILMIS (see section 6.3), questionnaires were first directed via the Royal College of Psychiatrists Research Unit to the consultant psychiatrists participating in the MILMIS study. Where no response was obtained from them, the same channels as for other Trusts were used.

Respondents were asked to complete the questionnaire for all mental health services provided for adults with mental illness within their catchment area, including those delivered by local authorities and by the voluntary sector. Where possible, the responses were recorded during a telephone interview, which gave the opportunity to discuss responses, although not all respondents could make time available for this.

The questionnaires were sent out between February and March 1996, but data-collection continued into July, as some trusts required several telephone and faxed reminders before a response was obtained. The Trusts who were slowest to respond received a letter from the chair of the Kings Fund London Commission to their Chief Executive, as well as letters from PRiSM. Finally a response was obtained from all 27 NHS trusts delivering acute mental health services in London.

One of our major aims was to compare service functioning and availability in the more and less deprived areas. The 27 Trusts were divided up according to Jarman's UPA score, calculated individually for each Trust on the basis of the Trust's stated catchment area for acute mental health services. The 13 most deprived Trusts, all with scores greater than 19, were grouped together as 'Higher Jarman' score trusts. The group of 14 'lower Jarman' score Trusts all had an UPA score of less than 15.5. Table 1 shows London Trusts and their UPA scores:

Table 1 London Trusts and their Jarman Under-Privileged Area Scores

Trust	Jarman UPA score
'Higher UPA score' Trusts	
Tower Hamlets	50.4
City & Hackney	43.3
Newham	40.6
Bethlem & Maudsley ('Camberwell' catchment area)	35.6
West Lambeth	35.0
Parkside	33.5
Camden & Islington	33.1
Lewisham & Guys	31.9
North West London	29.3
Haringey	28.5
Riverside	24.8
West London	22.7
Pathfinder	19.4
'Lower UPA score' Trusts	
Oxleas	15.0
Forest	14.5
Hounslow & Spelthorne	13.3
Redbridge	12.3
Croydon	11.1
Barnet	11.0
Hillingdon Hospital	9.6
Harrow & Hillingdon	9.6
Richmond, Twickenham & Roehampton	9.3
Enfield	6.3
Barking, Havering and Brentford	5.9
St Heliers	5.9
Kingston	2.2
Ravensbourne	-0.2

Although this grouping was made on the basis of deprivation rather than location, it approximates fairly closely to most classifications of 'inner' and 'outer' London, but has the advantage of grouping areas such as Newham and Haringey with the inner city Boroughs, which appears justified for our purposes in that they have deprivation scores as high as most of the adjacent 'inner London' areas.

8.2 Organisation of mental health services in the London acute mental health trusts

8.2.1 Sectorisation

Twenty-six of the 27 London Trust catchment areas have now sub-divided their catchment areas into smaller sectors: the only remaining Trust, Parkside, reports that only its small catchment area size has prevented this taking place. The Mental Health Task Force on London, reporting in 1994 (Department of Health, 1994a), believed that effective follow-up of patients by community health teams was being hampered by lack of clearly defined catchment area populations for these teams. Our data suggest that

Trusts have sought to clarify this and create clear sub-divisions for service provision. Figure 1 shows the ways in which this sectorization is organised in higher and lower Jarman score areas.

Figure 1 Sectorisation of mental health services in London catchment areas

A Higher UPA areas

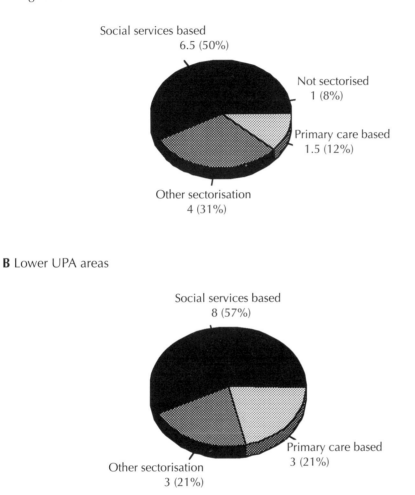

Social services based
6.5 (50%)

Not sectorised
1 (8%)

Primary care based
1.5 (12%)

Other sectorisation
4 (31%)

B Lower UPA areas

Social services based
8 (57%)

Primary care based
3 (21%)

Other sectorisation
3 (21%)

In both higher and lower UPA score areas, the largest group of Trusts have sector boundaries which are coterminous with social services catchment areas. This promises to be a good basis for the joint provision and planning by health and social services which has been vigorously advocated in a series of reports and policy documents including 'Building Bridges' (Department of Health 1995a) and the Mental Health Task Force's report (1994a).

However, an important dilemma for mental health Trusts is that co-terminosity with social services is achieved at the expense of basing catchment area populations on General Practitioners' lists, so that each GP is liaising with a single mental health team. As discussed in more detail in section 5.8 of this report, the latter system is likely to improve joint working between primary and secondary care and the maintenance of continuity of care. Primary care based sectorisation is less prevalent than co-terminosity with social services, having been adopted in 3 lower UPA score areas and in the whole of one higher UPA area and part of another. A recent study by Bindman et al (1997) in Camberwell suggests that involvement of GPs in the care of the severely mentally ill in the inner city is low, and that they are often inadequately informed about patients' care. A factor which may contribute to this finding is the fragmentation of the primary care structure in the inner city, with a large number of widely dispersed practices, often single-handed, responsible for the care of patients resident in each sector. This fragmentation may make basing sectors on GP lists a more complicated and daunting strategy – however, it also probably increases the need for such ways of improving joint working. It may be significant that health centre based sectors are a little more prevalent in outer, lower UPA score areas, where large health centres and fundholders are commoner than in higher UPA score areas. Further consideration is needed of the most effective ways of organising catchment populations so as to facilitate inter-agency work with both primary care and social services. In part of one Trust catchment area, mental health social services have now also adopted general practice based catchment areas – this promises to be a helpful solution to this dilemma.

Four higher UPA and 3 lower UPA areas have adopted some other form of sectorisation, generally geographical but not based on either GP lists or social services boundaries. This seems likely to be a wasted opportunity, as service organisation does not maximise integration with any other agencies.

Table 2 shows sector population sizes in the sectorized Trusts:

Table 2 Sector population size

Sector population sizes in Trust	Higher UPA Trusts (n = 11)	Lower UPA Trusts n = 14	All Trusts n = 25
All sectors: more than 75,000 population	1 (9%)	4 (26%)	5 (20%)
Mixture of greater and less than 75,000	4 (36%)	3 (21%)	7 (28%)
All sectors: less than 75,000 population	6 (55%)	7 (50%)	13 (52%)

Thus in much of London sector sizes are relatively small. There is some evidence of a tendency towards smaller sector populations in higher UPA trusts, which may reflect greater levels of need within a population of a given size in these areas.

8.2.2 The extent of development of community-based services

A major aim of this survey was to assess how far Trusts had now developed a suitable infra-structure for delivery of community based services. Basic organisational principles for developing community services have been identified as including: (i) sub-division of catchment areas into sectors (already discussed above) (ii) development of community mental health teams in which the major mental health professions work jointly to deliver a comprehensive service; and (iii) establishing community-based premises within sectors (often known as Community Mental Health Centres or Mental Health Resource Centres), so that services are geographically accessible to the local population and teams can readily work extensively in patients' homes within the sector (Strathdee and Thornicroft, 1992).

In order to assess the degree to which multidisciplinary community mental health teams now form the basis of community work in London, we asked Trusts what proportion of their community nursing staff now worked in such teams rather than in single discipline CPN services. Figure 2 shows the responses:

Figure 2 Proportion of Community Psychiatric Nurses who are members of a multidisciplinary mental health team

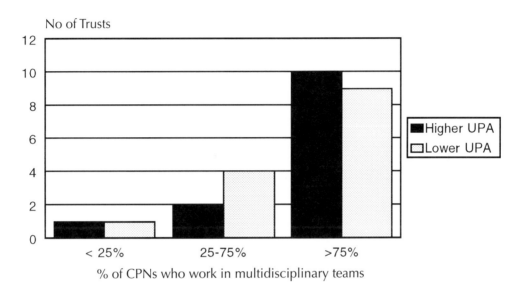

These data suggest that most London Trusts have made substantial progress in setting up multidisciplinary mental health teams, which are the basic service delivery unit favoured in recent national policy documents (Department of Health, 1995a) . We also requested information about the availability of community bases for such teams, referred to subsequently in this report as Community Mental Health Centres (CMHCs). Figure 3 indicates whether CMHCs are available throughout the Trust's catchment area, in parts of the catchment area, or not at all.

Figure 3 Extent of availability of Community Mental Health Centres

Higher UPA Trusts   Lower UPA Trusts

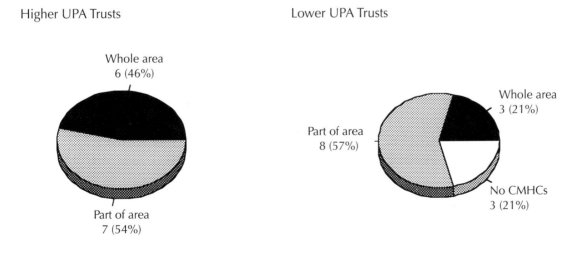

Thus CMHCs are being widely adopted in London, with only 3 Trusts indicating that they have no such facilities as yet. The more underprivileged inner London areas seem to have progressed further than the rest in providing CMHCs throughout their catchment areas. However, in many Trusts coverage is only partial, suggesting that many areas are still in transition to a fully community-based model.

A second indicator of the extent to which relocation to community bases has taken place is the degree to which out-patient consultations with medical staff now take place away from the hospital, in sites such as CMHCs and primary care health centres. Figure 4 indicates the proportion of out-patient consultations which currently take place on hospital sites:

Figure 4 Proportion of out-patient consultations with medical staff taking place at community sites

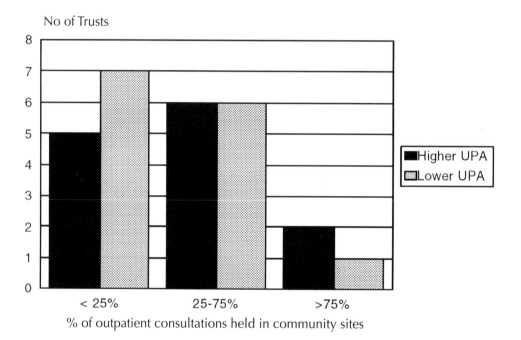

Thus much out-patient work still takes place on hospital premises rather than community sites. When the main elements of the structure required for community based care are considered, it seems overall that a geographical shift to community sites has not been achieved as extensively as sectorization or multidisciplinary team creation. This may be because reorganising staff into multidisciplinary sector teams may be done without extra expenditure, but providing them with a CMHC is likely to require significant initial outlay. Less deprived areas seem to have been slightly slower to move away from the hospital base: possible explanations might include a greater need for outreach services in deprived inner city areas, greater expenditure on mental health in the inner cities or a tendency to set up innovative services more readily in the major research centres, most of which are in inner London.

8.2.3 Mental health team organisation

Traditionally there has been some separation between acute and longer term services, at least for the purposes of establishing specialised rehabilitation services. Recently, some have proposed that community mental health teams should be a generic form of provision, combining acute and continuing care services in a single seamless service. Figure 5 shows how far acute and rehabilitation services are provided by a single mental health team:

Figure 5 Are acute and rehabilitation teams separate or integrated?

Higher UPA areas

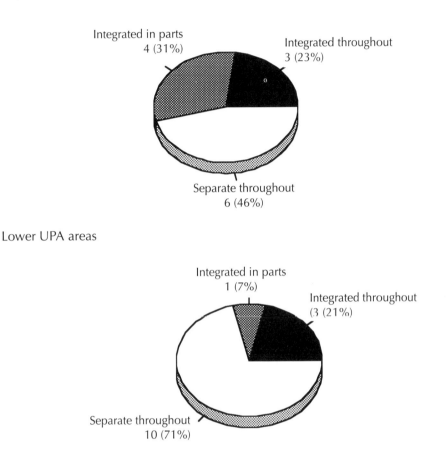

Integrated in parts
4 (31%)

Integrated throughout
3 (23%)

Separate throughout
6 (46%)

Lower UPA areas

Integrated in parts
1 (7%)

Integrated throughout
(3 (21%)

Separate throughout
10 (71%)

'Integrated in parts' indicates that some areas within the Trust catchment area have adopted a combined team model, others separate acute and rehabilitation teams.

Most Trusts seem so far to have favoured the retention of separate rehabilitation services. Further, 2 of the 6 Trusts who have integrated acute and rehabilitation teams throughout specify that in addition to these local teams they have a centralized rehabilitation service which provides a specialist service to the whole catchment area. Whether to retain separate rehabilitation services is a question on which little evidence or guidance is available to service planners. Most model programmes for which research evaluations have been carried out are integrated acute and continuing care services, so that London services are not in general adhering to these models. However, the separate team model may have advantages in terms of maintenance of specialist rehabilitation skills and prioritisation of long term care, an area which Cochrane et al's (1994) report for the Task Force suggested was neglected in London compared with other areas of the country.

8.2.4 Organisation of emergency services

Trusts were also asked to provide data about which sites were routinely used for assessment of patients referred to psychiatric services in an emergency within and outside usual office hours. Figures 6 to 8 show (i) how many Trusts identified each setting as **the site most frequently used to assess patients** referred for emergency assessments in the Trust catchment area (ii) how many Trusts rated each setting as **one of the three sites most frequently used** for emergency assessments: and (iii) how many Trusts rated each setting as **a site of which any use was made for emergency assessment**. When assessing how often the casualty department was used, respondents were asked to exclude assessment of patients who had initially presented to casualty officers and been referred on by them.

Figure 6 Sites for emergency assessment (i) most frequently used site

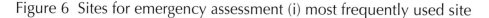
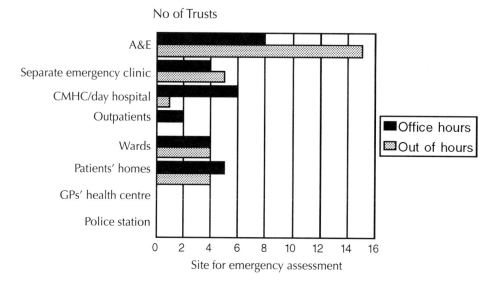

In 4 instances two sites were nominated as jointly the most frequent

Figure 7 Sites for emergency assessment (ii) three most frequently used sites

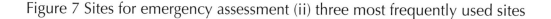
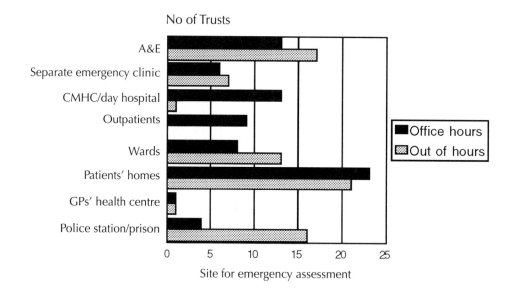

Figure 8 Sites for emergency assessment (iii) – sites of which any routine use is made

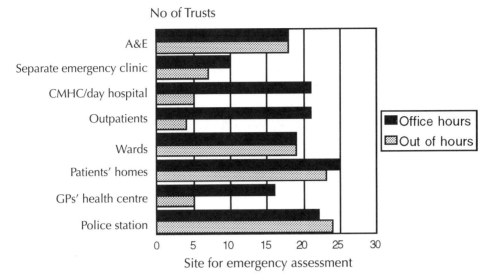

A concern expressed by the Task Force on London (Department of Health, 1994a) was that general hospital Accident and Emergency (A & E) departments often appeared inappropriate environments for the emergency psychiatric assessments for which they were in routine use. Aspects of A & E departments which tend to make them unsuitable for this purpose include lack of staff training, lack of appropriate security arrangements, poor staff training in the management of mental illness, and the impact on disturbed patients of being in a noisy, busy and highly charged environment. Our data indicate that A & E departments continue to be in widespread use in many London mental health Trusts. As in a national survey of emergency services (Johnson and Thornicroft, 1995), this seems especially to be the case out of hours, when they are the most frequently used emergency assessment site in 15 London Trusts. The appropriateness of this extensive use of casualty departments for emergency psychiatry needs to be considered.

A number of other sites on hospital premises are also in routine use for assessing emergency referrals. A minority of hospitals have separate psychiatric emergency clinics on hospital sites. Wards are used for assessments both in and out of hours, and the out-patient department is used in office hours in a minority of trusts. Police stations and/or prisons figure more significantly in out of hours services than during working hours.

With regard to assessments based in the community, CMHCs or day hospitals are first on the list in office hours in only 6 Trusts, but more often figure among the three most frequently used sites. However, their use is generally limited to office hours. In 5 Trusts, patients' homes are the sites where assessments most often take place, whilst in most Trusts they are among the top three sites both in and out of hours. Health centres are not frequently used for this purpose. Thus there is evidence that a substantial proportion of emergency assessment work does take place in the community, but this service seems to be taking place alongside hospital-based emergency provision rather than replacing it, and community-based work features more prominently in office hours provision than out of hours.

The degree to which emergency assessment is routinely multidisciplinary was also assessed. 17 of the 27 Trusts stated that emergency assessment by more than one discipline was part of routine practice throughout the catchment area, and 5 in parts of the catchment area. Five reported that multidisciplinary assessment was not usual (respondents were asked not to include assessments which involved both a doctor and an Approved Social Worker purely for the purpose of completing assessment for detention under the 1983 Mental Health Act). However, only 5 Trusts continued routine multidisciplinary assessment on weekday evenings, 4 during the day at weekends, and 3 on weekend evenings. Thus multidisciplinary emergency assessment is largely a feature only of office hours practice, probably reflecting 9 to 5 working hours of community mental health teams and CMHCs.

8.2.5 User participation in service planning

User participation in service planning has received increasing emphasis during the 1990s. We asked whether service users were routinely involved in planning catchment area services, and whether any funding was available to support this involvement. Table 3 shows the results:

Table 3 User participation in service planning

	Higher UPA n = 12	Lower UPA n = 14	All Trusts n = 26
Whether users involved in service planning	8 (67%)	11 (79%)	19 (73%)
Whether funding available for this involvement	8 (67%)	9 (64%)	17 (65%)

Thus the majority, though not all, report some form of user involvement in service planning. The form taken by such involvement included patients' councils, representatives on planning meetings, involvement in project teams and in service evaluation, and representation in planning via MIND. In most instances this was accompanied by some form of funding, although this was often limited to provision of a room and of refreshments – a few Trusts specified that they did pay for time spent at meetings, including one Trust where £15 per hour is paid for attendance at groups involved in planning and commissioning.

8.2.6 Provision for ethnic minorities

As chapter 3 has shown, one of London's dominant characteristics is its remarkable ethnic diversity, and, as discussed in Chapters 4 and 5.10, a series of reports and enquiries have emphasised the need for specific measures to be taken to provide appropriate services. Two approaches are available to increasing the appropriateness of services. Firstly, segregated services for a single ethnic group may be established. This has the advantage that these services can focus entirely on providing an appropriate service for a particular group, and can try to recruit staff who are all from that group. However, there are also substantial limitations to this approach (Bhui et al, 1995a;

Ismail, 1996). It is not likely to be possible to replicate every element in the service system for each ethnic group: particularly for specialist services and for smaller minority groups, some provision will necessarily be mixed. The local service as a whole therefore needs to become culturally sensitive, and this process may be impeded if the segregated services are perceived as fully dealing with the particular needs of ethnic minorities and if staff from ethnic minorities tend to go and work in these separate services. Further, members of ethnic minorities will not invariably want or benefit from segregation of service provision and ethnic matching of thereapists.

In order to study the approaches taken to meeting the needs of ethnic minorities, we asked Trusts both to list separate, specific services for ethnic minorities in their areas, and to describe more general initiatives aimed at making the generic services more culturally sensitive. Tables 4 and 5 show the responses.

Bethlem Royal and Maudsley and Haringey Trusts are omitted as they did not respond to this section. The answers to these question were often very brief notes, and it seems unlikely that they are fully comprehensive in all cases. However, they form a basis for some observations to be made on the ways in which services for ethnic minorities seem to be developing in London.

With regard to separate services for ethnic minorities, the predominant types of provision seem to be day centres, drop ins or support groups, with few residential services, vocational services or services working with patients in their homes. Thus even in those Trusts where services for ethnic minorities are relatively numerous, members of ethnic minorities will continue to rely on the generic services for most types of care, making it essential, as is discussed in section 5.10 of this report, for these generic services to become as culturally appropriate as possible. The very limited development of separate residential services may be a significant omission, as sharing accommodation long term with people with different values, customs and dietary habits may be particularly difficult for members of some ethnic and religious groups.

Some information is also available on who provides these services, although not from all Trusts. The voluntary sector has been identified as the main provider of services for ethnic minorities (e.g. Ismail, 1996), and our data suggests that it is an important source of such services, although there do also appear to be a substantial number of local authority day centres for particular ethnic groups.

In the more deprived areas, most catchment areas seem to have some form of specific provision for the ethnic groups which predominate there, with up to three different ethnic groups represented among the specific services of some catchment areas. This obviously makes some sense in terms of meeting needs, but it does mean that specific services are mainly available to those who live in areas where there is a high concentration of their particular ethnic group. Thus there is little specific provision available for Asians in Lambeth or for Black Caribbeans in Tower Hamlets, and no dedicated facilities for those groups who are significantly represented across London, but do not reach very high concentrations in any particular area, such as South Americans, Eastern Europeans or people from various Arab countries. Similarly, several of the less deprived areas, which have some residents from ethnic minorities, but often a smaller proportion than the inner areas, seem to be without specific services. These

Table 4 Provisions for ethnic minorities in London Trust catchment areas: Higher UPA Score areas

Trust	Specific ethnic minority services	Initiatives within generic service
Camden & Islington	(i) Social services day centre – black people with SMI (severe mental illness); (ii) Psychotherapy service – various ethnic minorities; (iii) joint NHS/ LA drop in – people with SMI, various ethnic minorities	(i) Ethnic minorities steering group with strong user representation – promoting access to services; (ii) advocacy service for ethnic minorities
City & Hackney	(i) Centre for Africans & Caribbeans with SMI (ii) Muslim day centre (iii) Vietnamese day centre (iv) Asian women's day centre	Clinical nurse specialist responsible for liaison with ethnic minorities
Lewisham & Guys	(i) Drop in for Afro-Caribbeans; (ii) Group for Afro-Caribbean women; (iii) Vietnamese group; (iv) Turkish group (All voluntary sector, funding from purchasers & social services)	(i) Needs assessment carried out to discover Afro-Caribbeans' experiences of mental health services (ii) Ethnically appropriate catering; (iii) positive recruitment for substance misuse worker from ethnic minority (iv) Clients asked ethnic preference regarding CPN (but cannot always be met)
Newham	(i) Social services day centre for Asians; (ii) Social services day centre for Afro-Caribbeans	(i) Outreach workers at the day hospitals; (ii) Positive recruitment policy in place; (iii) range of social services initiatives
North West London	(i) Social services day centre – Asians; (ii) Social services day centre – Afro-Caribbeans; (iii) Jewish residential programme (iv) Trust plans Afro-Caribbean crisis intervention service	None reported
Parkside	Black users forum – Afro-Caribbeans	Local authority has appointed a development officer to review targeting of ethnic minorities by services
Pathfinder	(i) Residential service & counselling – Black people; (ii) Day & advice centre – Black & Asian women (Both voluntary sector)	Intensive outreach worker project
Riverside	(i) Residential service, advocacy & counselling – Afro-Caribbeans with SMI; (ii) Women's group at Irish Centre; (iii) Namibian centre – people with SMI	*Did not respond to this section*
Tower Hamlets	(i) Day centre- Bengalis with psychosis; (ii) Day centre for Somalis with psychosis	(i) Bengali and Somali healthcare workers attached to community teams and wards; (ii) Research programme planned to examine morbidity
West Lambeth	(i) Residential service for Afro-Caribbeans with SMI (24 hour staff) ; (ii) Day centre for Afro-Caribbeans with SMI; (iii) Psychotherapy service for women from ethnic minorities; (iv) Residential alternative to hospital for Afro-Caribbeans with SMI	(i) Cultural awareness training; (ii) Ethnic food; (iii) 'Inreach' from local church and voluntary organisations
West London	(i) Group for refugees from Iran, Iraq & Bosnia; (ii) Group for Afro-Caribbean service users; (iii) Drop in for Asian people; (iv) Advocacy & resettlement – Asian people; (v) Asian women's group	Psychotherapy services

Table 5 Provisions for ethnic minorities in London Trust catchment areas: Lower UPA score areas

Trust	Specific ethnic minority services	Initiatives within the generic service
Barnet	(i) Day centre – Asians; (ii) Day centre – Jewish people with mental health problems; (iii) Day centre – Jewish people with mental health problems including dementia (*all voluntary sector*)	(i) 2 ethnic development workers, one Trust & one social services employed – liaison & education role; (ii) ethnically appropriate catering; (iii) staff training in cultural awareness
BHB	None reported	None reported
Croydon	(i) Workshop in Resource Centre – Asians and Afro-Caribbeans with depression; (ii) Vietnamese centre (voluntary sector)	(i) Interpreters available on all wards; (ii) Designated ethnic minority workers – one focuses on Asian men, one on Afro-Caribbean men; (iii) Policy on ethnic minorities available on all wards; (iv) Successful bid made for a series of seminars
Enfield	None reported	(i) Specific ethnic minority groups arranged within generic services – especially RSUs; (ii) Staff training in cultural awareness at Middlesex University; (iii) Research commissioned & report produced in 1995 on services available to ethnic minorities
Forest	(i) Day centre for Afro-Caribbeans with long term mental health problems; (ii) Day centre for Asians (elderly & adults) (*both voluntary sector*)	None reported (major changes in services taking place)
Harrow & Hillingdon	(i) Social services day centre – Asians; (ii) Voluntary sector support groups – Asians; (iii) Voluntary sector counselling service – Asians;	Specific social worker post
Hillingdon Hospital	Social services day centre – Asians	Consultation and training service for management of refugees with major mental illness – Health Authority
Hounslow	None reported	Attempt to recruit staff from variety of ethnic backgrounds
Kingston	None reported	None reported
Oxleas	(i) MIND network for Afro-Caribbeans with major mental illness; (ii) Voluntary sector Project for Vietnamese with major mental illness; (iii) Further services ('Afamba') for Afro-Caribbeans with major mental illness (nature not specified)	Under joint commissioning a report on needs of Afro-Caribbean people has recently been commissioned & received – working group set up to implement
Ravensbourne	Drop in for refugees with post-traumatic stress disorder	Joint strategy group including all stakeholders is considering how to improve access for ethnic minorities
Redbridge	(i) Meeting room in day centre for Asian women (ii) Day centre in Newham available to Afro-Caribbeans	(i) Nurse recruitment campaigns particularly targeting Asian women; (ii) Looking at ways to improve interpreting service
Richmond	None reported	None reported
St Helier	None reported	None reported

members of smaller or more dispersed ethnic minority communities may in fact have a greater need for culturally sensitive services, as they are likely to have less access than those in more concentrated communities to social support from others from the same background and to generic community resources for their group.

Increasingly, many Londoners are of mixed parentage and do not fit comfortably into the remit of any specific service. There are also often considerable cultural differences between newly arrived immigrants and UK born people from minority backgrounds, so that needs and wishes will vary considerably within ethnic groups. These are further reasons why, even where very effective and acceptable services have been set up for specific groups, their contribution to comprehensively meeting the needs of all Londoners from ethnic minority backgrounds is necessarily limited.

With regard to initiatives aimed at improving provision for ethnic minorities within the generic service, most Trusts except for the most prosperous outer London areas describe some form of action. In some instances, descriptions are rather vague, and it would have been necessary to ask more detailed and specific questions to get a clear sense of what is actually happening. However, a number of broad types of initiative may be identified, including:

- policy of positive recruitment or ensuring staff from particular ethnic backgrounds available (5 Trusts)
- appointment of specific workers with responsibility for developing appropriate services for minorities (4 Trusts)
- staff training programmes in cultural awareness (4 Trusts)
- groups set up to consider needs/access to services (4 Trusts)
- ethnically appropriate catering (3 Trusts)
- research to assess local ethnic minority needs (3 Trusts)

Most Trusts report one or two initiatives of these types, but few seem to have a comprehensive strategy which appears likely to make a major impact on local practice throughout the mental health services. Developing and implementing such a strategy throughout the generic mental health services is a considerably more complex task and is likely to require more resources than providing the specific separate services described, yet for the reasons we have discussed, bringing about such general change is of considerably greater overall importance.

8.3 Availability of services

The second main focus in this study was on service availability. As is discussed in chapters 7 and 10, attempting to count numbers of places provided or in use in various service types is of limited usefulness both because of poor information quality and lack of standardised methods of collecting data, particularly for non-residential services, and because in some facilities places may be largely occupied by long term users or residents, with very few places available for new referrals. We have therefore taken a different approach to assessment of whether Londoners' needs are currently met by services, and have asked Trusts to assess how available services of various important types can be delivered. The following three major indicators of service availability have been used: (i) frequency of service contact available; (ii) delays experienced gaining access to services; and (iii) proportion of those who would benefit from a service who can currently receive it. The most appropriate indicator or indicators were chosen for the measurement of availability of each type of service.

8.3.1 Availability of community-based treatment

Respondents were asked whether intensive home treatment was available, with home treatment defined as the provision of planned home visits to acutely ill patients at least on a daily basis during the working week. Table 6 shows the results:

Table 6 Availability of intensive home treatment – office hours

Availability of intensive home treatment	Higher UPA Trusts (n = 13)	Lower UPA Trusts (n = 14)	All Trusts (n = 27)
Usually available – whole catchment area	1 (8%)	1 (7%)	2 (7%)
Usually available – some parts of catchment area	3 (23%)	4 (29%)	7 (26%)
Available at times, but in practice only 25%-75% of time (demands on service too great at other times)	2 (15%)	0	2 (7%)
Available at times, but in practice less than 25% of time	2 (15%)	1 (7%)	3 (11%)
Not available	5 (38%)	8 (57%)	13 (48%)

The definition of intensive home treatment adopted here is a relatively minimal one compared with the model programmes reported in the literature (Stein and Test, 1980; Hoult and Reynolds, 1984; Dean et al, 1993; Muijen et al 1992; Burti and Tansella, 1995). Descriptions of these model services suggest that staff are usually available to spend several hours a day in the homes of acutely ill patients if required, and are on call for patients and their families 24 hours a day. Yet even by our rather minimal criterion, only two Trusts in London report that they are usually available to provide intensive home treatment for acutely ill patients in all parts of their catchment areas, whilst almost half report that such care is generally not available at all. It therefore seems that the 'care in the community' which most London services can currently provide is of a quite different and much less intensive type than the model services which published evaluations have shown to be effective alternatives to in-patient care. Home visits which cannot even be provided every working day seem unlikely to be an adequate substitute for many admissions to acute wards, particularly in the inner city where patients are often socially isolated or live in chaotic environments.

Trusts were also asked to specify the hours outside usual office hours when planned visits could be made to acutely ill patients. Figure 9 shows the results.

Figure 9 Planned out of hours home visits for acutely ill patients – availability in best served parts of Trusts

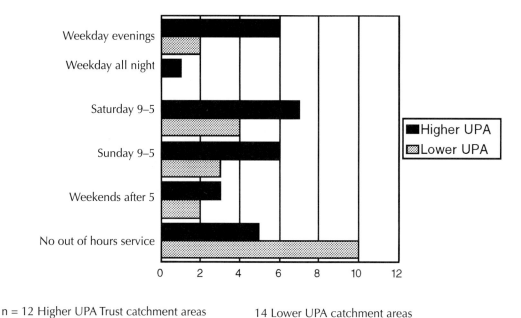

n = 12 Higher UPA Trust catchment areas   14 Lower UPA catchment areas

This figure shows service availability in the best-served parts of the catchment area. The out of hours service described was available throughout the whole catchment area in 3 of the 7 higher UPA areas who have some form of out of hours service and in only 1 of the 4 lower UPA trusts with an out of hours home visiting service. Thus some extended hours home visiting services are beginning to develop, particularly in the more deprived inner city areas, but their availability is still very patchy.

Another indicator used to assess the availability of community-based care was whether enough CPNs were available to meet all needs identified under the Care Programme Approach care plans. Figure 10 shows the results.

Figure 10 Whether enough CPNs are currently available to meet all needs identified under the Care Programme Approach

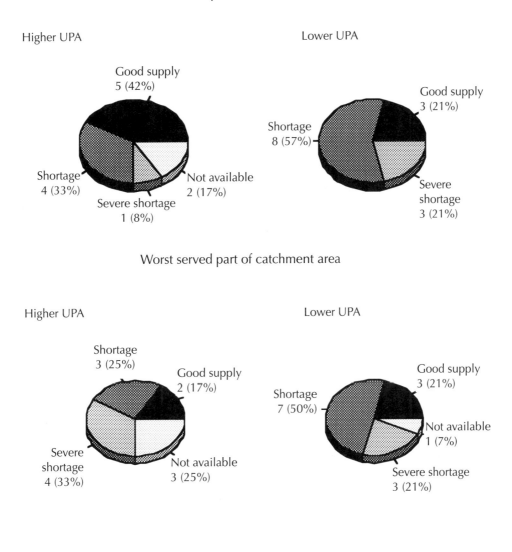

Best served part of catchment area

Higher UPA

Good supply
5 (42%)

Shortage
4 (33%)

Severe shortage
1 (8%)

Not available
2 (17%)

Lower UPA

Good supply
3 (21%)

Shortage
8 (57%)

Severe shortage
3 (21%)

Worst served part of catchment area

Higher UPA

Shortage
3 (25%)

Good supply
2 (17%)

Severe shortage
4 (33%)

Not available
3 (25%)

Lower UPA

Good supply
3 (21%)

Shortage
7 (50%)

Not available
1 (7%)

Severe shortage
3 (21%)

Good supply = can be provided for at least 90% of those who would benefit
Shortage = can be provided for fewer than 90% but more than 50% of those who would benefit
Severe shortage = provided for fewer than 50% of those likely to benefit
Not available = cannot currently be provided

Thus shortage of CPN services in relation to needs identified under the Care Programme Approach appears to be a significant problem in many areas, spanning both more and less deprived parts of London. Particularly among the more deprived Trusts, there is evidence of considerable variation within catchment areas, with a substantial difference between CPN availability reported for the best served areas within each Trust and the worst served.

A final indicator of the degree to which community services are able to meet identified needs in London is the delay which occurs before a CPN or a social worker can be allocated. Respondents were asked to report the average delay which occurred before allocation of each of these types of worker, and the longest delay of which they were aware in the past 6 months.

Figure 11 Delays in CPN allocation

Average delay – CPN allocation

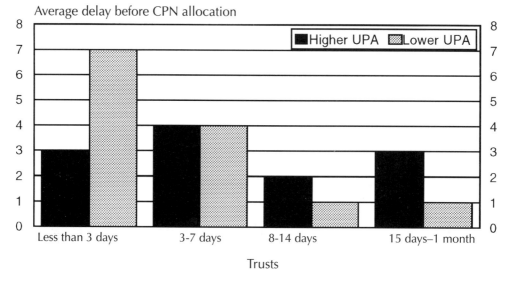

Average delay before CPN allocation

Trusts

Median estimates for 'average delay':
Higher UPA Trusts – 1 week   Lower UPA Trusts – 2 days
Median for all London – 1 week

Longest delay in past 6 months – CPN allocation

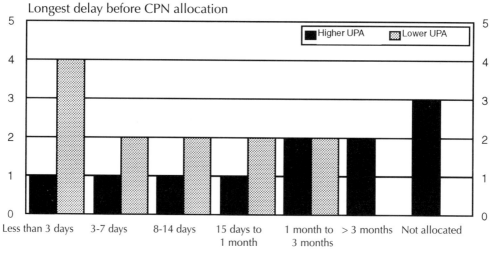

Longest delay before CPN allocation

Trusts

Figure 12 Delays in social worker allocation

Average delay – Social worker allocation

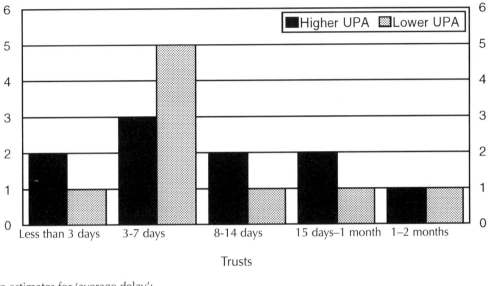

Median estimates for 'average delay':
Higher UPA Trusts – 1.5 weeks   Lower UPA Trusts – 1 week
All London – 1 week

Longest delay in past 6 months – Social worker allocation

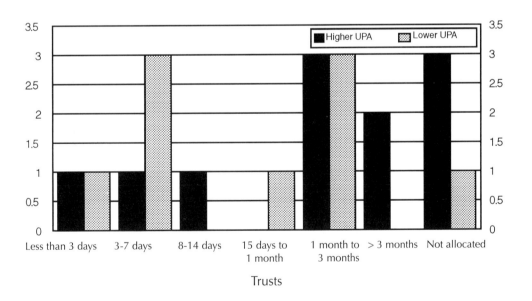

Thus these indicators again indicate some strain on community services in many parts of London, with many services appearing unlikely to be able to respond quickly and flexibly to all new presentations. There is some evidence of a tendency for greater delays to occur in the more deprived areas, but the picture is striking for the wide variations in speed of response within both higher and lower UPA score groups.

8.3.2 Hospital beds

The PRiSM survey complemented data collected in other studies on bed occupancy by taking a slightly different perspective on bed availability and requesting information on delays experienced in obtaining access for patients to acute, intensive care and Regional Secure Unit beds.

Table 7 Average delays before acute admission

Delay	Higher UPA Trusts (n = 12)	Lower UPA Trusts (n = 13)	All Trusts (n = 25)
Under an hour	3	4	7
1-4 hours	4	5	9
5-8 hours	0	1	1
9-12 hours	1	0	1
'hours'	1	0	1
'same day'	2	2	4
2-3 days	1	1	2
Median	4 hours	1.5 hours	

Table 7 shows the average delays reported for acute beds – as the table shows, some of the responses were too vague for very precise interpretation so that the results have not been represented graphically. Where a range of values is given by a respondent, medians have been calculated using a value at the midpoint of this range.

Figure 13 Longest delays experienced in past 6 months before acute admission

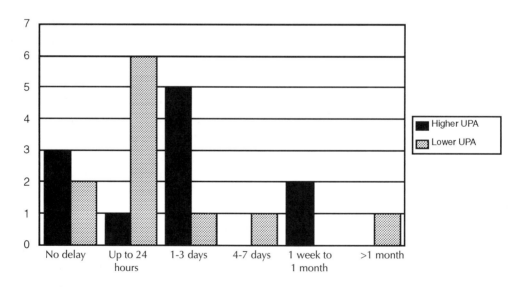

Thus again there are a very broad spread of responses, with some Trusts having apparently not experienced very severe delays at any time, and a few others reporting some remarkably long delays. In most Trusts it does generally appear possible to arrange admission to an acute bed within hours, although there is cause for concern about the Higher UPA Trust which reported an average delay of 2 days before acute admission, and the Lower UPA Trust which reported an average of 3 days. Figure 14 shows responses regarding delays experienced before an intensive care unit bed becomes available:

Figure 14 Average delay in getting access to intensive care unit bed

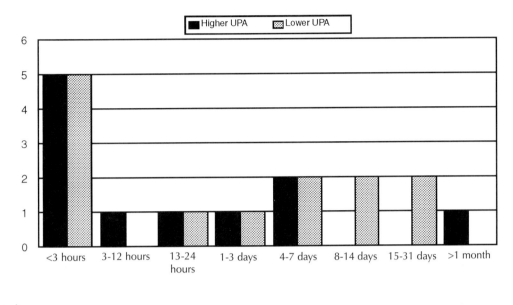

Median:
Higher UPA Trusts: 3 hours   Lower UPA Trusts: 24 hours
All London: 24 hours

The responses are remarkable for the very wide spread of responses, with some Trusts apparently having little difficulty getting access to this facility for patients and others experiencing delays which seem unreasonably long, particularly if patients are having to be managed in a less secure setting in the days or weeks which elapse before intensive care unit placement is possible. For this facility some of the longest average delays seem to be experienced in the less deprived areas, possibly because they are less likely to have substantial intensive care provision within their own services. An item on *longest delays experienced in the last 6 months obtaining access to intensive care facilities* were also included. In Higher UPA areas, 1 Trust reported no delays, one a 2 week delay and one a 3 week delay, whilst the remainder all reported delays between 2 and 5 days. For Lower UPA areas, 3 Trusts reported that no delays had been experienced and 1 Trust a maximum delay of 3 days. However, the other less deprived areas reported maximum delays between a week and a month, or in one instance a delay of 'months', with the need for an intensive care unit ending before a placement can be made.

Delays experienced in obtaining RSU placements was one of the areas where the response rate was poorest, with only 14 Trusts providing any information. Of those who responded among the Higher UPA Trusts, one reported a delay of 1 to 2 days and two others delays of less than a month. Average delays were greater than a month in the other 4 Higher UPA Trusts, with one outlier giving an average of one year wait for an RSU bed. One lower UPA Trust reported an average wait of 24-36 hours and three others waits of between 2 and 4 weeks. In each of the other three Lower UPA respondents, the wait was 3 months. Median values for the 'average delay' in getting access to an RSU bed were 5 weeks in 'higher UPA' areas and 4 weeks in 'lower UPA' areas.

8.3.3 Residential care

Availability of residential care was again assessed by asking Trusts to report average and longest times before local accommodation could be obtained. Figure 15 and Figure 16 show the waits reported for 24 hour staffed facilities and other supported facilities respectively:

Figure 15 Average delay in obtaining place in 24-hour staffed accommodation

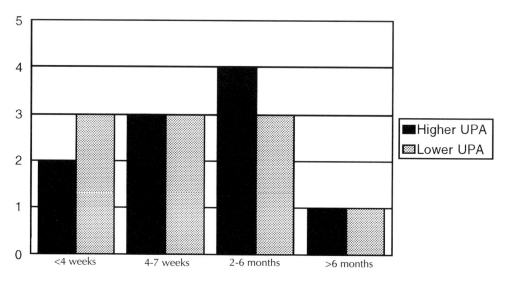

Median: Higher UPA Trusts: 2 months   Lower UPA Trusts: 6 weeks
All London: 7 weeks

Figure 16 Average delays for place in other supported accommodation

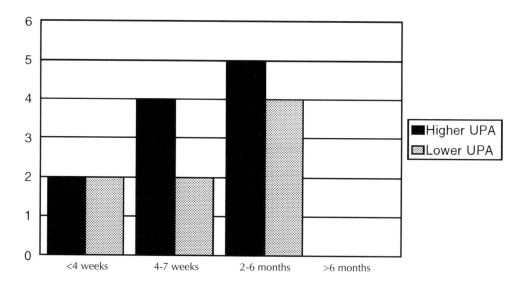

Median: Higher UPA Trusts: 6 weeks   Lower UPA Trusts: 2.75 months
All London: 2 months

Figures on longest delays indicated that for 24 hour supported accommodation waits of at least 6 months (and up to 3 years) had been experienced in 6 of the 7 Higher UPA Trusts who responded to the question and in 3 of the 9 Lower UPA responders. For other supported residential care, 6 out of 8 Higher UPA and 6 out of 8 Lower UPA responders reported delays of at least 6 months. Thus for both forms of supported care, substantial delays in placement appear to be frequent: in many Trusts waits of at least 2 months are usual, and certainly where patients to be placed are in hospital or in inadequate accommodation, this seems an unacceptable delay.

8.3.4 Day care

Indicators of availability were obtained for two forms of day provision: acute day hospital care and day or drop in centres. For day hospitals, Figure 17 indicates respondents' assessment of supply in relation to numbers of people likely to benefit:

Figure 17 Availability of day hospital places

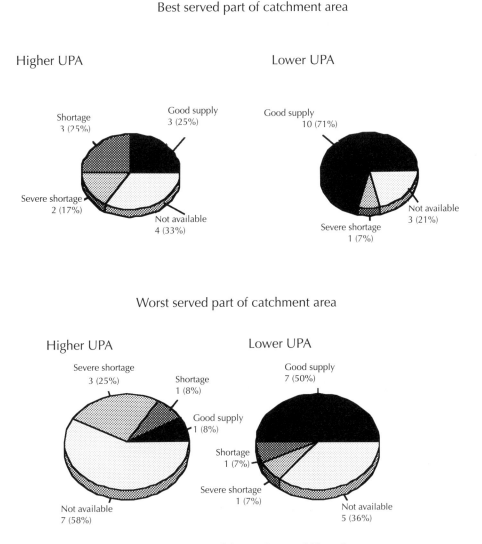

Good supply = can be provided for at least 90% of those who would benefit
Shortage = can be provided for fewer than 90% but more than 50% of those who would benefit
Severe shortage = provided for fewer than 50% of those likely to benefit
Not available = cannot currently be provided

The correct interpretation where Trusts report that no day hospitals are available is uncertain, in that in some cases the traditional functions of the acute day hospital may have been integrated into the service delivered by the community mental health centres, so that a similar form of care may be available in some of the Trusts which report they have no acute day hospital. However, overall these figures suggest that acute day hospitals are currently a more significant and readily available element in services in the less deprived areas of London. Information was also obtained on average delay before patients could be admitted to an acute day hospital. Among Higher UPA Trusts, 1 Trust reported that immediate admission was available, 1 Trust an average wait of 3 days, 2 Trusts waits of 1 week and 3 Trusts waits of between 2 weeks and a month. For Lower UPA Trusts, 5 Trusts reported that immediate admission was usual, 5 others that on average admission occurred within 3 days, 1 Trust a wait varying from same day to one week, and 1 Trust a wait of 2 to 3 weeks. The median for higher UPA Trusts was 1 week, compared with 2 days for lower UPA Trusts. Thus acute day hospital admission within three days appears to be possible in the majority of less deprived Trusts but in only 2 more deprived areas. This suggests that in many of the lower UPA areas, acute day hospitals provide a service which is capable of a swift enough response to be a feasible alternative to admission for some patients, but that this is uncommon in the more deprived areas.

As an indicator of the availability of long term day care, respondents were asked to assess the availability relative to identified need of day centre and drop in places.

Figure 18 Day centre and drop in place availability

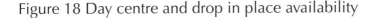

Best served part of the catchment area

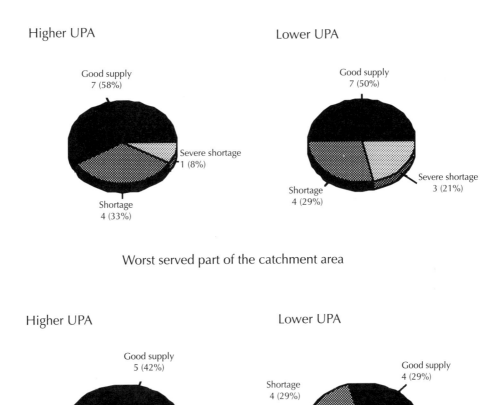

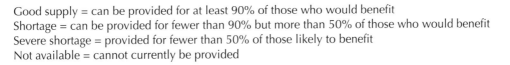

Worst served part of the catchment area

Good supply = can be provided for at least 90% of those who would benefit
Shortage = can be provided for fewer than 90% but more than 50% of those who would benefit
Severe shortage = provided for fewer than 50% of those likely to benefit
Not available = cannot currently be provided

Thus some shortages of long term day provision are reported in areas distributed across the more and less deprived parts of London, although within each group of Trusts around half report that at least the best served parts of the catchment areas have a good supply of such facilities.

8.3.5 Work-related services

Information about two forms of work related service was obtained: Figure 19 shows availability of sheltered work in settings specifically designated for the mentally ill, whilst Figure 20 shows availability of services providing training and opportunities for work in open market settings.

Figure 19 Availability of sheltered work in settings specifically for the mentally ill

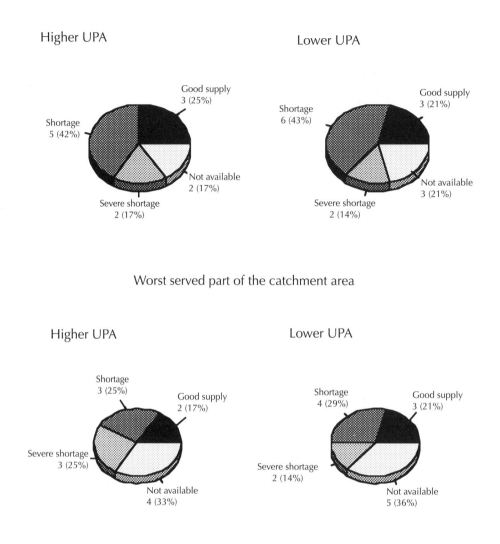

Good supply = can be provided for at least 90% of those who would benefit
Shortage = can be provided for fewer than 90% but more than 50% of those who would benefit
Severe shortage = provided for fewer than 50% of those likely to benefit
Not available = cannot currently be provided

Figure 20 Training and opportunities in open market employment

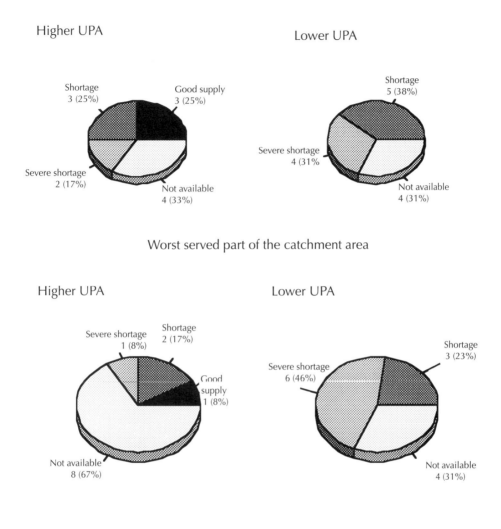

Best served part of the catchment area

Higher UPA

Shortage 3 (25%)
Good supply 3 (25%)
Severe shortage 2 (17%)
Not available 4 (33%)

Lower UPA

Shortage 5 (38%)
Severe shortage 4 (31%)
Not available 4 (31%)

Worst served part of the catchment area

Higher UPA

Severe shortage 1 (8%)
Shortage 2 (17%)
Good supply 1 (8%)
Not available 8 (67%)

Lower UPA

Severe shortage 6 (46%)
Shortage 3 (23%)
Not available 4 (31%)

Good supply = can be provided for at least 90% of those who would benefit
Shortage = can be provided for fewer than 90% but more than 50% of those who would benefit
Severe shortage = provided for fewer than 50% of those likely to benefit
Not available = cannot currently be provided

Thus both these forms of employment scheme are in short supply even in the best-served areas of London, and are completely unavailable in several Trusts or parts of Trusts. This supports the argument put forward in Chapters 9 and 10 that employment schemes do not appear to have been given a high priority in recent service planning and development, despite high levels of unemployment and lack of activity among the severely mentally ill in London (as discussed in Chapter 3). This situation contrasts with developments in the USA in the late 1980s and 1990s, where there has been a movement towards community programmes in which the central emphasis is on vocational rehabilitation and support in obtaining and maintaining competitive employment. This movement in the US appears to have been a result of users and carers expressing strong preferences for services which help them get a paid job and of a body of research which indicates that with appropriate support this is a feasible goal for a high proportion of the mentally ill (Drake et al, 1994; Hoge et al, 1992; Kasper et al, 1993).

8.3.6 Other major components of community services

Information was requested in the same format regarding six other important elements of comprehensive community services. These were (i) liaison clinics or attachments of secondary care staff in primary care; (ii) court diversion schemes; (iii) specific outreach and treatment services for the homeless (iv) family interventions and support for carers of the severely mentally ill; (v) interpreting services and (vi) advocacy services. The responses are summarised in Table 8 – this indicates for each of these services the number of Trusts in which the service was either not available or in severely short supply, according to the definitions used in the charts above. Data in this figure refer to the worst-served parts of catchment areas: discrepancies between best and worst served parts of catchment areas are not as great for most of these service types as for those previously discussed, perhaps because most are less likely to be provided on a sectorised basis.

Table 8 Availability of other major elements in community services
(All figures relate to worst-served parts of catchment areas)

Service	Higher UPA Trusts where service unavailable or severe shortage	Lower UPA Trusts where service unavailable or severe shortage	Trusts where service unavailable or severe shortage – all London Trusts
Primary care liaison/attachment of secondary care professionals	8/11 (72%)	6/13 (46%)	14/24 (58%)
Court diversion schemes	4/10 (40%) (& 'not applicable' in 1 Trust)	6/13 (46%)	10/23 (43%)
Specific outreach & treatment schemes for the homeless	2/9 (22%) (& 'not applicable' in 2 Trusts)	10/11 (91%) (& 'not applicable' in 3 Trusts)	12/20 (60%)
Family interventions & support for carers of the mentally ill	7/11 (64%)	7/14 (50%)	14/25 (56%)
Interpreting services	3/12 (25%)	4/14 (29%)	7/26 (27%)
Advocacy services	4/12 (33%)	6/14 (43%)	10/26 (38%)

Thus for three of these major service components, the service is reported to be unavailable or in very short supply in parts of the majority of London Trusts. For services for the homeless, the greatest shortages appear to be reported in the less deprived areas where less need would be expected, whilst respondents from the more deprived areas rate availability of this service fairly highly. However, it may be that in these outer areas there are small populations of the homeless mentally ill for whom no targeted services are provided.

The poor availability of interventions for families and support for carers is notable, given the demonstrated clinical efficacy of family interventions in psychosis and the repeated emphasis in central policy documents on work with and support for carers of the mentally ill. It is also remarkable that for 5 of the Higher UPA Trusts and 1 Lower UPA Trusts, it is reported that family work and carer support are not available at all in the worst served parts of their catchment areas.

8.4 Overview

The following general points about the current state of London's mental health services emerge from these data:

- London's mental health services appear to be in transition towards a community-based model. Elements in establishing community services which require no major initial expenditure, such as sectorisation and organising staff into multidisciplinary teams, have largely taken place. However, in many areas, community premises for service delivery are not as yet available.
- The general hospital A & E department still has a central place in emergency service delivery, particularly out of hours, despite some service delivery at community sites during office hours.
- Out of hours services are beginning to be developed in some parts of the city, but most community service provision is still limited to office hours.
- In most London catchment areas, acute home-based treatment services are not yet sufficiently highly developed for it to seem realistic to expect them to constitute an adequate substitute for admission. In some less deprived areas, acute day hospital response is sufficiently swift and available for it to appear likely that some patients can be diverted from admission using this facility – this is not generally the case in more deprived areas. Particularly in more deprived areas, CPN and social worker allocation appear too slow for the community service to be readily capable of a response which diverts admission. Thus overall our data suggest that in most parts of London community care has not yet developed to a point where it is likely often to be an adequate alternative to the acute ward.
- For most major aspects of care, there are very significant shortages and delays in many parts of London, so that few areas are likely to be available to deliver reliably the comprehensive 'spectrum of care' recommended in policy documents.
- For most service types, there is great variation between Trusts in availability. Londoners in different parts of the metropolis are likely to be experiencing very different supplies of major services. A small minority of London's Trusts do appear to be succeeding in delivering most major elements in care without serious delays and shortages arising.
- There are also large variations in service availability within Trusts. This draws attention to a need for researchers and planners to assess services in a detailed sector-by-sector way, as the view at the level of whole Trusts will miss many such variations. It also raises the question of whether an unforeseen consequence of sectorisation may be an increase in inequity – prior to sectorisation, most services within a District or Trust catchment area would presumably have been available to most residents, whereas now some small areas seem to experience great shortages of important services, despite their availability elsewhere in the catchment area.

Chapter 9

A functional approach to assessing services: the DISC framework

Helen Smith and Edward Peck

Summary

This chapter presents a conceptual model to assist planning and providing mental health services. The DISC (Developing Individual Services in the Community) framework identifies:

- the major categories of need of people using services
- the corresponding service functions – what the service needs to *do* to meet needs
- examples of good practice which fulfil each of these functions.

The framework is based on six major categories which structure information on need:

- access and information
- needs related to ordinary living and long term support
- personal growth and development needs
- needs in crisis
- needs for individual planning
- needs for treatment and support with mental distress

A comprehensive service will include the following components:

- a range of supported housing
- employment schemes
- advocacy and involvement
- crisis services
- services for mentally disordered offenders
- services for ethnic minority groups
- services for women

This chapter provides examples of the application of the framework to London's services.

9.1 Introduction

In previous chapters, the mental health needs of Londoners have been discussed and the services which currently attempt to meet these needs described. Conclusions so far suggest that provision is patchy, with identified need apparently exceeding supply in many parts of the city. This applies not only to services in the already hotly debated area of acute bed provision, but in a range of essential aspects of care, from intensive home support to support with employment and family intervention.

Whether sufficient resources are currently allocated to London's mental health care is obviously a question which must be addressed in considering how a better match may be achieved between needs and services. However, purchasers and providers in both health and social services also need strategies for planning comprehensive services. A number of structural and organisational obstacles may prevent the development of clear overall plans for good practice in local areas. These organisational obstacles to service improvement are discussed in depth in Chapter 12, which describes CMHSD's survey of obstacles to good practice currently facing London mental health managers.

Apart from these organisational obstacles, a further important impediment to service improvement is where planners lack an overall conceptual model on which to base development. The main focus of this chapter is on such a model, the DISC framework developed by CMHSD, which has been already been applied in a variety of settings. This is a needs based framework which for all groups of service users identifies:

1 The major categories of need of people using services.
2 The corresponding service functions – that is, what the service needs to do meet needs.
3 Examples of service responses which appear to fulfil each of these functions.

In this chapter, the framework and its conceptual basis will first be outlined. Its application to an analysis of purchasing plans throughout London will then be described. On the basis of this analysis, examples of existing and emerging practice which seek to fulfil major service functions are identified, and a commentary is made on the overall effectiveness of services in meeting the mental health needs of Londoners.

9.2 Background to the DISC framework

A key influence on service development in the 1980s and early 1990s was policy on needs assessment, usually emanating from the Department of Health. In the health service, the purchaser/provider split located responsibility for needs assessment and service delivery in purchasing and providing agencies respectively. Local authorities were directed to assess need through community care plans. However, it remains an imprecise science. Epidemiological assessments, community morbidity surveys, the use of social indicators (such as the Jarman UPA score), Diagnosis Related Groups (DRGs), indicators of service use all gather information about needs, yet this information is not generally in a format which allows conclusions to be drawn directly about what services should be developed. For example, information of this type may allow planners to calculate that in an area with a population of 30,000, about a hundred people (0.4%) are expected to have a diagnosis of functional psychosis and one in seven (4/5,000) will have neurotic disorder. Admission to hospital will be in the order of 5.71/1000 population, and so on. However, this is not information about peoples' needs: for example, how many of the people admitted actually need respite from an unbearable family situation, a skilled sympathetic ear, physical help to alleviate intolerable symptoms, help in shopping and caring for themselves adequately or in finding decent accommodation?

A further limitation of such models of needs assessment has been a tendency to think of responses strictly in terms of particular service types: for example a need for some form of meaningful daytime activity may be construed as 'they need a day centre place'. This limits service development to a small range of service dominated responses, when there may in fact be many other appropriate ways of meeting that need. Thus it is important that needs and service responses be separated, as failure to distinguish between the two will mean that solutions will almost always be defined by what already exists, rather than thinking of creative new ways of meeting particular needs.

A contrasting approach which has also emerged during this period was service planning based on 'getting to know' individual service users, an approach advocated particularly in the field of learning disabilities (O'Brien, 1987) This was a step forward in making a qualitative assessment of individual needs. However, it did not provide sufficient information to plan for a range of services, and tended to produce a long 'wish list' of needs which, being too long to ever be resourced, was quietly disposed of.

Another significant influence on service development in the late 1980s was the raised profile of health service management. This was particularly important in mental health services where, with a few notable exceptions, innovation in different models of response (as opposed to treatment) has been largely led by non-clinicians. Their influence was felt in the growing emphasis on creating a vision, involving a range of stakeholders and setting up dynamic, planning processes which recognised the evolving nature of mental health services as individual and community needs change. This approach was aided by the growth of user involvement – a movement supported by growing political pressure to expand consumerism in the health service as a whole.

A final important influence on service development has been the use of demonstration projects. In an attempt to show that community care works, the government funded a range of demonstration projects in mental health and learning disabilities services. However, there are serious pitfalls in assuming that such demonstration models can necessarily be transferred into service clinical settings, in that they may have succeeded because of charismatic leadership, exceptional staff commitment, ring-fenced funding, short timescale, or the freedom to determine whom they will select and how they will offer a service.

However, none of these approaches seems to have led to widespread development of services which users and carers feel meet their needs. As yet, few purchasing agencies have an understanding of what a comprehensive service would look like for their population, across the statutory and independent sectors. Still less have they grasped the necessity of developing a range of service options, *within each service area*, to meet the range of users' needs. For example, within a single service category such as crisis response, people's needs differ greatly (Smith, 1996): the long term user with a diagnosis of schizophrenia will have very different needs from the depressed mother who urgently needs a break from the demands of her family, from the adolescent admitted to A&E after taking an overdose and from the black homeless person admitted on section 136. Services need to provide a range of care settings and treatment approaches in order to deliver effective local services to such a variety of users.

As yet there have been few specific guidelines on what would constitute a comprehensive mental health service, based on user preferences and research evidence. MIND's *Common Concern* (MIND, 1983) was an influential document which attempted to define a comprehensive service, although the long lists of necessary services worked against its aim of being a 'manifesto for a new mental health service'. Purchasers and providers continue to be left to look at isolated examples of good practice, without a clear idea of how the model would function in the context of local history, strengths, weaknesses and values.

One solution to these difficulties is to view service development in terms of the service *functions* required to meet needs, and to adopt a *functional* approach to service development. In the mid-70s, the National Institute of Mental Health (NIMH) looked to develop a unified vision of a comprehensive mental health service. Subsequently, they have organised a series of conferences where the major interest groups with a stake in mental health (users, families, managers, professionals, researchers, planners and policy makers) have been brought together to encourage dialogue about the question 'what do people want from the service?'. NIMH have defined the major functions which should be components of a comprehensive service and require each state to develop services which can deliver each function. Examples of these functions include client identification and outreach, case management, rehabilitation, housing, peer support and crisis response services. Local mental health services are given the responsibility of organising this range of components into an integrated system. The value of this approach is that it does not impose a national 'blueprint' for services, but rather defines what they should be achieving and leaves it to local discretion to decide how these achievements should be delivered.

Recently, a number of UK initiatives have tried to describe an effective mental health service. The Mental Health Task Force (1994) produced a framework for purchasing services for people with severe mental health problems which identified the components of a 'well organised local system of support' across health and local authorities. This covers five areas: information, service planning and co-ordination, treatment, accommodation, individual support and development, and user, carer, staff and community involvement. It is intended as a checklist, to help purchasers see whether essential needs are being met.

More recently, the Spectrum of Care (Department of Health, 1996a) sought to summarise 'the components that make up the complete spectrum of care that should be offered to people with mental illnesses on a local level'. However its focus on health care deflects from the wider spectrum of social care and the role of the independent sector in meeting many health and social care needs, and its emphasis on models of care may detract from its application in local services.

Turner-Crowson (1992; 1993) in a study of mental health policy in the US and its implications for Britain, described the NIMH service framework, which was also subsequently recommended by the Audit Commission (1994a). Strengths of this framework are the emphasis on user outcomes and the integration of activities throughout the service system. The framework has been influential in the NIMH development of the DISC framework, described in the following section.

9.3 The DISC (Developing Individual Services in the Community) framework and the stakeholder approach

The tables which conclude this chapter describe all the major categories in the CMHSD's DISC framework (Developing Individual Services in the Community) and selected examples of services which fit into each of its categories: the full version of DISC is available from the authors. The framework is based on six major categories which structure information on need. These are: Access and Information; Needs related to Ordinary Living and Long Term Support; Needs for Treatment and Support with Mental Distress; Personal Growth and Development Needs; Needs in Crisis; and Needs for Individual Planning. The categories were conceptually derived from the NIMH framework as well as O'Brien's (1987) Balanced Service System, and the framework has developed, in practice, out of CMHSD's work in over 45 health authorities, 60 Trusts, and with the majority of regional offices over the last five years, and from extensive consultation exercises with stakeholders.

A full range of service functions have been defined in relation to these needs, where 'service function' refers to what a service actually needs to *do* to meet people's needs. To achieve a comprehensive service needs in each category need to be addressed. Configuring mental health services in this way means that the service 'map' looks rather different to the usual map of in/outpatient services, day hospitals/ centres, CMHTs, supported housing and so on. Traditionally, services have been described in terms which may not clearly indicate what they actually do, beyond imprecise descriptions. The strength of this functional approach is that the outcomes to be achieved and the needs to be addressed by each service are explicitly stated. This allows, for example, the evaluation of the extent to which the local day centre is meeting all the various needs local users have for personal growth and development, and what gaps remain in addressing these needs.

The framework takes into account the specific needs of particular groups of users, incorporating particular key service functions required in services for children adolescents and young people, substance misusers, mentally disordered offenders and older people.

A further aspect of need which is not assigned a separate category but should be considered throughout in applying the framework is the needs of women and people from minority groups. Although only specifically referred to at points throughout the tables, all 'Descriptions of Need' should be taken to include consideration of the needs of women and/or people from minority groups, including people from a range of ethnic and religious backgrounds, those who have migrated from other countries, lesbians and homosexual men. In each service, meeting these needs in full will require models of assessment and treatment based on an understanding of the social contexts in which service users live, choice of female/black workers, effective policies on equal access and on discrimination and abuse and the availability of separate women/black-only provision. Needs for childcare provision must also be considered, and workers require training in their responsibilities under the Children's Act. All services defined in the framework need to meet the needs of people for whom English is not a first language and people with sensory deficits.

9.4 London services in the context of the framework

The tables which conclude this chapter show:

(i) the needs categories and service functions which make up the DISC framework
(ii) examples of ways in which innovative services across London are responding to the needs identified in this framework.

The 'descriptions of needs' in these tables are a summary of those from the full version of the framework, while the service examples are a selection from a substantially larger number identified. The full framework and paper on service examples are available from the authors at CMHSD. The tables are based on information gathered by CMHSD from agencies' purchasing intentions, community care plans, mental health strategy documents and trust annual reports, research literature and good practice directories of London services, as well as from CMHSD knowledge of London services. Inclusion in the tables does not, *in any way*, indicate the quality of a service. Similarly, non-inclusion is due solely to the number of other illustrative services already noted or the authors' lack of knowledge of the service. These documents are not likely to provide a comprehensive view of actual provision in a health or local authority – such a picture is currently very difficult to obtain, which is likely to be a significant obstacle to planning. However, some general trends in London service provision may be identified.

9.4.1 Overview of London's services

Despite the limited information available, it appears clear that no London services are comprehensive in the way defined by the framework; that is, are offering a range of appropriate service responses which meet all major needs identified through a stakeholder process. The involvement of the independent sector appeared often to be *ad hoc* and not a planned 'management of the market' by health and social services, working in partnership to identify gaps in service provision and/or identify those needs best met by the voluntary and private sectors (the exception is probably advocacy services). Voluntary sector services in general tend to find partnerships with the statutory services problematic and uncertain, due partly to the opportunistic nature of their being funded in the first place – funded because they are there and seem to be a 'good thing', rather than as part of wider planned development of the service.

9.4.2 Alternatives to inpatient care and long term support

Some residential alternatives to inpatient care have been developed, and most services state that they offer some form of crisis service. However, it is not clear how far these crisis services have the capacity to maintain people actively in their own homes rather than acting simply as a speedier and less traumatic pathway to the admission ward. Treating people with dual diagnosis in crisis was rarely mentioned, despite the prominence of this issue on London's inpatient wards.

People's needs for long term support in ordinary living are being addressed by most authorities, although it is not clear how much emphasis is placed on ensuring that people have their own long-term tenancies, whatever their needs for support at home. There are a few services which do try to provide people with long term needs both with their own flat and with a high level of intensive support. However, most services link the provision of housing with support, thus forcing users to 'climb a ladder' of different kinds of accommodation as their care needs change, rather than allowing them to receive varying levels of support in their own permanent homes, as indicated by their current needs.

The significant presence of voluntary sector supported housing in London (particularly MIND) gives a welcome diversity to the range of services available. However, it is striking that many mental health agencies are unable to state what level of support users actually receive in the different residential establishments in their area. More worryingly, given the acute bed crisis, few agencies identified a comprehensive set of protocols and procedures for links between mainstream mental health services and independent sector care. Some local authorities continue to have large-scale hostels (20 places and above) where the quality of the building and internal environment, if not the care as well, is poor.

There are still very few services seeking to provide long term and active support for people the framework describes as having:

> a substantial history of severe mental health problems [and] complex needs which require specialist treatments, immediate support in frequent crises, high levels of practical support, help to integrate into their local community, overcome social isolation, etc. A major characteristic is a chaotic lifestyle, antisocial behaviour, due both to mental health problems and general demeanour, difficulty in forming relationships and high risk of homelessness and/or involvement in petty crime; medication is often of limited value … Users may be difficult to keep track of and are unlikely to attend usual service settings. This small group of challenging clients may only accept a service from a small number of staff whom they know well.

They require a service which can assertively maintain contact and offer a highly structured 'total' service, so that individuals need not access other services where they may be at risk of ending up in a locked ward. Yet service responses remain overwhelmingly ward-based which, while clearly appropriate for some people at certain times, should not characterise the service received by this group. The drain they make on the ECR budget alone in London, aside from their use of inpatient facilities, amply justifies seeking other forms of service response.

9.4.3 Employment and activity

People's needs for meaningful employment (work and leisure) are still seen as an 'optional extra' to many authorities, despite the central importance such activities hold in most of our lives. There are some excellent schemes, but, overall, the picture is one of 'more of the same', gardening projects, pottery courses, etc., with little imagination in relation, for example, to the success of Clubhouse Transitional Employment Schemes in the States. The low priority such services seem to have in resource allocation is remarkable in view of the good research evidence for the effectiveness in improving clinical and social outcomes (Torrey et al, 1995), and of users' and carers' strong and clearly expressed wishes for these services.

9.4.4 Advocacy and user involvement

Independent advocacy services are now provided in many places, although it is unclear how far they are seen as integral to the service system and how far they fall victim to year-on-year funding. Few services had a strategic approach to developing advocacy by, for example, including the role of the advocate in all user-focused policies and procedures. However, many services have funded outreach advocacy workers to work in hospital services.

All statutory services have some form of user involvement, although this still seems to be largely at the stage of consultation and feedback, rather than involvement in actually setting the agenda for service development. The most frequently voiced criticism from users and their families, – and some staff groups and voluntary agencies – is that they feel passive recipients of someone else's plan. Many mental health strategies/community care plans, etc. are written to meet the needs of users, as perceived by planners and managers, distributed to a range of people and amended in light of comments. Those most significantly affected by the service are always responding to someone else's ideas about what should be on offer. As a result, many users and carers feel that their views hold little real influence. This is particularly true for women users and carers and, to a lesser extent, people from minority groups. Notable exceptions were those London services which had adopted a stakeholder approach to service development.

9.4.5 Community mental health teams

All localities either had, or were planning, community mental health teams (CMHTs). However, the public documents surveyed generally gave no details about how these teams were to translate the principles and objectives on which they are apparently based into practice. Thus, how would the CMHTs know, for example, whether their objectives for equality of access to services, promotion of individual rights and support for a lifestyle of the user's choice had been met? Few documents go beyond a description of services: for example, they often state that the Care Programme Approach will be implemented or that a crisis response will be offered, but do not indicate how this will be achieved for individuals. There is likely to be wide variation in the work of different teams, even within a single London district.

Many CMHTs in London are not fully constituted teams, with an identified manager, etc., but are rather networks of individuals. The presence of the teaching hospitals seems to affect the operation of CMHTs, but in diverse ways. Where hospital-based models of psychiatry are still dominant, fledgling CMHTs may be paralysed because psychiatrists continue in their old ways of working and the teams are forced to attempt to operate without medical commitment. On the other hand, teaching hospitals may attract doctors at the leading edge of their profession and many community-based innovations have been led from the front by medical staff who have often had the power to overcome organisational obstacles that other professions are not able to negotiate.

Stronger operational management is needed in many places to overcome the sometimes entrenched positions of the disciplines and to deal, in inner London in particular, with the lack of medical input due to shortage of psychiatrists.

9.4.6 Services for mentally disordered offenders

For mentally disordered offenders, there were some small highly innovative projects, such as the placement of a CPN in three inner London police stations and Lambeth's 'street level' workers, although most services sought to divert from court, rather than any earlier. The future shape of court diversion schemes is uncertain, given that the majority of these projects are currently funded through the Home Office. A gap is in the provision of Section 136 suites in London's hospitals. A recent study in inner London found that 'persons placed on section of the Mental Health Act at the station have been detained for up to four days in custody because of lack of beds, especially if a secure bed is needed'.

9.4.7 Services for ethnic minority groups

Many health and local authorities had taken account of the needs of people from minority groups, but the comprehensiveness of their response is in doubt, especially for crisis care and employment needs. A national DoH-funded study of local minority groups found that their specific needs are still poorly understood and catered for by purchasers (Office for Public Management, 1996). There seem to be more specific services available for Black Caribbean people than for Asian people or other minority groups.

9.4.8 Services for women

The needs of women appear very significantly under-recognised and unmet. With a tiny number of exceptions, there is no women-only provision, in any part of the service, or even recognition of the childcare needs of many women. There is evidence that many women using mental health services have a history of sexual and physical abuse, yet this is rarely addressed within mainstream mental health services and there appears to be significant abuse within mental health services (Rose et al, 1991; Nilbert et al, 1989). The range of service responses needs to take account of many women's needs to leave their home, particularly if victims of sexual or racial harassment, thus, for example, home-based care as the only alternative to inpatient care is an insufficient response for these women.

9.4.9 Service planning

Variability of services is still great. Within districts, excellent innovative projects may be found alongside very traditional hospital-based services, indicating that the influence of particular forceful and committed individuals on service development is probably still the most important factor. Despite some very thorough quantitative macro-level needs assessment, there is little evidence of an integrated health/social services approach to the qualitative assessment of need, based on user-defined parameters. Collaboration between health and social services is in evidence everywhere to a greater or lesser extent. What is less in evidence is creative collaboration in terms of, for example, CPNs having access to care management moneys, or, more imaginatively, CMHTs having joint control over care management funds.

There is also little use of evidence-based service development – or even evidence-based care. For example, the strong evidence in support of the effectiveness of home-based care (Dean et al, 1993), has not translated into practice on the ground. Users and carers are now highly vocal and articulate in stating what works and what doesn't in relation to their care, yet their wishes are still largely ignored or, more insultingly, written off as being what they 'want', rather than what they 'need'.

9.4.10 Conclusion

The planning of London's mental health services needs both to be capable of responding to expanding knowledge about how to help people with mental health problems and to achieve stability of *direction* through a programme of long term transformation which combines realism about mental health services and vision about what could be achieved. Cultural change is needed in the relationship between services and their users. Currently, services feel under pressure to make short term responses to policy demands. Yet this may be at the expense of the long term organic development of the service through increasing user-determination, matched with professional expertise. Developing a framework for services that is responsible, dynamic and respectful requires strategic judgement and committed action – London as a whole needs to rise to this challenge if users of mental health services are to receive a high quality, effective service.

London's Mental Health Services in the context of the DISC framework: Summary tables[1]

Table 1 Access and Information

Service Function	Description of Needs	Examples of London Service Responses (current or planned)
Access into services	Factors which make access to services a particular issue in London include: • The presence of groups who have not traditionally sought help, such as the homeless, refugees, and young Black Caribbean men. • The transient nature of the population, which means many are not aware of local facilities, and have no GP. • The presence of many individuals who do not speak English. Access to London services thus needs to be facilitated by active identification and outreach.	• Funding given to a user group to provide an information officer to improve access to services (Harrow). • 24 hour helpline for use by users, carers or professionals wanting to know how to obtain help (Merton). • Interpreting service provided after local minority community leaders highlighted difficulties where people could not contact services because of language difficulties (Barking & Dagenham). • Outreach workers who establish contact with the homeless and facilitate access to services (City and East London).
Information about the needs of the local population	Planning a service response requires good quality current qualitative and quantitative information about the local population, a particularly important task in London given the complex demography.	• Funding for a research worker to survey the social and healthcare needs of local families from ethnic minority backgrounds (Kingston Social Services). • Long term case register, annually updated, providing valuable information about people in long term contact with services (Pathfinder Trust). • Networking of social services information database to the community mental health team (Richmond on Thames). • Specialist staff employed to identify gaps in provision for people from minority ethnic communities and to make recommendations for development (Barnet).
Information about services	In some areas of London the large number of local voluntary services makes it difficult for individual users and staff to be aware of the range of services available: for example, LSL Health Commission has about 700 voluntary organisations within its boundaries.	• Joint information system terminal in various public places with information about local services (Harrow). • Information on care management produced for users and carers in Braille and on tape in five languages (Camden Social Services). • Production of 'Good Mental Health Guide' with information for users, carers, and agencies about statutory and independent sector services (Newham). • Library with books, journals and tapes relating to race and mental health available to professionals and for the black community in general (Forward Project, Hammersmith & Fulham).
Prevention/Health Promotion	A basic awareness of the symptoms of mental distress and how to recognise the need for help is important for many health and social care staff and for the public in general. This is especially the case for non-mental health workers who come into contact with at risk groups – for example, district nurses and health visitors.	No specific examples in this area identified by this London Survey. Examples of service responses might include health promotion campaigns on issues such as stress at work, education in recognising mental health problems for all health and social care workers, and information for employers on addressing the mental health needs of their workforces.

1 Please contact Helen Smith, CMHSD, King's College London, Campden Hill Rd, London W8 7AU for a complete version of the framework.

Table 2 Needs for Individual Planning

Service Function	Description of Needs	Examples of London Service Responses (current or planned)
Individual Assessment of Need	All individuals require rigorous assessment of mental health, and also physical and social care needs and needs associated with race and gender. Social and physical needs are a particular issue in highly deprived sections of London. There is also a major challenge for the assessment process where there are many different ethnic groups, each with culturally unique needs (for example, in Newham there are over 40 ethnic groups).	• Plan to give CMHT staff access to health and social service budgets for commissioning individual care packages, based on a unitary assessment procedure for community care (Redbridge and Waltham Forest). • Procedure for ensuring health professionals support other agencies in providing more effective services for older users, with a move of skills so that routine cases may be assessed in a primary care setting (Harrow).
Care Planning	This should be based on assessment and incorporate all sectors including primary care and the voluntary sector. One identified worker should have an overview of each care plan, and co-ordinate and monitor care.	• Plan to involve users in developing their own care plans, with a group to be set up involving both users and providers, to discuss what information and support users will need for this (B&G Health). • Consultant commissioned to work on a pilot 'Shared Care' scheme, aimed at improving contact between secondary services and GPs (Westminster).
Maintaining Contact	In London, keeping in touch with a mobile population may be particularly difficult. In inner London service users who are homeless, or who have chaotic lifestyles because of substance abuse and/or mental illness, easily lose touch with services. Some may need constant 'assertive outreach' in order to maintain contact.	• Social Worker post to be created to work with mentally ill men in hostels for the homeless, developing packages of care and support for people out of contact (Ealing). • Asian outreach project in conjunction with Wandsworth Race Equality Council (Wandsworth).

Table 3 Meeting Needs in Crisis

Service Function	Description of Needs	Examples of London Service Responses (current or planned)
Emergency care	Needs in crisis are diverse and include accommodation; brief assessment; prolonged assessment; medication; respite; problem solving or advice; rest and safety; or detoxification. Some pose a risk to themselves or others, and may need to be sectioned under the Mental Health Act. People whose behaviour puts them at risk of homelessness or crime figure prominently in London's population; their needs for immediate assessment and access to appropriate services are still more urgent. Needs in crisis are compounded by large numbers of single person households, unemployment and poor housing, leading to, amongst other things, a greater risk of suicide. Access is needed to a range of inpatient services with different levels of support, including access to women only inpatient care and segregated services focused on the needs of black people. For people with severe long term needs, appropriate service settings may be different for those without a substantial psychiatric history. The needs of long term users in crisis are often not well met on acute admission units. They need to keep close links with ordinary routines and living environments. Their medical treatment is probably well established and may be a routine, if lengthy, process. However the maintenance of independent living skills through this period is a major need. Therefore, early identification of and response to crises is essential if these long term users are to have maximum opportunity of maintaining independent living.	• Women's Crisis Centre – alternative to admission with 12 places plus facilities for up to 4 children under 5, for women requiring short-term intensive support (Camden and Islington). • Residential alternative to hospital for black mental health service users in crisis (Impapo, West Lambeth). Multi-disciplinary crisis intervention with psychiatrists, CPNs, counselling co-ordinator, and social workers – always have social workers from Black Caribbean, Asian and Somali communities. Open referral system and can provide intensive help, reducing the need for hospital admission (Newham). • 24 hour crisis intervention service, with a crisis card system for all users who are on the supervision register, subject to Section 117 Discharge Arrangement, or have more than one mental health professional involved in their care. Ensures that appropriate treatment is given if there is an urgent problem outside working hours (Ealing). • Emergency reception centre which provides an easy access point for assessment and admission without a wait in the casualty department, open 24 hours a day, (Haringey). • 24 hour crisis phone line with advice available from a qualified CPN (Croydon). • Independent organisation providing a crisis residential service and out of hours drop in for people with mental health problems (Umbrella, Islington).
Emergency care with significant physical component	Those who in addition to the needs above have a significant physical problem include people who have harmed themselves, people who need treatment for a medical condition and also have a mental health problem, and people who need acute detoxification.	• Acute Centre for elderly people which links physical and mental health care (Redbridge).
'Step-Down'/Sub-Acute Care	This is a 'step down' from emergency care, and serves those who are no longer so acutely unwell that they are a risk to themselves or others, as well as those who are not thought to require emergency admission but still need active treatment and high levels of support to prevent relapse.	• 12 bedded follow on ward for those who are no longer acutely ill but need further rehabilitation (Haringey). • Pilot home nursing team providing intensive short term support to people in their own homes to prevent re-admission to hospital (EHH).
Respite/Asylum	People may need respite from their current domestic situation because of intensive environmental stress resulting in a disruption of usual social roles. These are individuals who can care for themselves with minimum assistance, but would be at risk of admission without some short term support. Needs for this form of care are likely to be greater in inner city areas where there are few community supports or stable social networks.	• Pilot schemes providing a crash pad/respite care service, offering an alternative place to live for a short time for people in crisis or needing some escape from a situation which contributes to their distress (Westminster City Council). • Respite facility for Black Caribbean people in crisis (Hackney).

Table 4 Needs for Treatment and Support with Mental Distress

Service Function	Description of Needs	Examples of London Service Responses (current or planned)
Time-limited treatment of less severe mental health problems	People who require short-term treatment for psychological distress but can maintain independent living without significant difficulty.	• Mental health specialists appointed to develop links with GPs in order to identify people with mental health problems at an early stage and prevent the need for admission into mainstream mental health services (Redbridge). • Psychotherapeutic service to City workers and residents (the Inner City Centre, Corporation of London). • Counselling project for women with mental health problems (The Bridge, Hammersmith and Fulham). • Counselling services for Cantonese and English speaking Chinese people (Chinese Mental Health Association). • Psychotherapy and behaviour therapy services for people within the Asian Community, available in Asian languages (Ealing).
Specialist time-limited treatment for people with severe mental health problems.	People with needs significant enough to disrupt their day to day social functioning, although they can maintain personal safety and live independently. Usually specialist treatment and support are required. Diagnoses associated with such needs include agoraphobia, major depression, post traumatic stress disorder, obsessive compulsive disorder, and eating disorders. This group has traditionally been referred to secondary services. They may now fall outside the 'severe and long term' criteria, but their needs can rarely be dealt with within primary care.	• Plan to develop specialist day facilities with multi-disciplinary staff for people with eating disorders (North Essex Health Authority) • Specialist trust delivering psychotherapy services. Where people have more severe psychiatric disorders, they contribute to care in combination with other mental health services (Tavistock and Portman NHS Trust). • Day hospital offering specialist psychotherapy for the treatment of severe personality disorders (Haringey).

Table 5 Needs for Ordinary Living and Long Term Support

Service Function	Description of Needs	Examples of London Service Responses (current or planned)
Long term personal (practical and emotional) support to people with severe and long term problems living in the community	Support for people who are capable of independent living, but require help in maintaining or learning daily living skills, using community resources and overcoming social isolation. Practical support needs to be complemented by emotional support and long term monitoring, possibly over many years.	• Community support team offering practical support to people at home, including cleaning, shopping, laundry etc. (Kensington and Chelsea). • MIND project providing support at home to people who have a tenancy, and who do not wish to share accommodation or have problems too severe for them to be supported in shared housing. Includes a mobile maintenance workshop and a voucher scheme operating in various shops and gas and electricity services (Hammersmith and Fulham MIND). • Flats all situated in the same block for 14 people who all have very high levels of need and are visited on a daily basis. Includes people who have continuing psychotic symptoms requiring episodic inpatient care. One of the flats in the block serves as a staff base (TULIP, Haringey). • Support service for people with mental health problems in their own homes which include evenings and weekends (Umbrella and Flexicare, Camden).
Accommodation (District-wide co-ordination of housing provision for people referred from specialist services).	A long term strategic approach needs to be taken to planning and providing a range of accommodation, from 24 hour staff to occasional support in own home, encompassing independent and statutory sectors. The idiosyncratic characteristics of the London housing market may further complicate this difficult task. Support may be provided by the same or different agency as housing. Other than for people requiring intensively staffed housing, people need their own tenancies with sufficient support, separately provided, to enable them to live in their own home and choose who, if anyone, lives with them. Recent guidance states that 'shared housing can be highly inappropriate and creates management problems which could be avoided by, for example, housing in a scheme of self contained small flats grouped into a block with the staff present'. Shared accommodation may be particularly unsuitable for younger people with severe and long term mental health problems, especially those from ethnic minorities. If acceptable housing is not provided, users become more at risk of not engaging in a care plan, increasing the risk of homelessness and contact with the police.	• Central housing bureau proposed, which will provide a single point of access to a range of supported housing, maintaining an on-line database for vacancies (Bromley). • Joint work between housing department and locality community mental health teams to ensure that appropriate support is available and to develop good neighbour and concerned tenant schemes based on neighbourhood housing offices (Hackney). • Housing support workers offering practical help to people in danger of losing tenancies because of mental health problems (Haringey). • Project planned providing semi-self-contained accommodation for 10 people including some communal space and 24 hour staffing – planned to address a gap in existing provision (Wandsworth).

Table 6 Needs for Ordinary Living and Long Term Support – continued from Table 5

Service Function	Description of Needs	Examples of London Service Responses (current or planned)
Treatment of – and support with – long standing and recurrent symptoms	Some individuals have long term distressing symptoms such as hearing voices and/or loss of drive and motivation. Such people and their families and friends need to be helped to cope with these symptoms, and periods of crisis when they worsen need to be managed with as little disruption as possible to independent functioning.	• Short term emergency placements available within adult placement scheme (Bexley). • Proposal that community mental health teams continue to be responsible for users with severe mental illness through periods of hospital admission or day care (B & G Health). • Outreach teams and an out of hours helpline for case managed and outreach clients and carers (Ealing).
Active Rehabilitation	People who have lost important independent living skills may need a medium-term intervention, aimed at helping them regain these. The focus should usually be on supporting people in their own environment, with inpatient rehabilitation only rarely indicated.	• Two mental health trusts are working collaboratively on rehabilitation by contributing to a large team providing an intensive program linked to Department of Health research funding, comparing intensive rehabilitation with standard models (Parkside and North West London Trusts).
Specialist treatment and support of a small group of people with long term and complex mental health problems who are unable to adequately use existing services.	A small sub-group of service users are characterised by chaotic life style, antisocial behaviour, difficulty in forming relationships, and high risk of homelessness: medication may be of limited value. Services have often had great difficulty meeting their needs, leading to mutual mistrust. This group may be difficult to keep track of and often do not attend usual service settings. They require specialist treatments, immediate support in their frequent crises, high levels of practical support and help integrating into their local communities. They may only accept services from a small group of staff whom they know well. They need a service which is assertive in maintaining contact and offers a highly structured 'total service' including long term and short term crisis residential care, so that these individuals need not access other services where they may risk ending up in a locked ward. London contains a disproportionate number of such people, through the effects of 'urban drift', separation from family and social deprivation.	• Identified community mental health team members with explicit responsibility for provision of assertive outreach for those people whom it is particularly difficult for specialist services to reach and engage with (Barnet). • Long term 'street level' case work scheme for people with very severe difficulties for whom contact with services has been difficult to maintain (Lambeth, Southwark and Lewisham). • Community psychiatric nursing staff and other services as required in centres for the homeless. Acutely mentally distressed people assessed on the street by consultant psychiatrists if required (Corporation of London).

Table 7 Services to Promote Personal Growth and Development

Service Function	Description of Needs	Examples of London Service Responses (current or planned)
High support setting for occupational activities	Some individuals can only find a meaningful occupational in a highly supported setting with staff with significant knowledge of mental illness. There is generally some flexibility about usual work expectations. May include other types of support such as social outings and creative non-work activities.	• Work rehabilitation service run by Trusts with placements including car valeting, horticulture at a garden centre, carpentry and refurbishment, picture framing and printing (Ealing). • Community business which offers training and employment in property maintenance, and which offers a property maintenance service to local customers with special needs. Includes work toward NVQ qualification (Hammersmith and Fulham MIND). • Voluntary organisation-run cafe and associated work projects. MISG funds three placements per year to which people with severe mental health problems are referred by local community mental health teams (Hackney).
Assessment and preparation for work	People with mental health problems may need career guidance to determine their work interests and skills, and will need assessment and help with skills such as job seeking, application forms, interviews, and also interpersonal, self care and personal safety skills related to work. A work plan should be drawn up individually and include details of support and training needed to achieve full work potential.	• Resource centre provides employment training, education and advice to people with mental health problems, especially Black Caribbean people. Each user is assessed for job potential and the service then works jointly with Brent Job Search who offer additional training, counselling, and job finding services (Brent). • Two employment worker posts to be created to help people with severe mental health problems get access to training, and employment and to support them through this process (Islington).
Low support work setting	A more demanding work environment, where people are expected mostly to conform to usual work expectations, but are supported by some level of understanding about mental health problems. Even in parts of London where unemployment is high, there is often a high turnover in manual jobs, such as waitressing or cleaning. This can mean that employers' needs for a stable workforce may be met by innovative work schemes, such as transitional employment schemes, where a 'clubhouse' secures a post through the open market and supports members in doing this job.	• Transitional employment schemes being developed through user run clubhouse, which is funded by health and social services jointly (West Lambeth). • Council-funded work programme, which provides a structured day for trainees, during which they carry out routine tasks for companies, usually local businesses (Bexley).
Open employment	Self employment or work in an unsupported setting where colleagues may/may not know about psychiatric history. This will require active outreach into the employment market to identify appropriate work settings and work with local employers to encourage recruitment of ex-users.	• Brent Job Search provides an employment placement service for people with disabilities in Brent. Almost 500 people with disabilities receive services, and its placement success rate is over a third.
Ongoing support in open employment	Ongoing support may be necessary for both worker and employer in order to sustain open employment.	• No London examples identified. Schemes of this kind might include mental health employment liaison schemes, which work with employers to promote mental health awareness, particularly in relation to changes in the work environment, and to offer support with and for workers who are users or ex-users.

Table 8 Services to Promote Personal Growth and Development – continued from Table 7

Service Function	Description of Needs	Examples of London Service Responses (current or planned)
Informal support for service users	People need informal support, social contact, and access to staff without having to make a prior appointment. Particularly those who are socially isolated or who require help with independent living, need a welcoming place where they can 'drop in' to meet other users and staff, have a meal and perhaps gain access to specialist advice on issues such as welfare benefits and housing problems.	• Group of drop-ins which are available outside usual office hours, offering informal counselling and support, with all users allocated a key worker. (Brent). Transport home for women available on two evenings during winter. • Development manager and activity organisers employed to stimulate and develop groups and activities at local venues, with an emphasis on younger users. To include a befriending scheme to support users participating in mainstream activities (Barnet). • Day centre with range of advice and support available to homeless people, particularly those with alcohol, drug or mental health problems, with walk-in primary health care available daily (Arlington Housing Association, Camden). • Group for gay men and lesbians with mental health problems (Hackney Mental Health Team and Hackney MIND)
Leisure and recreational activities, including Adult Education	Users should have access to the usual range of leisure activities including hobbies, adult education, cultural pursuits and simpler activities such as going for walks. Activities should be appropriate to their cultural background, occur at the usual time for the activity (eg. theatre visits in the evening) and be offered in the usual setting. Users may need support in gaining confidence to use local leisure facilities. Low incomes may be a difficulty, although inner London in particular, has a good range of local leisure activities, many catering for people on low incomes.	• Social Services funding for local further education college to provide social leisure and recreational courses for adults with special needs (Newham). • Voluntary sector organised holidays for users at the National Schizophrenia Fellowships New Forest Centre (Hillingdon). • Mental health integration project encouraging users to take up educational opportunities (Lewisham).
Support with Welfare Benefits	Most people using mental health services over a long period will be on welfare benefits, and specialist help may be needed to ensure they receive their full entitlement.	• Lisson Grove computerised package for assessment of benefits available on public access computer system (Brent). • Mental health workers attached to community mental health teams who offer help and advice with money matters and can accompany people on visits to the Job Centre, Citizens Advice Bureau or Social Security offices (Kingston)
Advocacy	Some people need support in exercising choice about their lives, ensuring that they are listened to, and being treated by statutory and other agencies as individuals with the same rights as most citizens. Advocates and their user partners may address any issue regarding services from statutory or voluntary sectors, including the full range of local authority services. Various types of advocacy may be resourced by statutory agencies to act independently of their services.	• User empowerment worker appointed from joint finance to assist users who have difficulty expressing their needs and wishes, information worker to be recruited who will be based on the inpatient wards (MIND in Kingston). • Advocacy service to be provided for long stay hospital residents who have no relative or carer and come from Harrow (Brent MIND). • Provision of Black Caribbean advocacy worker (MIND in Haringey). Advocacy project based in a psychiatric hospital has extended its services to include citizen advocacy, which involves a training program enabling users to act on behalf of other service users (Assert, Islington). • Proposed advocacy project to represent the interests of mentally disordered offenders and their families and of people being considered for the supervision register (Barnet).

Table 9 Services for Mentally Disordered Offenders

Service Function	Description of Needs	Examples of London Service Responses (current or planned)
Specialist response in a crisis, when an individual is in contact with the Criminal Justice System or mental health services	Ideally, potential offenders with mental health problems should be diverted from the criminal justice system before formal contact can occur. Once in contact they need access to a specialist assessment service which diverts into the mental health services as early as possible. Immediate access to a 'place of safety' (not a police station) will facilitate assessment and treatment. A range of options needs to exist for diversion, and it is important for local inpatient services to have intensive care accommodation, so that people do not need to be referred to out of district secure facilities.	• Home Office funded police liaison community psychiatric nurses in 3 of Central London's largest police stations. Identify and divert mentally disordered offenders in to the mental health services (covers Charing Cross, West End Central and Marylebone Police Stations). • Specialist community liaison nurse providing a link to courts and probation services (Barnet). • Daily assessment clinic in HMP Wormwood Scrubs, and 14 bed inpatient locked unit specifically for male remand prisoners who need a mental health assessment (Ealing). • Diversion scheme for 4 courts with sessional input by a consultant psychiatrist, central co-ordination by a CPN funded from Home Office money (Kingston). • Specific needs assessment suite proposed within the planned new Hendon Police Station (Barnet).
Medium term residential care which seeks to actively treat and rehabilitate MDOs	For those who need medium level security, it is important that ordinary living skills and social networks are maintained as far as possible, and that services are as local as possible. Access to women only units or at least safe space in mixed units is important, particularly as women are often greatly outnumbered and often have a history of sexual abuse.	No specific London example found in this category. Appropriate service responses might include rehabilitation services within secure facilities, women only facilities, supported voluntary sector befriending schemes which take account of race, gender and sexual orientation, and support for the involvement of external advocacy groups such as Women in Special Hospitals (WISH).
Long term practical and emotional support to enable people at high risk of serious re-offending to live in the community	Long term highly structured support is needed by some to maintain independent living and prevent re-offending. Some will require specialist support including ongoing expert assessment of mental state. As much use as possible should be made of mainstream services. Ideally there should be immediate access to specialist 24 hour staffed residential care which provides 'asylum', reducing the risk of offending.	• Specialist nursing, medical and psychology teams providing a consultation and liaison service to local community agencies (Bexley and Greenwich, and Lewisham and North Southwark).

Table 10 Needs Related to Substance Misuse

Service Function	Description of Needs	Examples of London Service Responses (current or planned)
Prevention, advice and information, including prevention of infectious disease and further drug-related harm.	Awareness of substance related issues needs generally to be increased in the community, and users allowed to make informed choices about their substance use, with a focus on harm minimisation.	• Needle exchange which uses street workers and has peer education projects and satellite work with probation officers (439 Project Bethnal Green). • Voluntary sector organisation aiming to reduce harmful affects of drug use by providing accessible, free and confidential services for people with drug related problems, and by offering drug awareness training to community groups and support to other professionals (The Angel Drug Project, Islington). • Outreach staff employed by drug and AIDS counselling and advisory service to recruit people who would otherwise not receive help, including female sex workers (Wandsworth).
Assessment and early intervention.	Specialist services should have a very low access threshold, as substance misuse should be tackled as early as possible so as to prevent further dependence.	• Healthy Options Team offering specialist work with homeless injecting drug users and drug users with HIV provides a range of services targeting 'hard to reach' populations, including HIV counselling, general counselling, help with prescribing and legal advice (East London and City Health Authority).
Detoxification and intensive therapy/ treatment, to encourage motivation to change and provide long term support.	Intensive physical and psychological treatment may be needed for withdrawal from substance use, with further long term support in maintaining a substance misuse-free life. People with chaotic life styles need support which takes into account their possible unwillingness or inability to seek help and use services in the usual way. Treatment may need to be offered in places where people live, or through short term hospital admission. Clear policies and care protocols are also needed for people with 'dual diagnosis'.	• 19 bed drug project which will accept users who are continuing to take prescribed drugs (Turning Point, Hammersmith). • House for women treated for alcohol problems who need further rehabilitation before independent living (Greenwich). • Group of rehabilitation houses, including ones that will take people on parole and on 'condition of residence' orders (Cranstoun Project, Wandsworth).

Table 11 Services for Children, Adolescents and Young People

Service Function	Description of Needs	Examples of London Service Responses (current or planned)
Identification of potentially serious problems; management and/or referral as appropriate	Accurate recognition is needed of emotional and behavioural disorders which can be helped and/or may persist. Child health surveillance by trained staff is needed by all children, and it is particularly likely that children from highly mobile populations may miss out on this, for example, if they are living in temporary accommodation, are missing school or are homeless. For young people access to services may require confidential self referral services including telephone advice and helplines.	• Promoting school mental health initiatives, run in collaboration with school health service (Barnet). • Youth counselling service (West Surrey).
Preventive interventions to children and young people at risk.	Children and young people in certain situations are known to be at high risk, for example, where their home backgrounds are characterised by discord, chronic ill health, alcoholism, violence or homelessness, or where children suffer neglect or abuse, have disability or learning difficulties, in trouble with the police, or in local authority care. Parents, teachers and other people working with this group need support and education from specialists.	• Service for mothers of sexually abused children run by a health visitor (Croydon). • Anti-bullying programs in schools (Islington). • Joint statutory and voluntary sector parents support initiative for depressed mothers and their babies (Camden)
Management and treatment of EBDs	A range of skills from child health, mental health, social work, education and youth justice may be needed for adequate assessment of childrens' needs, with a variety of elements in management. Young people need to be able to contribute to decisions about their own needs.	Specialist psychologists working in primary care to support and consult GPs. Advise on appropriate referral and do case work (Wandsworth).
Emergency assessment & placement.	Speedy and skilled assessment and treatment is needed for seriously disturbed psychotic or dangerous young people.	Many districts have difficulty providing full emergency cover by the local child and adolescent psychiatrists, and young people are admitted to adult facilities.

Table 12 Needs of Older People with Mental Health Problems or Dementia

Service Function	Description of Needs	Examples of London Service Responses (current or planned)
Emergency physical, psychiatric and psychological assessment	Older people need rapid access to skills assessment taking into account social and clinical factors. Both physical and social complicating factors are particularly common in older people, and close liaison is needed with geriatric medical services and local authority services.	• Out of hours team providing an emergency night service which is intended to prevent inappropriate admissions to hospital or residential care (Barking and Dagenham).
Specialist Treatments/ Interventions	A range of specialist treatments and interventions are required to maintain physical health and cognitive functioning, and close monitoring may be needed for limited periods. Service responses should be delivered in various settings, including residential and day services.	• Plan for 'dementia centre' incorporating a day facility, respite and long term residential care (Barnet). • Multi disciplinary day services provided with emphasis on integrated care and treating mental health problems outside the hospital setting (Harrow).
Support to remain in own home	People need a range of supports to enable them to remain in their own homes for as long as possible. Analysis of social, clinical and environmental needs to be carried out for each individual, and practical help put in place to address these.	• Specialist home care workers in each social services area, providing an intensive service to people with dementia. Care workers have skills to provide extensive help with every day tasks (Barking and Dagenham). • Home treatment service providing intensive support to people in their own home as an alternative to admission or means to early discharge (Riverside Trust). • Dementia home support service offers advice and emotional support to service users, their families and their informal carers, from 8am to 7pm, 365 days a year (Newham). • 'Alone at home' scheme providing support for elderly people with dementia living at home in the community (Hackney). • Culture specific home care for Black Caribbean, Greek and Turkish Cypriots, Irish, Chinese, and Asian elders (Satellite Consortium, Haringey).
Respite for carers	Carers need to have access to respite, including residential options, respite care at home, and day respite.	• Night centre for support and respite for carers of people with dementia. 7 beds including 1 emergency bed available 3 nights a week, between 8pm and 8am, with transport to the centre provided (Bexley Association for Carers of the Elderly). • Weekend respite care scheme and care attendant scheme for older people with dementia (Ealing). • Respite care and personal care provided at home through Crossroads care attendance scheme (Redbridge). • Day care on Saturdays and Sundays for people with severe confusion who have carers (Merton MIND). • Plan for respite care beds at a local authority resource centre (Harrow).
Residential care	Adequate residential and nursing care and clear criteria for access to both are needed in a high quality service. Health and local authorities need clear criteria for access to different forms of care and clear definitions for eligibility for continuing care.	• This area is not addressed as part of this project.

Chapter 10

London in close-up: the spectrum of care in three London catchment areas

Thomas Becker, Sara Bixby, Sonia Johnson, Rosalind Ramsay and Graham Thornicroft

Summary

In order to provide a more detailed view of London service provision, the full range of statutory and independent sector services for adults aged 18-65, for children and adolescents, for substance misusers and for the elderly in three London Trust catchment areas were studied. Major conclusions emerging from this exercise include:

- Accurate information about the full range of services available in local catchment areas is difficult to obtain, with particular obstacles including lack of uniformity in the way different agencies collect data; variations in provider catchment areas, with independent sector services in particular often taking referrals from a wide area; difficulty in judging how much provision is really available where some services have a very low turnover or are appropriate only for quite a limited client group; and lack of centralised data collection encompassing health service, local authority and independent sector facilities.

- There is great heterogeneity in the precise service models adopted by catchment areas as they move towards a more community-based model of care. Little evidence or guidance is available to local planners about, for example, whether to integrate acute and rehabilitation services, which services to offer on a centralised and which on a sectorised basis, or whether to base sector catchment areas on social services areas or on General Practitioners' lists.

- In all the catchment areas, a mixed economy of care seems to have developed across the sub-specialities, although private sector providers figure prominently only in the suburban catchment area and do not appear to have entered the market in the inner city to any significant degree.

- The voluntary sector is a major service provider for day and residential care in each catchment area. It also plays a very significant role in provision of substance misuse services.

- Local Authorities deliver some services but do not appear to be taking the lead in provision of any type of general adult service in any of the catchment areas. They are more prominent in services for the elderly.

- The NHS has become a substantial provider of long term as well as acute day care in all the catchment areas, taking on some traditional social services functions. It has not become a very significant provider of community-based residential services. In one of the areas, most work rehabilitation services are also health service provided, whilst in the other two areas, availability of employment schemes is limited.

10.1 Introduction

Previous sections have given an overview of overall service functioning and of quantities of residential provision. In order to obtain a more fine-grained view of the range and functioning of London mental health services, the care provided for mentally ill adults (18-65) within three catchment areas was studied in greater detail, with approaches to all services delivering residential, day, community or out-patient care within the areas. This was complemented by a study of the major provisions for elderly mentally ill, children and adolescents and substance misusers in each area. In this chapter, the patterns of service provision found are summarised and discussed: the appendix which follows the chapter contains more detailed tables describing the services. The data refer to the state of services in the first quarter of 1996, when the survey took place.

Recent reports on the range of general adult services which need to be provided for the severely mentally ill in local catchment areas have included those of the Audit Commission (1994a), the Clinical Standards Advisory Group (1995) and the Department of Health (1996a). Central considerations for service planning which emerge from all these documents include:

- Planning for a local area needs to be based on comprehensive information about provision by health, social services, voluntary and private sectors, and plans for development should include all these sectors.
- Each catchment area should have adequate access to a comprehensive range of services including acute hospital, day and home-based care, long term domiciliary, residential and day care, employment schemes, and long term care management.
- Within each service category, a range of different types of facility should be present so that the diverse needs of patients may be met: for example, residential care available outside hospital should include flats and group homes with some visits from staff, hostels with daytime staff and with staff sleeping on the premises at night, adult placement schemes and hostels where nursing staff are awake and available 24 hours a day. An unmet need for the last of these has particularly been emphasised in recent reports.

Chapter 5 has discussed specific considerations for sub-speciality services: however, many of the considerations about gathering comprehensive information about needs and services, planning for all sectors jointly and providing a wide variety of types of services so as to meet a wide range of needs apply to all mental health specialities. This chapter will discuss the different ways in which a range of services has developed in each area and the degree to which services in each area constitute a comprehensive spectrum of care of the kind recommended in these recent reports.

10.1.1 Method

Data collection took place between January and April 1996. Initially a letter was sent to the Trusts, Social Services and Health Commissions covering each area explaining the purpose of the research and requesting co-operation. Permission to proceed with the survey was given by the Trust chief executives and directors of social services in each area. Telephone contact was then made with purchasing authorities, Trusts, social services, Community Health Councils, Voluntary Services Councils and major voluntary agencies such as MIND, with a request for help in identifying all the significant providers of mental health services in the catchment area. They were also asked to send copies of any reports and directories relating to local service provision, and to provide details of any other useful local informants. In Croydon, a major information source was a survey carried out in late 1995 and early 1996 of Croydon's mental health services by David Turner and Dr Jeremy Broadhead at PRiSM.

For general adult services, we designed a questionnaire for administration to each service provider, requesting details of services provided, target populations, staffing, capacity, activity and catchment area. Because of the short timescale, data collection generally took place by telephone: all major service providers in the area were contacted and asked either to give the information by telephone or to send it to us. Up to three follow up telephone calls were made to each service provider to attempt to obtain complete information. Where the service providers did not respond fully, local directories and key informants were used to fill in the gaps as far as possible.

For substance misuse, old age and child and adolescent services, medical staff or clinical managers working in each speciality in each of the three areas were contacted and visits arranged. A structured questionnaire similar to that used for the general adult service was taken to these appointments, although it again proved difficult to fit the information obtained into this fixed format. These key informants were also asked for their views on gaps between local need and current service provision, and on how local services need to change. Further information was obtained from the available written literature about services, such as Health Commission and Trust reports and Social Services community care plans. In each of the areas, some services were visited. The final text was sent to the major informants in each service for them to check its factual correctness.

Finally, draft versions of both the sub-speciality and the general adult section were sent to the chief executive and director(s) of social services in each area, with a request for the text to be checked for any errors. Revisions requested were incorporated. The text was then circulated to these individuals again, with a request that they contact us with any further modifications needing to be made before publication.

10.1.2 Limitations of information obtained

The quality of the information obtained is limited in several respects:

- Although surveys of various types of provision had been undertaken at various times in each area, none appeared to have a mechanism for routine, comprehensive centralised information collection about mental health service provision in the area. This was particularly marked for voluntary and private sector providers, about whose activities there is often little detailed information available within the statutory sector.

- The time available (four months for planning, collection and collation of data) significantly limited the quality of information obtained, as responses were often very slow to arrive and there was very little time to make personal visits: where such visits could be made, they seemed to result in greater co-operation and fuller information. Most of the data collection took place in the final three months of the financial year, and it appeared that time pressures on managers at this time made co-operation more difficult to obtain.

• Many services are undergoing major changes and are uncertain of their plans: this both made it more difficult to obtain an accurate view of current provision and also seemed to make staff more reluctant to respond to our survey.

• There is great variation in how respondents monitor and record their service activity: their information often could not be fitted into the standardised ways in which we hoped to record it.

• In some voluntary sector organisations, we encountered some reluctance regarding the recording of information about clients and activities, particularly where this was seen as involving 'labelling' clients (e.g. staff were sometimes reluctant to state whether or not they provided services for people with psychotic illnesses).

• Where information was obtained from more than one source about the same service, it was not always consistent.

For these reasons, it must be borne in mind that the description of services in the three areas is based on what we judged to be the best available information that we could obtain in limited time – there are substantial uncertainties about its reliability.

10.1.3 Characteristics of the three sites

The three NHS Trust catchment areas selected for detailed examination were **Ealing**, **Camberwell** and **Croydon**. The Ealing catchment area is the London Borough of Ealing, for which services are provided by West London Healthcare NHS Trust. 'Camberwell' is the former Camberwell District Health Authority, which now forms the catchment area of the Community Directorate of the Bethlem and Maudsley NHS Trust. It spans the southern part of the London Borough of Southwark and the eastern part of the Borough of Lambeth. The name Camberwell is not now used to refer to the Trust's catchment area, but will be retained in this chapter as no suitable brief way of describing this catchment area has replaced it. However, it should be noted that one of the five sectors into which this catchment area is divided is also now called Camberwell – this smaller area is referred to below always as the 'Camberwell sector', rather than simply 'Camberwell'. The Croydon catchment area is the London Borough of Croydon, and has mental health services provided by Croydon Mental Health Services (which merged with the Bethlem and Maudsley NHS Trust in April, 1995). The three areas were selected for representativeness of London as a whole: Camberwell is an inner city area, Ealing represents 'middle London' and Croydon is a more affluent outer suburb. Ealing has a total population of 280,000, with 209,000 in Camberwell and 319,000 in Croydon.

10.2 Services for adults aged 18 to 65 years in the three areas

10.2.1 Organisation of the three catchment areas

Each area has sectorised its catchment area on a geographical basis. Camberwell has five sectors and has the smallest sector populations, ranging from 39,000 to 46,000. Ealing has five sectors, with total populations ranging from 50,000 to 80,000. Croydon has three 'localities', with between 65,700 and 77,950 inhabitants in the 15 to 64 age group each. Each of these localities is sub-divided into two or three smaller 'patches'. The Trust catchment area is co-terminous with the local authority in Croydon and Ealing, but not in Camberwell, where the Trust catchment area encompasses parts of two Boroughs (Lambeth and Southwark). Sector boundaries are co-terminous with social service area boundaries in Camberwell and Croydon, but not in Ealing. Ealing has been sectorised for twenty-five years – this is a very long period compared with most UK areas (Johnson and Thornicroft, 1993), so that Ealing is of particular interest as an opportunity to observe the longer term sequelae of sectorisation in an urban area. However, the number of sectors has changed over the years from 4 to 5, then back to 4, and now again to 5, with 6 proposed, so that boundaries have shifted frequently. Referring to the data on the structure and functioning of London's mental health services reported in Chapter 8, Ealing is also of some interest in that, unlike most of the other inner and outer London Trusts, ready availability of most services is reported, and West London is one of only 2 inner London Trusts where acute and intensive care bed admission and CPN allocation are apparently all available on the day of referral. The data returned thus suggest that Ealing's mental health services may currently be functioning relatively well, and this is also the impression given by various of the Trust's documents and by informants from the Trust who suggest that they believe that most local need is now being met by Ealing's long established community mental health services.

10.2.2 In-patient service organisation

In **Croydon** in-patient beds are divided between two wards at a large psychiatric hospital which is in the final stages of closing and is located some distance from the areas where most of the population live, and a ward in the local District General Hospital. There has been much local criticism of the physical environment in the old asylum, and the closure of both these units is planned, with reprovision in a single unit at the Bethlem Royal Hospital, on the edge of the catchment area. In **Camberwell** the in-patient units are all situated at the Maudsley Hospital, a specialist psychiatric hospital which is situated centrally in the catchment area, adjacent to the District General Hospital. In **Ealing** the acute wards are in the John Connolly unit and refurbished accommodation in St Bernard's wing, which now share the site with Ealing Hospital Trust (the general hospital). In each of the areas, acute in-patient care is sectorised to some degree, but the nature of links between in-patient and community services varies:

Camberwell has one in-patient ward per sector, and links between ward and community are fairly close, with a single sector clinical manager covering both. However, ward and community nurses are clearly distinct groups in most sectors, with no rotation between the two settings.

Croydon in principle has links between localities and particular wards, but in practice beds are frequently allocated elsewhere in the service and the management structures for the two services are distinct.

In **Ealing** there are substantial links between in-patient and community services. Each ward is linked to a particular sector. Within sectors, there are separate in-patient and Community Mental Health Resource Centre managers (although the area has two locality managers, who each cover both in-patient and community services in two or three of the sectors). There are regular meetings for communication between managers of the two services in each sector. A number of procedures have been set up to ensure continuity of care between the two services: two sectors have link nurses who work part-time in the ward and part-time in the community, and who attend ward rounds, assist in discharge planning and attend CPA reviews. The other sectors have either rotas or designated workers for ward round and CPA review attendance. Community keyworkers keep in contact with those on their caseload when they are in-patients.

Patterns of secure provision in the three areas are as follows:

Ealing has a large forensic in-patient service, which includes provision for patients from Ealing along with people from outside the catchment area. It has two intensive care wards – Blair Ward caters for people for stays of less than three months, whilst Bevan Ward has recently opened and aims to provide stays of 3 to 6 months. Barron Ward offers rehabilitation for stays up to two years in a secure setting for difficult to place patients. In 1996/7, 8 beds on Blair ward, 3 on Bevan and 9 on Barron ward are contracted for residents of the purchasing authority, Ealing, Hammersmith and Hounslow. Bentham Ward was a remand unit with a mixture of intensive care and Regional Secure beds – this was commissioned as a two year pilot scheme, and is due to merge with the Three Bridges Regional Secure unit, also part of the Ealing forensic directorate, in 1996/7.

Croydon has a single intensive care facility, which is the Farleigh Unit at Warlingham Park Hospital. It does not provide any Regional Secure beds, but purchases 3 per year at Springfield Hospital (Pathfinder).

In **Camberwell**, the Maudsley has an intensive care ward on which there are 14 beds for the catchment area. The Special Care Unit is a 9 bed 'challenging behaviour' unit for people in need of longer term care and rehabilitation. The Dennis Hill Unit at the Bethlem Royal Hospital is a Regional Secure Unit on which there are 12 places for the South Southwark part of the Camberwell catchment area. Eight medium secure beds were provided at Cane Hill for the East Lambeth part of the catchment area up to April 1st 1996, but were due to be transferred to the Dennis Hill Unit.

Ealing has a number of other wards which provide specialised forms of care within the general adult service. Osterley ward is a pre-discharge ward which frees up beds on the acute wards. Dean ward is a rehabilitation and resettlement ward, which has served former long-stay patients of St Bernard's Hostel, and will shortly close. Drake Ward provides a programme of care for 'revolving door' clients who appear to need a more intensive rehabilitation service and a longer hospital stay than is provided on the acute wards. Denbigh ward provides treatment for people with concurrent brain injury and psychiatric illness. Most of these specialised wards take people from outside the catchment area as well as having a number of designated Ealing beds.

Croydon has a ward (Beatrice Ward) which provides beds and a limited rehabilitation service for people leaving its intensive care ward. Apart from the secure facilities described above, **Camberwell** does not appear to have beds with differentiated, specialist functions within its general adult service for the local community.

There is thus considerable variation in the degree to which the three areas have developed a range of different types of in-patient care. Ealing has much the most extensive group of specialist services supplementing the generic acute wards, with both a variety of types of secure care and several non-secure models available. The mode of organisation of most of these services is the provision of a substantial number of beds designated for Ealing within a ward which takes referrals from a wider area. In Camberwell, the more limited development may be in part attributable to the provision of a wide range of specialist in-patient services within the Trust's national directorates, which may be seen as readily accessible even if they do not make specifically designated provision for the catchment area.

10.2.3 Community mental health centres

All the catchment areas have to some extent adopted the model of providing a range of services from community team bases (referred to here as Community Mental Health Centres or CMHCs) located within the sector. In Ealing, each sector has a single CMHC (known locally as Community Mental Health Resource Centres) located within the unit. Croydon has one CMHC for each of two of the sectors and two in the third. In Camberwell the pattern varies: two of the sectors share a CMHC, one sector has a single CMHC within it, and two sectors have two team bases each. Some of the arrangements in Camberwell are intended to be short term only.

10.2.4 Community Mental Health Team Organisation

As in London as a whole, there is some variation in the organisation of community teams, and in particular in whether acute and continuing care teams are separate or integrated and in which facilities are provided on *centralised* basis, with a single team serving the whole larger Trust catchment area, and which on a decentralised, sectorised basis. There is also variation in the degree to which service provision is homogeneous through the catchment area – Camberwell has a variety of different models of team organisation, whereas in Ealing patterns of provision are similar throughout the area. The models found in each area are as follows:

Camberwell has:
- one sector in which there are separate acute and continuing care teams, each with its own teambase
- two sectors which are each served by a single integrated team delivering both acute and continuing care
- one sector which has been divided into two smaller catchment areas on a geographical basis, with an integrated team for each small catchment area, but some staff and facilities shared between the two sub-sectors

- one sector which has two integrated teams with allocation between the teams based on which GP the patient is registered with.

Croydon has:
- division of the larger 'localities' into two or three smaller 'patches' on a geographical basis, with one integrated team for each patch providing acute and continuing care, but not rehabilitation
- in two of the localities, day care staff are shared between all the patches in the locality
- a centralised, specialist rehabilitation team serving the whole of Croydon – this supports people who live independently, but require more care than is usually available from a CPN.

Ealing has:
- an integrated team providing acute and continuing care in each of the five sectors
- a centralised crisis intervention service serving the whole of Ealing – this is a new service, which picks up crisis work from the sector teams during the day and provides an out of hours service for existing service users.

There are a number of centralised services for all of Ealing, including an eating disorders team based at one of the CMHCs, a psychotherapy service, a rehabilitation team with a caseload of 40 patients who had repeated admissions and require assertive outreach and three CPNs who specialise in cognitive behavioural therapy.

10.2.5 Community mental health team staffing

Table 1 shows the number per 100,000 population of staff of various types working in community services in each of three areas. The figures provided by the three areas thus suggest very different patterns and levels of staffing. Camberwell has the highest levels of staff of most types, which may at least in part be a reflection of the fact that it is the most deprived of the three areas. The presence of a major post-graduate training hospital and research institute in the catchment area may also contribute. Croydon and Ealing have fairly similar overall numbers of nursing staff, but it is striking that in Ealing, they seem to be concentrated almost entirely at the higher grades, whereas the majority in Croydon are more junior. It appears that in Ealing resources are concentrated on employing a relatively small number of nursing staff who have particularly high levels of skill and experience.

Some degree of differentiation of role among nurses occurs within the teams. Croydon has some staff dedicated to day care and some to community work within each locality. In Ealing, around half the community nurses are outreach nurses, working primarily at people's homes, whilst the others work principally in the Community Mental Health Centre. In Camberwell, three sectors have a specialist forensic CPN attached to the sector team.

Table 1 Community mental health team staffing in the 3 areas

Type of staff (all health service)	Camberwell (Whole time equivalents **per** 100,000) (Includes members of community teams in five sectors)	Croydon (Whole time equivalents **per** 100,000) (Includes community and day staff in all locality teams & outreach team at rehabilitation unit)	Ealing (Whole time equivalents **per** 100,000) (Includes CMHC staff & Crisis Intervention service, eating disorder, cognitive therapy & rehabilitation teams)
Nurses – H & I Grade	5.7	0	3.6
Nurses – F & G Grade	20.6	4.8	12.2
Nurses – D & E Grade	6.4	8.9	1.1
Total Nursing staff – D Grade and above	**32.7**	**13.7**	**16.9**
Nurses A to C Grade	4.1	1.8	0
Head OTs	1.9	0.5	0
Other qualified OTs	4.7	1.6	0.4
Total qualified OTs	**6.6**	**2.1**	**0.4**
OT technicians & assistants	0	1.8	0.5
Art, dance & music therapy, yoga	0	0.1	0.3
Consultant psychiatrists	3.6	2.2	1.3
Senior Registrars	3.8	0	0
Registrars/SHOs	2.4	3.2	0.6
Clinical Assistants/ associate specialists	0	0.5	1.4
All medical staff	**11.6**	**5.9**	**3.3**
Psychologists	3.9	0.3	1.4

10.2.6 Mental health social work teams

This is an area in which information was particularly difficult to obtain. The social services mental health teams in the three areas appear to be as follows:

In **Ealing**, 20 social work staff, 18 of them Approved Social Workers, are based within the West London Healthcare Trust Mental Health Unit, and work jointly with Trust staff in the hostels and in mental health resource centres. In Acton Town Hall, there are two social work staff who support residents in the social services group homes (see below). A team of seven community support workers are also based at Acton Town Hall, and provide support and practical help to people living in the community – they have caseloads of about 20 each and help clients to acquire and sustain the skills needed for independent living, such as shopping, dealing with bills and keeping appointments. In addition, there is a team of social workers and probation secondees working with the forensic directorate teams.

In **Croydon**, there are case management teams in which social workers are attached to locality teams, an Independent Living Team, and an Adult Placement Team. The Independent Living Team staff appear to resemble community support workers, and mainly provide outreach to people in independent accommodation. The Adult Placement Team supports Croydon's adult placement service (see below under residential care), which was established in 1962. In this scheme, people in the community provide food and lodging for people with mental illness or learning disability in return for a payment of a little over £100 per week. The team also supports some group homes and provides link workers for Croydon's substantial private registered home sector.

Camberwell bridges two local authorities. **South Southwark** mental health service team serves three of the sectors, providing each with a senior practitioner and four social workers. There is also an out of hours team for Southwark, which covers the whole of the Borough. We were unable to obtain clear information regarding the **East Lambeth** social services team, currently in some disarray as a large budget deficit is leading to large cuts in social services resources and staffing in the Borough of Lambeth. As well as duty services, the Mental Illness Specific Grant has funded in Lambeth a 'Street Level' Team, which is based in Brixton and keeps in touch with users who might be lost to follow up without assertive outreach, and five 'Community care officers', who offer befriending and practical support to people with mental health difficulties, living independently or in accommodation with low levels of support. In their 1996 Mental Health Strategy, they reported that they aim in future to develop joint health and social services community teams in the two East Lambeth sectors. Lambeth and Southwark each also have a specification for single homeless persons.

10.2.7 Residential care

Tables 1 to 3 in the appendix to this chapter show details of the main providers of residential care for the mentally ill situated within each of the three areas. Some important difficulties are encountered in trying to assess how much supported residential accommodation is available for people with mental illnesses in each area:

- Voluntary and private sector accommodation often does not have a fixed catchment area, so that a listing of services situated within a particular catchment area is not necessarily helpful in judging what places are available to residents of the area.
- Where Trust boundaries and local authority boundaries do not coincide, as in Camberwell, it is also difficult to ascertain how much local authority accommodation is in practice available to residents in each Trust.
- Some residential accommodation has a very slow turnover, with places in practice very rarely available, particularly when the accommodation was opened as part of the resettlement of long term patients of the asylums. For example, documents from Southwark's Housing Department indicate that most local 24 hour staffed accommodation was established as part of asylum reprovisions, and still largely houses this group, so that availability of 24 hour accommodation in the Borough is poorer than it first appears.
- In some instances, it is probably more appropriate to see residential services situated within a catchment area as a source of added demands rather than as a resource for the local mental health service: this will occur where most of the residents of a facility are referred from outside the catchment area and begin to make use of the area's mental health services following transfer.

Thus surveying the services present in a catchment area provides an initial indication of what may be available for patients. In order to obtain a clearer picture, it would be useful to study the local options which are available when placements are sought for particular patients: this may be a helpful methodology for future assessment of service availability. However, some observations may be made about the patterns of care in the three areas.

Encouraged by central policies aimed at creating a market in health care, the last five years have seen a national trend towards a decrease in residential care provision by local authorities, and an increase in independent facilities, particularly private ones (Department of Health, 1995). It has been estimated that nationally most of the growth in non-hospital accommodation following the closure of the large mental hospitals has been in the private sector (Davidge et al, 1993), but it has also been suggested that such growth has been less marked in urban areas than in rural and mixed ones (Knapp et al, 1995; Faulkner et al, 1992). Patterns of care in the three areas appear to support this conclusion. In Croydon, the private sector is one of the major care providers, with a substantial number of places funded by the Borough in private registered care homes within the Borough. Ealing, the 'middle London' area, has a much smaller number of such places locally, whilst we are aware of no such facilities in inner city Camberwell (although West Lambeth, the part of the Borough which falls outside the Camberwell catchment area does have a number of such homes and these may in part be in use for Camberwell residents).Thus whilst in the suburban area private providers are entering the local care 'market' as envisaged by the Government, non-statutory provision in the other areas is dominated by housing associations and mental health charities, suggesting that it is unlikely that market forces can be relied on to produce suitable amounts of provision in these areas. A survey of residential care facilities by Lelliott et al (1996) suggests that the private sector is notable for providing the majority of high-staffed facilities (70%) and is also the largest provider of medium and low staffed hostels. The lack of growth in this sector in the inner London areas may partly account for the dearth of 24 hour staff facilities.

In each area, a large variety of independent organisations are involved in care provision, with the statutory sector providing only a minority of places. This creates a risk that regulation of care and training standards may become excessively complex. However, some reassurance may be drawn from a recent report by Shepherd et al (1995), which is discussed further in Chapter 6: their study of 20 residential facilities in Greater London suggests that the private and voluntary sectors (as well as facilities jointly commissioned by health trusts and housing associations) provide better physical and social environments than local authority accommodation, and that patient quality of life and interactions with staff are similar. This study also found that patient quality of life, environment and satisfaction were strikingly better in all these facilities than in long term hospital wards. However, Lelliott et al (1996) indicate that there are few staff with formal care qualifications working in such settings, and that links with mental health services are very limited, so that their capacity to manage severely disabled residents is likely to be limited.

Only in Ealing has the health Trust so far become a major non-hospital residential accommodation provider. Provision of hostels with 24 hour care by nursing staff has been encouraged nationally (Department of Health, 1996c). Ealing has a large 24 hour staffed nursed home of this type. In Croydon, there is also a health service 24 hour staffed unit, but literature provided by the Trusts suggests that this has to a large degree been in use as part of reprovision for former long-stay asylum patients, rather than for newer referrals to the mental health services. In Camberwell a number of properties have been acquired and some schemes initiated, in some cases using joint provision between the Trust and a housing association, a model which appears to be increasingly prevalent nationally (Faulkner et al, 1992, Shepherd et al, 1995). However, not all these schemes have thus far been successful: difficulties have been encountered in staffing projects, and a paper from Southwark's Special Needs Housing Department suggests that these schemes have not always been precisely targeted to meet local needs and have not always been based on adequate consultation with local bodies more experienced in the field of housing (Shiress, 1996).

With regard to the range of residential care provided, a variety of types of facility is present in each area, but there is considerable variation as to which types of accommodation predominate.

As well as the substantial private sector already referred to, a distinctive form of care relied on to a substantial degree in Croydon is the Adult Placement Scheme. Although supported lodging schemes of this type has been developed rather more extensively in the US and some European countries, and such schemes are alluded to in "The Spectrum of Care" (Department of Health, 1996a), they have not been much described or discussed in UK literature. It is a form of care which has the potential to provide real integration into the community to a greater degree than most forms of supported housing, as placements are "ordinary" families. However it may be difficult to find families who are able and willing to take on this role, particularly in the inner city, and it has been suggested that such schemes are mainly appropriate for older and more settled patients.

In **Ealing**, one of the main elements in the range of local residential provision is supported tenancy. This way of providing residential care has also not been very prominent in recent UK reports and published literature and services, to the extent that it is not one of the specific categories in the MINI (see chapter 7). However, the survey of residential provision reported in Chapter 7 indicates that it is becoming common in the care provision of a number of Boroughs. Tenancies of this kind may receive varying levels of support. Sometimes a flat will only occasionally be visited and will have some support on call, whilst for other schemes the flats are grouped around an office where a full-time member of staff is based and is able to offer a relatively high level of support for tenants. Such schemes are sometimes purpose-built or, otherwise, may be based in flats which are part of mainstream Local Authority or Housing Association housing stock. One feature of many schemes is that the tenancy is permanent so that if contact with staff is no longer needed this support is withdrawn but the resident remains in the flat. Such schemes thus promise to be an effective way of fulfilling the recom-mendations of the Audit Commission (1994a) that residential care should provide privacy, autonomy and a "home for life". This type of housing may particularly be appropriate for younger people who, unlike members of the previous generation who had been long-term hospital inpatients, are unused to communal living and to the shared rooms which are a feature in many of the older hostels. It may not fulfil the needs of those that require staff attention 24 hours per day. However, it may well be an appropriate alternative to care in a day staffed hostel, where residents in any case have to function sufficiently well to be left alone overnight and through the weekend.

In **Camberwell**, there are some supported tenancies available but the predominant form of provision appears to be in staffed hostels. A report from Southwark Housing Department (Shiress 1996) suggests that many of these hostels have residents who have been there for a very long period and who are now ageing. This report comments that some of the hostels have difficulty filling vacancies, particularly when rooms are shared, drawing attention to the need for there not only to be adequate quantities of residential care, but for it to be acceptable to patients from a variety of backgrounds and generations, so that types of housing which were acceptable to those discharged from long-stay wards, who were accustomed to a lack of privacy and autonomy, may be less acceptable to a new generation who have never experienced prolonged institutionalisation.

In general most of the accommodation in most of the catchment areas is longer-term and none have very extensive facilities for crisis or respite admission outside hospital.

10.2.8 Day care

Again in the area of day care, comparison of the three areas illustrates the wide variety of service models making up the range of facilities in London. Tables 4–6 in the appendix to this chapter show the main facilities available for day care in each of the three areas. These tables indicate that each of the Boroughs has a mixed economy of day care, with health, social and voluntary sector providers. The picture also departs strikingly from the traditional distinction made in government policy papers between day hospitals provided by the health service, where the focus is on intensive acute *treatment* to avert admission or aid readjustment to the community following admission, and day centres, which are provided by local authorities and by the voluntary sector and meet needs for *support and long term contact* (Shepherd, 1991). The major shift from this model seems to be that in each of the three Boroughs, the health service is providing not only acute treatment, but a wide range of other forms of day treatment, including rehabilitation, recreational activity, drop in facilities, welfare advice and a range of other services which might be seen as more the traditional province of the Local Authority Day Centre. Further, in both Ealing and Camberwell, the health service sector facilities seem, in terms of both numbers and range of provision, to have become the main providers of long term day facilities. This tendency is rather less marked in Croydon, where the voluntary sector appears to be a more substantial provider, with a MIND day centre which provides a service for a large number of people. In the Borough of Lambeth in particular, there has been a notable lack of development of voluntary sector facilities, in mental health as in other spheres of community care provision, and this has left the mentally ill resident in the Borough especially vulnerable to the severe cuts in local authority provision currently taking place in response to Lambeth's large budget deficit.

10.2.9 Work facilities

Table 7 in the appendix to this chapter shows the main sheltered employment facilities and work training schemes serving each area. Reports from at least two of the three areas (Camberwell and Croydon) suggest that lack of such facilities is a significant problem, and the range and volume of opportunities provided does not seem great when the high proportion of unemployed people among London's mentally ill is considered (see Chapter 3). As commented on in Chapter 8 it does not appear that the development of work opportunities has been a very high priority. It is also notable that the range of types of employment available in sheltered employment schemes is relatively narrow, and the industrial and manufacturing work which is prominent at least in Camberwell and Croydon may not be a particularly good preparation for employment in the open market when London in general has very little remaining employment in manufacturing industries (Travers and Minors, 1995). Another potential gap in the range of care provided is in longer-term support in open employment: whilst some short-term training schemes are available there does not seem to be provision for supporting people in maintaining long-term functioning in an open work setting. It is notable that although the Audit Commission's "Finding a Place" (1994a) observes that "Having the opportunity to work is very important for most people", its report, in common with others such as "The Spectrum of Care", provides no specific discussion or recommendation on how to develop an effective local structure of employment schemes.

As with residential and day-care patterns of who provides care are rather different in each catchment area. In **Ealing**, the major provider of work opportunities is the Health Service, which plays little part in this sphere in the other two catchment areas. As noted before, community mental health care is relatively long established in Ealing, and it appears that a system has evolved where the Health Service is a major provider of a full range of community based services, including facilities such as long-time day care and work, which would not traditionally be seen as mainly the province of the Health Service.

10.2.10 Emergency services

Table 2 shows the main facilities dealing with people referred as emergencies. During usual office hours (9–5pm, Monday–Friday) in each area the local mental health team staff are major providers of daytime emergency care. However, none of the areas maintains such sectorised acute care out of hours, and in each are care by sector teams is supplemented in some way during working hours. This illustrates a dilemma for emergency provision in a community based system which has been extensively discussed in literature on emergency care (Katschnig and Konieczna, 1990; Katschnig, 1995). Where integrated sector community mental health teams which seek to provide comprehensive long term care have been developed, emergency care has often been seen as one of the range of functions which they should take on. However, there are some disadvantages to this decentralised non-specialist form of emergency care provision. For sector teams, emergency care competes with and may disrupt a variety of other functions. A more serious problem arises out of hours when very few districts in the UK maintain community-based emergency care (Johnson and Thornicroft, 1995). This is likely to be because the expense of maintaining night-time cover for each sector team individually is likely to be high, and an individual sector may not have enough out of hours emergencies to warrant this expenditure. These problems seem to have led to some form of centralised emergency provision persisting or being instituted in each of the three areas, alongside the sector teams:

In **Camberwell**, the Emergency Clinic has been established for over 40 years as a walk-in 24 hour service, this continues to function and to provide the only major alternative to the local Casualty Department at night and at weekends.

Table 2 Emergency care

	Camberwell	**Croydon**	**Ealing**
Office hours (9–5, Monday–Friday)	• Emergency clinic • Sector mental health teams in 4 of 5 sectors	• Crisis team consisting of one CPN rostered from each locality for each shift • 24 hour one number crisis line (staffed by CPNs from localities during day) • Rehabilitation team covers its own patients	• Sector mental health teams – each offers three appointments per week for crisis assessments. • Crisis intervention service – offers 9-5 assessment service complementing resource centre service. • Duty ASW service
Out of hours	• Emergency clinic • Mental health teams in 1 out of 5 sectors only, where: • Acute team available 9–5 seven days a week, by phone 24 hours. • Continuing care team available 24 hours to its clients	• Crisis team operates 8am–8pm Monday–Friday • 24 hour crisis line (own permanent staff at night) • Rehabilitation team on call for its 30 patients • Accident and emergency dept. at General Hospital	• Crisis intervention service 24 hours (provides 'crisis card service' – for existing patients only, no medical staff out of hours) • Accident and emergency dept. • Social services emergency duty team

Ealing and **Croydon** have both very recently developed specific crisis services to supplement sector team provision. In both instances, these were established in 1995 and are to a large degree a response to demand from users and carers locally, for whom various surveys have shown out of hours crisis care to be a high priority (Rogers et al, 1993). In Croydon, the specific crisis service takes the form of a 24 hour phone line staffed by CPNs. In Ealing the provision is rather more elaborate. A crisis team has been established which works alongside the sector teams during the day and continues to provide both a telephone service and visits at night. The daytime service is intended for new referrals, whereas the evening and night time service is purely for existing clients, who have "crisis cards" indicating plans to be followed in an emergency. It is notable that such a centralised service has been developed in Ealing despite its very long history of sectorised care. Some problems have arisen with this service: there are some difficulties assigning and co-ordinating work between this service and the sector teams, some doubts about the appropriateness of some of the use made of the service, and the service organisation was being reconsidered early in 1996. A particular question was whether the service served a useful purpose after midnight: there were very few visits made after midnight, but where they were requested all patients needed assessment by a psychiatrist (not available within the Crisis Team), and admission was frequently required, so that the usefulness of a service with no psychiatrist within it was uncertain.

10.2.11 Summary points: services for adults aged 18 to 65 years

One of the most significant issues arising from this more fine-grained examination of London Services is the difficulty in obtaining good information. Obstacles to obtaining a comprehensive view of mental health services available to the population of each area include the large number of providers and variety of ways in which they collect information, the lack of regularly updated centralised reviews of service availability, variations in provider catchment area, the need to assess turnover in order to know how available services really are and the difficulty in fitting a great variety of models of care into a fixed set of categories. In the absence of good quality information about current service provision in every catchment areas, it is difficult to see how rational planning of a comprehensive range of services can take place. Some conflict may arise between this requirement and the need to avoid overloading hard-pressed mental health staff with an excess of paperwork. However, this makes it all the more necessary to ensure that the information which is collected about services is really useful. Each of the areas would benefit from the development of standardised ways of collecting information from all statutory and non-statutory providers within the area and from a central mechanism for regular collation and review of this information. Such a strategy is needed to ensure that service planning for a local area is consistently based on up-to-date and interpretable information about current service provision.

Comparing the three areas demonstrates that there is considerable variety in the models which may be adopted for development of community services. All three areas are at various stages in the adoption of a broadly community-based model of care, in which sectorisation and Community Mental Health Centres play a major part. However, the precise ways of organising services vary considerably. Examples of questions about how to provide care which have been resolved in different ways in different areas include whether to separate acute care from rehabilitation, how to deliver out of hours emergency care, which models of residential care should be adopted, and whether to develop specialised models in inpatient care such as rehabilitation wards and pre-discharge wards. There may well be differences in effectiveness and acceptability between these various ways of developing community care, but very little evidence and guidance is currently available to those trying to choose between different strategies.

There is also some variation in the degree to which a homogenous service is provided throughout the catchment area. Ealing, with its old established sectorised system and tendency for the Health Service to be the major provider of social care, appears to have a broadly similar service model in all parts of the catchment area, whereas in Camberwell there are substantial differences between the functioning of services in different catchment areas. Thus in some areas obtaining a detailed view of local service availability will involve not only enquiring about services offered at a Trust level, but examining individually the services available in each of the sectors within the catchment area.

Finally, there are also substantial differences between catchment areas in who provides which form of care. The Health Service seems to be a major provider not only of acute, but also of long-term day care in each of the areas, and in one area has also become a significant work rehabilitation provider. The voluntary sector appears an important provider in all areas, especially in residential care, where the Health Service is less important. Local Authority provision is present but does not seem to be predominate in any sphere in any of the catchment areas. The suburban area Croydon, is the main one in which private sector provision plays a very significant part.

10.3 Old age services in the three areas

Needs for care

The elderly account for a substantial proportion of mental health service utilisation, with the age structure of the population, social deprivation, physical health and physical risk factors each affecting the actual level of need. In London, the population is relatively young, which may diminish needs for old age services, but the high levels of deprivation will increase needs.

The availability of carers is another particularly important issue, where the mobility of London's population and the higher rates of people living alone may work to make people particularly dependent on statutory services. Many older carers have health problems of their own, and the majority of both older sufferers and older carers are women (Livingston and Blanchard, 1996).

Population structure

The estimated population aged over 65 in Camberwell (the area covered by former Camberwell Health Authority) is 27,505, including 2,411 over 85; 36,207 in Ealing including 3,620 over 85; and 43,000 in Croydon. These represent 12.5% of the total population in Camberwell, 12.9% in Ealing and 13.7% in Croydon.

Trends over time

In each of these three areas an overall decrease in the numbers of over 65s is predicted with 'slight decreases' predicted in Ealing and Croydon, and a 9% decrease in Southwark, up to the end of the century. However, there are likely to be increases in the numbers of over 75s in all three areas, and increases are predicted in the very old in Camberwell and Ealing. There is also a predicted increase in the number of elderly people from ethnic minorities in Camberwell and Ealing. As those who settled in the UK as young people in the post-war period reach old age, a need for ethnically appropriate services for the elderly is arising on a large scale.

Prevalence of mental illness

Both Ealing and Croydon can identify the number of people with dementia in their catchment areas, with an estimated 2,392 sufferers (7% of the population over 65) in Ealing including 718 with severe dementia, and 3,800 (8%) in Croydon including a third with moderate or severe dementia, of whom 450 are likely to need 24 hour care.

Service provision

Community mental health teams

As with the general adult services, each areas has adopted a sectorised model, with community mental health teams based at community bases – Camberwell has five such teams, whilst Ealing has four and Croydon two, one of which is sub-divided into two parts. Team organisation is as follows:

- In Camberwell the teams consist of CPNs, and the service appears to be rather more closely integrated with primary care than the general adult services, with out-patient clinics provided at five primary care sites (health centres and general practices), as well as on the Maudsley hospital site. There is also one community mental health centre from which outreach is provided. The psychology service is a centralised Trust-wide service.
- The **Ealing** team also works closely with GPs to provided community based assessment and treatment. The medical staff and CPNs are allocated to particular sector teams, and have access to Trust-wide services for psychology, occupational therapy and physiotherapy, with sessional input from a dietician, an occupational therapist and a hairdresser.
- In **Croydon**, community mental health centres are the sites for out-patient consultation and are the bases for the mental health teams. One of the Croydon consultants has responsibility for liaison with the geriatric medicine services.

Social services and independent sector community support

- **Southwark** social services provide personal care packages (enabling people to continue living at home) to 1400 people, and purchase 800 more through independent sector providers, although it is uncertain what proportion of these clients are mentally ill. They also provide meals on wheels and a specialist nursing service for people who are incontinent. There are a variety of volunteer-based schemes run by voluntary and religious bodies, providing befriending and practical support. A worker employed by the Alzheimer's Disease Society can provide information and links with local support networks.

- In **Ealing** the social services-employed support workers accept referrals for elderly people with functional mental illness as well as for younger adults. Elderly people also have access to the specialist money advice and benefits service which is available to all mental health clients. There is a multi-ethnic meals on wheels service and a seven day home care service available to all client groups, although this service is limited and has a waiting list.

- **Croydon** also has a generic home care service for the elderly, with home helps and meals on wheels.

Day care

Day hospital provisions are as follows:
- **Camberwell** has a day hospital at the main hospital in-patient unit, and some day care is also provided on the in-patient wards. A community base provides 20 day

hospital places. The Health Commission (Lambeth, Southwark and Lewisham) provides two day hospitals for short term assessment and rehabilitation, with stays typically less than six weeks – one of these day hospitals is within Camberwell and has 18 places.

- In **Ealing**, there are three day hospital sites in the community with a total of 30 places available for the assessment of patients with organic brain disease, and 16 places for the assessment and treatment of patients with a functional mental illness such as depression.
- Day care is also available at the community mental health team bases in **Croydon,** although there are no separate day hospital facilities.

The following day centre provision is made:

- In **Camberwell,** Southwark social services provide six generic day centres for the elderly with 300 places throughout the borough and also fund another two voluntary sector day centres with 70 places for the elderly. There are 65 places in specific local authority day centres for elderly people with mental health problems.
- The Borough of **Ealing** provides 65 places in day centres for elderly people with mental health problems. These are at two day centres, one of which is for people with dementia, the other for both younger and older adults with functional illness.
- In **Croydon** there are 79 social services funded places for people with mental health problems over the age of 40, with the majority of attenders in fact over 70. There are also several luncheon clubs, centres and pop-ins for the elderly, although these do not generally cater specifically for people with mental health problems.

In-patient care

The areas have the following in-patient facilities:

- **Camberwell** has 50 in-patient beds at the Maudsley hospital. It also has a community-based ward facility with 24 continuing care beds and 12 respite or intermediate care beds for people with severe dementia and behavioural problems.
- **Ealing** has a total of 40 in-patient assessment and treatment beds and eight in-patient respite beds within the catchment area. The purchasing authority (E.H.H.) has also made available a small number of beds in West Middlesex and Wembley hospitals (outside the catchment area), but this option has often been turned down by patients and relatives. There is also within the catchment area a nursing home with 53 beds for people who have been discharged form E.H.H. long stay wards – however, this cannot admit people with severe functional disorders such as schizophrenia or with dementia. Throughput in the acute wards has been affected by a local shortage of continuing care places.
- In **Croydon,** there is a 20 bed mixed ward providing assessment and respite care at Warlingham Park Hospital, and two other wards providing a total of 47 continuing care places. Bed occupancy is reported to be 127% for the assessment ward, but 75% and 87% for the two continuing care wards.

Residential care

- **Southwark** has a total of 757 units of sheltered housing with 293 beds in residential care homes. Again this appears to be a figure for provision for a variety of client groups. Southwark Age Concern is contracted to provide long-term residential nursing care for people with continuing mental health needs. Twenty Camberwell residents are in out of borough placements.
- In **Ealing** there are six residential homes, each of which offers respite care. Three of the homes have specialist facilities for Asian and Polish elderly people.
- **Croydon** has three residential care homes designated for elderly people with mental health problems. There are also six designated respite beds in residential homes. There is also a substantial amount of private sector residential accommodation in Croydon, some registered to provide care for the elderly mentally infirm. However, there is no continuous nursing care for people with severe challenging behaviour.

Casemix

Casemix data is available for Croydon mental health teams, and indicates that the most frequent diagnosis for treatment episodes is dementia (32%), then depressive disorders (27%) and schizophrenia (12%).

Gaps in service provision

In each area, possible gaps in provision of a full spectrum of services could be identified, some of which are to be addressed in future service plans:

- **In-patient and residential care**: In Croydon, the assessment ward has very high occupancy and is at Warlingham Park, where inadequacies in the physical environment are the subject of considerable local concern. This will be addressed by the building of a new elderly assessment and treatment unit at the Bethlem Royal Hospital. The continuing care facilities will be replaced by inviting tenders from private sector providers. In Ealing there is a shortage of a range of continuing care places. In Croydon also, there is a lack of places for those with severely disturbed behaviour despite a range of private nursing home places being available.
- **Community and home services support**: Unlike the general adult services, community teams still appear to be largely CPN based, rather than having fully integrated multidisciplinary teams – development of full multidisciplinary teams is seen as an important target in Camberwell. In Ealing local consultants consider that some of those referred to social services mental health day centres in fact require high levels of care and have high rates of physical as well as mental disability, so that their needs are in reality too great to be met by day centre placement. These inappropriate placements are believed to reflect a lack of intensive home care and of long term day hospital placement. In each of the areas, the long term elderly mentally ill appear to be rather dependent on generic social care provisions, rather than having available very intensive and specific home support services.
- **Cultural appropriateness**: As the proportion of older people who belong to ethnic minorities rises, this is becoming a major issue for all services for the elderly mentally ill, particularly in Ealing and Camberwell. As yet there are relatively few specific initiatives, but purchasing plans suggest a high level of awareness of the need to make old age services more ethnically sensitive.

- **Carer support**: As previously noted, this is a particularly crucial aspect of services for the elderly mentally ill, and in both Camberwell and Croydon local key informants note that levels of carer support appear inadequate. In general, this aspect of provision appears largely to be left to the voluntary sector, rather than being the focus of co-ordinated and comprehensive initiatives from the statutory sector.
- **Integration with medical geriatric services** appears limited, and is also likely to be an important aspect of meeting the complex needs of this group.
- **Catchment area populations**: In Croydon, the sectors are large, and one consultant looks after a population of more than 22,000 people over 65, where the college guideline is that there should be one consultant per 10,000.

10.4 Child and adolescent services in the three areas

Needs for care

The overall prevalence of mental illness in the child population is estimated at up to 25% with 7 to 10% having moderate or severe problems, and disabling problems present in 2.1% of children (NHS Health Advisory Service, 1995). Factors which will affect parents' ability to provide a consistent supportive home for their children are those normally associated with deprivation, such as being a single parent, an economically inactive head of household, poverty and homelessness. These factors are prevalent in London in general and in inner London in particular, and population-based rates of children looked after are higher than in England and Wales as a whole (see Chapter 5.2).

Population characteristics

Croydon has a relatively young age profile while in both Camberwell and Ealing there are rising numbers of children under 16. For example, in Camberwell, the group of under fives is twice the size of the group of 10 to 14 year olds. Camberwell information also indicates that the proportion of under 16s who are from ethnic minorities is around 25%.

Prevalence of mental illness

An estimated 3,500 to 7,000 children in Croydon may have mental health problems, but only a small number of these children will be referred to child and adolescent mental health services. The majority of children seen as in-patients follow self harm episodes, with an increase from 20 per 10,000 child population in 1991/2 to 80 in 1993/4. There has also been an increase in the number of children excluded from school, for example currently 180 pupils in Croydon, while educational psychologists and school nurses have reported a rise in the number of pupils with emotional and behavioural problems at primary school. There are high levels of child abuse and neglect found in Camberwell, and the number of cases on the child protection register in Croydon is four per 1,000, compared with three, the national average.

Service provision

Community teams

Service organisation varies between the three areas.

- In **Camberwell,** there are multi-disciplinary teams for community services at two child guidance clinics in the community and also at a department in the general hospital. Some Camberwell children are also seen in the specialist out-patient clinics of the national services at the Maudsley hospital.
- In **Croydon**, the child and adolescent service is based in the community with three separate sector multidisciplinary teams operating from one community-based premises.
- In **Ealing** the children and families service is based on the main hospital site. Some clinics are held in the general hospital.

The multidisciplinary teams in the three areas each include a range of professionals: psychiatrists and child psychotherapists, with some additional staff: child psychologists (Camberwell, Ealing), family therapists (Camberwell, Ealing), clinical nurse specialists (Camberwell, Croydon), an art therapist (Croydon) and attached social workers in Camberwell and Croydon, and can provide a variety of therapeutic skills. The community teams in Camberwell and Croydon each offer therapeutic help and support to children and their families from the catchment area, with a variety of available treatment approaches including individual, family and group work. The commonest interventions in Croydon are counselling and support for the referred patients or family, with family therapy used in 24% of all cases.

Community teams in Camberwell and Croydon offer liaison and consultation services to other agencies including paediatric services, primary care, education services, and social services. Due to the demand on the service in Ealing, there is a waiting list and duty service run by experienced members of staff who allocate a degree of priority to cases.

Emergency services

In Camberwell there is a multi-disciplinary emergency service for adolescents who have attempted self harm and are admitted to the emergency department at the general hospital during office hours, with a specific child psychiatric on call rota for the accident and emergency department and wards out of office hours. In Ealing there is an agreement that the paediatric unit will admit children and adolescents admitted to the general hospital after self harm, and a member of the child and family consultation service will carry out an assessment within 48 hours.

Specialist services

Some specialist services are also available in all three sites, including specialist out-patient clinics for research projects in Camberwell, a specialist service for abused children and their families in Camberwell and Croydon, assessment of complex cases for court in Camberwell, and a neurodevelopment and under fives service in Ealing.

Ealing also has a specialist community service for 16 to 20 year olds who are not seriously mentally ill, offering various models of psychotherapeutic work and psychiatric assessment, and including domiciliary and GP liaison visits.

One of the Camberwell child guidance clinics offers a parents' support group at a specialist autistic unit.

In-patient services

- **Camberwell** has separate units for children (nine beds) and adolescents (14 beds) on the main psychiatric hospital site, but this is a national facility for which admissions take place through a Department of Health Research and Development contract.
- **Croydon** does not have its own in-patient facilities but may occasionally negotiate admissions individually to the Camberwell units. Croydon also has a block contract with a specialist unit in the area for the under 12s, and to an adolescent unit with 12 beds in Epsom.
- **Ealing** has no in-patient facilities in the area, but there are contracts with an in-patient unit for children, and two separate in-patient adolescent units.

Non-statutory provision

Each area has a variety of youth counselling services, Croydon and Ealing each have counselling services available for young people, the service run by MIND in Croydon also offering counselling for parents under stress.

Gaps in service provision

Possible gaps identified in this range of provision include:

- **Residential provision**: Currently young people over 16 in Croydon have to use the adult services if admission is required, and a young people's in-patient service is seen as an important requirement.
- **Inter-agency working**: In each of the areas, aspects of joint working with other agencies are seen as requiring reinforcement. Child Guidance Clinics have shifted to become health service rather than local authority based, and there has been a withdrawal of involvement from education authority employed staff. In Camberwell in particular, this has been problematic: the removal of Education staff in 1995 led to the closure of the Camberwell Child Guidance Centre's walk in service and under fives project, and has weakened links with schools. In Ealing, improving liaison with paediatric services is seen as an important requirement.
- **Community outreach services**: Whilst there are community-based clinics, there is relatively little capacity in any of the services for outreach and work in homes, and this is seen as one of the priorities for future development in Ealing.
- **Day facilities**: Generally specific child and adolescent day facilities have not been developed, and this is seen as a priority in Ealing and in Croydon.
- **Crisis facilities**: Only in Camberwell is there a specific 24 hour emergency service staffed by child psychiatrists, so that use has to be made of paediatric and/or general adult services for this purpose in the other areas, particularly out of hours.

10.5 Substance misuse services in the three areas

Needs for care

A third of people making contact with substance misuse services in the UK are reported to be in London, the number of admissions to services in the capital growing between 10 and 20% per year. This is a mobile population, and many are only in contact with services for a short period, and there are particular problems in the homeless population, prison population and the mentally ill, so that assessing local need is difficult.

The regional drug misuse databases have notifications from 611 residents in Southwark (approximately half of whom live in Camberwell), 1,683 residents in Ealing and 806 in Croydon. However, these databases are believed to indicate only a relatively small proportion of the overall prevalence – in Camberwell the estimate is that 20% of local drug misusers appear on the database. In Ealing and Croydon drug users are most frequently in the 25 to 29 age group, with men accounting for 67% of cases in Camberwell and 73% in Ealing. In each area, the drugs most commonly misused among those recorded on the databases are heroin (81% in Southwark, 32% in Ealing) and also cannabis. Other drug misuse reported includes stimulant drugs such as crack cocaine (Southwark, Ealing), and benzodiazepines and methadone in Ealing.

There is less information available about levels of alcohol misuse in particular areas, but a survey in Southwark suggests 7,000 residents drink alcohol in excess of safe limits. Ten to 15% of these people seek help each year.

Service provision

Community teams
All three areas have community drug services.
- The community service in **Ealing** provides outreach and also day care, with detoxification, methadone prescription, one to one counselling, group therapy, a well person clinic and one GP session per month. Methadone treatment is provided by approximately 10 local general practices. Community team staff make domiciliary visits and conduct satellite clinics at general practices, community mental health centres, and for the homeless. Ealing has two social workers who specialise in substance misuse.
- The multi-disciplinary community drug team in **Croydon** assesses new patients and offers specific help with harm minimisation and HIV prevention, relapse prevention and liaison with GPs.
- In **Camberwell** the teams can provide community detoxification and some day services. There is a GP liaison service and a separate methadone maintenance clinic.

Each of the three areas also has a community alcohol team:

- In **Ealing**, the community alcohol team is based in Ealing hospital, and offers out-patient detoxification and support from the Community Mental Health Resource Centres, including assessment of GP, hospital and casualty department referrals, family and couple work, and relapse prevention groups. Most referrals can be seen within a week. For dual diagnosis, joint work is undertaken with mental health teams.

- The team in **Croydon** is based at the same site as the community drug team. The Ealing and Croydon teams offer detoxification and prevention work. The Croydon team also offers supportive home visits, group therapy and an out-patient clinic.
- In **Camberwell**, the community alcohol team shares premises on a local high street with the community drug team, and can provide services including detoxification and liaison with primary care.

In-patient services

- In-patient provisions for **Camberwell** are part of provision made for the Lambeth, Southwark and Lewisham catchment area as a whole. This larger catchment area has a combined drug and alcohol in-patient acute assessment, detoxification and stabilisation service (four beds drug misuse, six beds alcohol misuse) on the hospital site in Camberwell. There is also an acute in-patient alcohol detoxification service at the Bethlem Royal Hospital, as well as eight in-patient beds for drug misuse patients from Lambeth, Southwark and Lewisham. The Bethlem also has longer-term in-patient rehabilitation, provided as part of a research and development programme.
- For **Croydon**, five detoxification beds are available for alcohol and three for drugs. Further regional and national detoxification beds can sometimes be accessed, but individual negotiation is needed, and waiting times are sometimes lengthy.
- In **Ealing**, an in-patient ward in Ealing hospital provides two to three week detoxification, with 13 beds for alcohol users and 2 to 3 beds for drug users.

Residential provision

- In **Camberwell**, social services purchase a range of residential care home placement from voluntary sector organisations in London and the rest of the country. However, Lambeth in particular is currently experiencing a major funding crisis and is unable to find funding for rehabilitation places. Crisis intervention services are purchased for alcohol misusers from a voluntary sector centre in Lambeth and for drug misusers from one in Islington.
- **Croydon** funds extended placements of around three to six months in two residential care homes within the Borough, one of which is managed by the Richmond Fellowship.
- In **Ealing**, there are 12 short term and rehabilitation places for alcohol misusers in a voluntary sector centre, with some then moving on to the same organisation's rehabilitation facility. Chaucer House is a voluntary sector provider located on the premises at Ealing Hospital and providing detoxification and residential rehabilitation to people with alcohol dependence – this is apparently the largest voluntary sector provider for this patient group in the UK. Placements with various out of borough drug rehabilitation services are funded through social services.

Day care and community support – voluntary sector

- In **Camberwell,** two voluntary agencies concerned with drug misuse (Community Drug Project and Stockwell Project) offer direct access, drop-in services providing counselling, day care, support for families and friends, help with getting medical treatment, assistance with benefits, and a needle exchange facility. In the voluntary sector, there is also a day treatment programme for people with alcohol problems, drop-in facilities include one which targets the black community and a counselling service which works through sites including GP services.

- In **Ealing**, a large Drug Advisory Service is funded by the health authority and local authority jointly and is managed by a voluntary sector organisation. It is a community and outreach service with 400 clients in regular contact, with a range of services including a community detoxification team, health assessments, drop-in facility and needle exchange. It takes referrals from other professionals and self referrals, seeing new clients within 72 hours. There are also smaller drop-in facilities run by other organisations such as Narcotics Anonymous and Cocaine Anonymous in Ealing, and out of Borough places are bought from organisations including a crisis intervention service for drug users, a service for people dependent on tranquillisers, and one for chaotic drug users in crisis.
- In **Croydon**, local voluntary sector services do not appear to be as extensive as in the inner areas, but a voluntary organisation offers a telephone helpline and community support for drug users and another organisation offers counselling and referral for detoxification.

Gaps in service provision

- **Services for ethnic minorities**: In Camberwell there is concern that members of ethnic minorities make use of substance abuse services little, so that there is a need for attention to be paid to developing services which appear accessible to members of these communities – this is likely to apply in other areas also.
- **Services for women**: A further priority in Camberwell is the development of services for women with children.
- **Services for non-opiate drug users** – The AIDS epidemic has led to relatively high levels of funding for services for injecting opiate users, but services for users of other drugs remain less developed. Crack cocaine is a particular problem in Camberwell. In Ealing a need for services for benzodiazepine users has been identified.
- **Integration with mental health teams and treatment of dual diagnosis**: In Ealing there is some integration of substance misuse with community mental health team work, allowing joint working where there is comorbidity, and in Camberwell such specific attachments to sector teams have been initiated. However, specific provisions for the management of dual diagnosis of mental illness and substance abuse remain very limited.
- **Pressure on services and lack of resources**: Both in Ealing and Croydon, statutory services are reported to be stretched and to have limited resources. Voluntary sector provision, at least for drug users in the inner areas of London, seems to be fairly extensive, but, as with the current lack of funding for rehabilitation places for residents of Lambeth, an important obstacle to meeting needs is lack of resources to fund placements.

Appendix: Details of service provision for adults aged 18–65 in the three areas

Table 1 Principal providers of residential care in Camberwell (as reported first quarter of 1996)

Health Service	*Voluntary & Private Sector*
Camberwell sector: – hostel with temporary accommodation for **8 people** – owned by Bethlem and Maudsley Trust, managed by **South London Family Housing Association** **Nunhead sector.** **4 beds** in a house for respite & diversion from admission – visited by staff at least daily. **4 recently purchased Trust properties were unoccupied in early 1996**	**24 hour staffed, waking:** **Brixton Circle Projects** – Cavendish House – Provides **21 beds** for African and Black Caribbean men and women. Rehabilitation programme, move on within 18 months. 80% from Camberwell. **Hexagon Housing Association** – registered residential nursing home with some Trust funding. Originally for resettlement of long term in-patients – low turnover of residents – **10 beds**. **24 hour staffed, sleeping in at night:** **St Vincent's Family Housing Association: 12 bed** home for women with mental illness. Help with daily living skills, emotional support. Most are very long-term residents **Southside Partnership** – house with **5 beds** for vulnerable people – mainly people with mental health problems. **Nserroma House** – **10 beds** for Black Caribbean men and women, skills training, help in finding long term accommodation. Recent management change, and future is uncertain. Referrals from wide area **Day staffed** (usually with out of hours on call system) **Advance Housing** staffed 10-8, 10-4 at weekends. **8 beds** for people with long term mental health problems. **Camberwell Community Support:** Staffed 8am-8pm. For people with long standing mental illness who need social support and help with daily living, indefinite stay. **8 places,** referrals from Maudsley hospital and Southwark **Southwark Caring Houses Trust: 34 beds** for men over 30 – most have mental health problems & history of homelessness. Intensive support from staff, but no structured programme -encouraged to use community facilities. Indefinite stay **Effra Trust: 38 beds** in various houses for ex-offenders, 80% with mental health problems. Some funding from probation service. Many do not originate from Camberwell. **Windsor Walk Housing Association** – **8 bed house** with staff 8-5, all referrals from Camberwell. **Lower support hostels and flats:** **Camberwell Community Support: 7 beds** permanent accommodation in visited house for the long term mentally ill **Eddie Brindley Project: 10 places for mentally ill in permanent accommodation, 22 for people in housing need in temporary –** **approx. 50% mentally ill.** Staff available 9-5, but move round sites or based in office. **5 places for Peckham sector,** otherwise referrals from anywhere. **Brixton Circle Projects:** 6 places for African/Caribbean women, with mental health problem or fleeing domestic violence. Most go to Fanon day centre. Support worker visits. **Camberwell Supported Flats: 16 independent supported tenancies** for mentally ill – 1-2 visits weekly. Support withdrawn once not required, client remains in flat. Referrals generally from Southwark **Carr-Gomm** – association provides houses for people with various needs of support, sometime mentally health. In March 1995, approx. 38 residents in Southwark and 8 in Lambeth had mental illness. Staff pop in or in some cases may be available 9-5. **Hummingbird Project** – jointly set up by Hyde Housing and Maudsley Hospital, **6 places** for single homeless mentally ill men in visited house. **South London Family Housing Association:** 5 places in visited flats. Housing Dept has nomination rights for 50%. **Camberwell Circle Project: 10 beds** in supported flats for mentally ill women (Talford Road). **Lorrimore Centre – 4 short term beds** (up to 3 months)

Table 2 Principal providers of residential care in Croydon (as reported first quarter of 1996)

Health Service	Social Services	Voluntary and Private Sector
24 hour staffed, waking staff **Westways Unit:** Has trained nursing staff, Occupational therapist, medical cover. Patients are a mixture of 'new long stay' and former patients of the local large asylum where reprovision is taking place. **30 beds.** Hostel for rehabilitation of Mentally Disordered Offenders. Trained nurses and medical cover. **10 beds.** **Group homes:** Group home for long-term rehabilitation, daily support from Westways Unit. **3 beds.**	**London Borough of Croydon** **24 hour staffed with sleep in** **Ashburton House:** men and women up to 40, rehabilitation programme, 2 year time limit **10 places** **Emergency Assessment Unit,** – for homeless persons vulnerable because of mental illness – referred by Housing Dept. **10 beds** **Glazier House** – men & women 26-65, no time limit **8 longer stay places, 2 planned respite** **Day staffed:** **12 hostel places** supervised by Social Services Adult Placement Team **5 places** are provided in a house near the Emergency Assessment Unit, supported by same staff **Group homes:** Social services owns three small homes, visited at least weekly, total of **12 residents** **Supported flats** – **6 bedsitters**, training programme for independent living, max. one year **Social services adult placement scheme** – lodgings with families, paid for and supported by social services – **approx 50-60 used by mentally ill people**.	**Hostels** **Hostel run by South London Churches organisation:** Linked with health service hostel for mentally disordered offenders, run by South London Churches. **Registered care homes:** Croydon has **190 places** in registered care homes, of which **113** were purchased by Croydon Social Services during 1995. Apart from a 24 bed home owned by the Mental Aftercare Association, these are all privately owned. Most have staff sleeping on the premises at night, and all are required to have some form of 24 hour staff cover. No legal requirement for staff to be trained, but Social Services Adult Placement Team provides link workers – **52 people in Croydon, 8** out of Borough supported in private homes by such linkworkers in Feb. 1996. **Group homes** MIND has two group homes with a total of **12 places** There are three other group homes provided by various housing associations with a total of **14 places.**

Table 3 The main providers of residential care in Ealing (as reported first quarter of 1996)

Health Service	Local Authority	Voluntary Sector
24 hour nursing staff **'The Limes'** Nursing home with around 60 places for younger long term mentally ill people (opened around five years ago).	**24 hour staffing, sleep in** **Rehabilitation Hostel with** rehabilitation programme, individual care plans, skills training, various groups. **16 places** **Rehabilitation Hostel: 15 places,** including some respite & assessment **Group homes** 13 properties visited at least once a week, out of hours contact team. **47 places.** **Supported flats** **Housing department** – owns **30 supported flats** in four permanent mental health supported housing schemes with some staff contactable and popping in at times.	**24 hour staff, sleep in** **Richmond Fellowship:** therapeutic community with intensive programme. **16 places but no current resident from Ealing.** **St Mungo's Trust:** For homeless people nominated by housing dept, at least 90% have mental health problem. Support with daily living, no resources for activities. **20 places.** Trust manages second 24 hour staffed hostel for people with long term mental illness, with **8 places.** Residents generally from Ealing. Ealing Consortium – 24 hour care home for people resettled from long-stay wards **Private registered nursing homes:** these include **Rainbow Lodge,** where there are **20 places,** and **30 further** places at 15 other small residential homes. Many placements are from outside Ealing. **Day staffed hostels:** **MIND project** for women. Staffed until 7pm weekdays, weekend afternoons. **7 places,** for Ealing residents only. **St Mungo's Trust** manages a hostel for people of Asian origin, staffed 10-6 7 days. Rehabilitation, daily living training. **8 places.** **George Doyley House:** For young Black Caribbean people with various special needs. In Ealing, but only 3 current residents from Ealing, none mentally ill. **Group homes:** **2 MIND group homes:** weekly visits by staff – **9 places,** all for Ealing. **Supported flats:** **Somerset Road Project (MIND):** For people to re-establish themselves in the community Resettlement officer available for clients to drop in 9-5, checks on clients at least twice weekly. **9 independent flats, Ealing residents only** **Central and Cecil Housing Trust:** provides some support, skills training, co-ordination from staff member on site working hours. Permanent tenancies. **6 supported flats** **Ealing Family Housing Association:** 2 supported flat projects, staff available Monday to Friday. **56 flats, though not all necessarily used by mentally ill.** **Ealing Consortium:** independent tenancies for people resettled from St Bernard's long term wards, staff from adjacent hostel available. **Generic provision:** The **YMCA hostel** is a significant non-specialist provider of accommodation for mentally ill – c. 35 mentally ill people – 24 hour waking staff

Table 4 Day care in Camberwell

Health Service	Social Services	Voluntary Sector
• **Brixton & Norwood sectors** – shared day site. 10 sessions weekly. Rehabilitation & acute care, drop in, wide range of structured activity, welfare advice, medication supervision – **40 rehabilitation attenders and 40 users of drop in services, capacity for 60 in rehabilitation service.** • **Camberwell sector** – sector core day site, 10 sessions per week. Acute care, rehabilitation, drop in, wide range of structured activity, welfare advice. **32 attend each day, capacity for 50 per day, 112 on register.** • **Nunhead sector** – sector day site offers acute care and rehabilitation, range of activities, welfare advice, medication supervision. **25-30 attendances per day**, 120 on register • **Peckham** – main day care site open 5 sessions a week, range of structured activity (but currently limited by staff shortage), drop in, advocacy. **30 patients attend regularly, 86 on register.** Some additional day care at teambases of each sector team – one has **4-5 regular drop in attenders,** and the other has **10-15 attenders each day, with a daily maximum capacity of 20.**	**Three of the sectors make up part of the Borough of Southwark, whilst the other two are part of Lambeth** **London Borough of Southwark** • **Ivydale Mental Health Resource Centre** -open four short days as day centre, two as drop in. Limited programme of groups, help with daily living problems. **6 to 8 regular day centre attenders, 10 regular drop in attenders, 20 to 24 on drop in register.** also African/Caribbean pop in one session per week – **20-25 each week.** • **Castle Day Centre**: For long term mentally ill. 10 sessions weekly. Substantial structured group programme, daily living help, welfare advice. **20-25% of clients are from Camberwell, total average daily attendance 26, daily capacity up to 30. 72 are on register.** **London Borough of Lambeth** **Borough has very large deficit, great uncertainty about future of services** • **One day centre already closed.** • **Effra Road Day Centre: Closed to further referrals.** Four sessions weekly. Some groups, daily living help, welfare advice, but no individual programmes. **30-46 attend daily, with 100 on register** – approx. **50% are from Camberwell catchment area.** • **Riggindale** – 10 sessions weekly, one evening. Previously structured activity & group programme, but now only one support group weekly. Individual counselling, daily living help, welfare advice & individual care programmes. **35 clients attend each day, 80 are on register.**	<u>Southwark</u> • **Crossways day centre** Run by independent charity. 10 sessions per week plus one evening and Sunday drop in. Groups throughout day, daily living help, welfare & housing advice, ethnic minority development worker. **30 attend per day, 67 on register, 50 places bought by Southwark (rest by Guys)** • **Lorrimore Centre** 24 hours during week, 6 hours on Saturday. Drop in, some groups, welfare advice. **30 clients attend 2-3 times weekly 142 on register, Southwark & Lambeth** • **48 Club**: 27 hours per week, 7 on Sunday. People with at least one year's mental health service contact. Very informal, some creative groups & welfare advice. Funding from Trust, and Health Commission, numbers not available. • **Copleston Centre** – community centre not specifically for mentally ill, but with some groups for mentally ill (input from local sector teams) **Day care for particular groups: The Fanon day centre provides day care for members of ethnic minorities, including a women's project. St Giles' Day Centre provides for homeless people, many of whom are mentally ill.**

Table 5 Day care in Ealing

Health Service	Social Services	Voluntary Sector
No day care in Trust's contract with purchasing authority, but extensive day care provision for people with long term mental illness at the Community Mental Health Resource Centres Opening is 10 sessions per week plus small number of early evening groups, with a weekend service for those specifically referred by keyworkers. Day care at each centre includes a full daily programme of therapeutic, activity and social groups, individual support & counselling, drop in service, music, drama & art therapy, a women's group, psychoeducation, carer support & education . **At one of the five centres (Avenue House), approx. 300 patients attend for a full group programme and 200 use the drop in. service.** Detailed figures not available to us for the other four, but services offered are similar.	**London Borough of Ealing** **Carlton Centre:** 10 sessions per week. Offers rehabilitation, aims to keep clients in the community. Range of structured activities, individual care plans. Some specific facilities for Asian clients. **45-55 attend daily, capacity up to 55, 100 on register (but approx a third of clients are over 65)** **Solace Centre:** 4-8pm weekdays, 12-8 weekends and bank holidays. Drop in, aiming to become 'user-led'. **60-70 clients use, varying attendance.**	**MIND Ivy Club:** 5 sessions weekly. Informal day centre for 'lonely people and those with emotional and nervous difficulties'. Leisure and creative groups, some organised outings. Average **27 attenders per day, capacity up to 40, 70 clients currently in contact.** **MIND Sunday Club:** 10am-4pm Sunday, informal drop in for those who feel isolated on Sunday. Lunch and some groups. **9 attend each Sunday, 20 members in total.** **Facilities for specific groups:** **Southall Mental Health Support Project (Lotus Centre)** provides a drop in service which targets Asian people – 3 days per week. **Emmaus House** is a facility for the homeless with a substantial number of mentally ill attenders.

Table 6 Day care in Croydon

Health Service	Social Services	Voluntary Sector
Each of the three localities has one or two community resource centres which provide day care. The resource centres are all open 10 days per week. offer acute care, individual care plans, creative and therapeutic groups, help with daily living problems and welfare advice. **Central locality:** Queens Resource Centre has **30-35 daily attendances and 55 on register.** This includes places for up to 5 *intensive care patients*, who attend all sessions for up to a fortnight and are nursed at all times, and for 12 *extra care patients*, who attend 3-5 days per week, with a higher than usual level of input. **North Locality:** Westways has **15 attendances per day and 38 on the register.** It can also provide intensive care, although not always with nursing at all times. **South Locality:** Crescent Resource Centre has **30 attendances per day and 40 to 50 on the register.** Purley Resource Centre has **12-21 daily attendances and 40 on the register.** A distinction between intensive and sessional care is not made at these two centres.	**London Borough of Croydon** **Bensham Day Centre:** Clients aged **55 and over.** 10 sessions per week. Individual programmes, social and creative groups, light work. **20 attendances daily, 47 on register of whom approx 28 are under 65.** **Lantern Hall Day Centre:** For people with mental health problems. 10 sessions per week. Individual programmes, recreational and social activities, daily living skills. **55 places.** **Informal day care projects:** 8 informal day care projects are run by social services social development team for people referred by care managers, CPNs or psychiatrists. Aim is to provide mutual support, social and recreational activities at local bases. Aim to be user led. These projects provide a total of **145 places.**	**Fairfield (MIND):** 10 sessions per week plus weekends and evening opening on three days. Social activities, range of informal groups. **Approx 270 current members, daily attendance approx 40-60** **Enterprise House (MIND):** This is a day centre where the main focus is on providing a structured work-oriented programme for those who wish to return to full employment. It has **12 places available a day, with 30 on register.** There are also a number of **drop ins** are including: **Rainbow Club** – one evening a week, run by Association for Pastoral Care of Mentally Ill with approx **30 attenders** **The Bridge:** Sunday afternoon drop in. **8-9 each week, 30 on register** **Open Door Club:** one evening a week, average of **12 attenders, 45 on membership list.** Drop in for attenders of Westways Rehabilitation Unit – one day per week

Table 7 Work facilities

Camberwell	*Croydon*	*Ealing*
Health service: • **Melting Pot Cafe** – established by staff from one of mental health teams. Has **17 employees.** **Local Authority** • **Choices Course** – 6-week course, one day per week, for people with mental illness to consider work, education & leisure options. (*Southwark Adult Education*) **Voluntary sector:** • **Camberwell Resettlement Association:** Light industrial work 10 sessions per week, for people with long term mental illness **12 employees on wages, 35 rehabilitation places, currently 26 filled – all usually Camberwell area:** • **Southside Rehabilitation Association** – operates a group of small businesses, offering sheltered work to people with long term mental illnesses. **Approx 100 users in Southwark, Lambeth & Croydon – no. from Camberwell uncertain** • **PECAN:** Charitable company run by local churches which runs courses to help people get back to work, including specialist course for people with mental health problems. • **Blackfriars Work Centre** – range of activities which develop and improve work skills, including printing, woodwork, sewing, clerical work, word processing. Pay – 50p per session. **24 places a day, attendance at least three days a week required. Catchment area – Southwark.** • **Lambeth ACCORD –** for people with mental illness (& other disabilities) – 4-week assessment programme 1-year training programmes in office & catering skills	**Local Authority** • **Crosfield Industries** – provides for all people with disabilities, proportion of mentally ill not known. **65 disabled people** employed in a unit with fully open market working conditions, **35 more sheltered places** for people not able to reach these expectations. **Voluntary sector:** • **Enterprise House (MIND)** is a day centre offering a structured work programme, with **30 people attending 1-3 sessions per week.** Some outside opportunities such as light removals & voluntary work. (*Also listed under day care*).	**Health Service:** • **Work Rehabilitation Unit** of Trust – provides work assessment and either advice on other opportunities or placement in one of Trust's units, where there are **110** places in a range of activities including horticultural, commercial and carpentry. Some allow attenders to obtain Level 1 National Vocational Qualification. **Local authority** • **Ealing employment rehabilitation service:** large centre mainly catering for physically disabled, but accepts some mentally ill people for work at centre or on external contracts. **Voluntary sector:** • **MIND Support Training & Resource Team (START)** – training scheme and counselling for entry into work. **In six months – 35 interviewed, 16 attended courses, 3 placed in work** • **MIND Shop:** 14 places for workers in shop which is also fund raising venture

Chapter 11

Mental health services in London: costs

Daniel Chisholm, Ana Lowin and Martin Knapp

11.1 Introduction

Mental health care policy in the UK has undergone unprecedented change over the past decade, the impact of which has been felt in all aspects of mental health planning, delivery, funding and evaluation. Proponents of reforms to the organisation and delivery of mental health care provision have emphasised the desirability of moving from a hospital to a community-based service, organising services within a more contestable (competitive) environment, and focusing more explicitly on the needs of people with mental health problems, in particular those with severe and enduring mental illness.

Fuelled by a series of tragic incidents involving former psychiatric inpatients, critics of the current system have pointed to the fragmentation and lack of coordination surrounding existing financing and delivery arrangements. These difficulties can be exacerbated in metropolitan and inner city areas where there are often concentrations of mental health needs but not the range of services available to meet them. There has been widespread discussion as to whether the provision of mental health services in London is particularly or differentially disadvantaged in terms of a lack of resources to meet the particular needs of its population.

Aims and objectives

The agreed objectives of the economic component of the London Commission mental health project were to inform the London Commission of the costs associated with both the current provision of a range of mental health services in the capital and the level of provision required to meet (measured) local mental health needs; to comment where possible on the efficiency with which resources are being used in different sectors and localities in London, including examination of the resource implications associated with supplementation or substitution of innovative services that are indicative of 'good practice' into the existing balance of provision; and to provide a clear description of the costing methodology adopted and to develop (brief) guidelines for future use by commissioners in their own respective areas.

Scope and limitations

The activities required to meet these objectives follow a progression of stages, some of which are dependent on the output of other King's Fund commissioned work such as data on current service activity, so that cost comparisons could be afforded between actual and predicted levels of provision. One particular requirement for the resolution of issues around the relative efficiency of services (our second stated objective) was consensus on a) the elements that together constitute a 'reasonable and safe' local mental health service in London and b) the substitutability effects of any innovative elements on existing models of delivery. This consensus proved elusive, as a result of both the heterogeneity of particular service responses in different parts of the capital, and the absence or paucity of concrete evidence upon which to base estimates of effectiveness and/or substitutability. The absence of a baseline or benchmark against which to assess local practice and performance has constrained our ability to comment on the key question of how efficiently mental health resources are being targeted across London. We have nevertheless presented a number of (unsubstantiated) service scenarios as a basis for discussion and for further development.

A further objective considered by the mental health support group – but not covered by this study – was to explore the *sufficiency* of current resource allocations (and their associated formulae) to meet and predict current and required levels of mental health service provision and need in London. The relative extent to which problems with mental health services, and particularly those found in large conurbations, are attributable to the (in)efficient use of existing resources as against the (in)sufficiency of resources made available is an extremely complex question to resolve. However, one contribution at the London level would be to compare findings relating to the resource implications of (various) full service configurations with the resources actually allocated by current national funding formulae (see Carr-Hill et al, 1994; Smith et al, 1996). Such analyses might provide a useful empirical platform upon which to comment on the adequacy of current allocation formulae with respect to mental health care in London.

It should be noted, however, that attempting to compare or reconcile aggregated, top-down expenditure figures and bottom-up cost estimates of service provision is liable to be fraught with difficulties, not least in trying to reach a basis for like-with-like analysis. For example, the cost analyses presented here are based on a limited set of service components, to which uniform and economically defined unit costs have been attached. By contrast, year-end expenditure figures or financial returns are based on activity or performance data which contain considerable variations in terms of definitional and operational criteria as well as local modes of delivery and contract prices, and which in any case closely reflect initial annual allocations arrived at by formulae which are acknowledged to be incompletely sensitive to mental health need (Smith et al, 1996).

11.2 Policy context: is London different?

Key issues

Chapter 4 has provided an overview of national mental health policy developments and their differential impact on service delivery in London, and these have also been summarised by Knapp et al (1995) under three heads:

• *Reprovision of services:* The move away from in-patient hospital care to community-based care has, in some areas, been argued to have resulted in numbers of long-stay or other hospital places being reduced at a faster rate than new community or hostel places are being made available. Whether or not this is the case, the shifting locus of care is raising substantial new challenges for mental health care agencies, as well as for people with mental health problems and their families.

- *Reorganisation of services:* The promotion of market forces in the mixed economy of health and social care and the extension of greater responsibility for purchasing community care to social services departments (which have traditionally been neither major providers in or major purchasers of mental health services) have not yet produced clear or distinctive organisational roles for the main stakeholder organisations.

- *Financing of services:* Changes to the funding routes, particularly the shift from means-tested social security payments to needs-based local authority contractual payments, have complicated the purchasing side of the new mixed economy. The increasing pluralism of provision has added to the complexities.

In relation to the 'London question', there has been no shortage of commentary and debate, but a conspicuous absence of firm evidence to support or inform this debate. The shortage of evidence has been particularly acute in relation to costs and cost-effectiveness. The main financial question with respect to London is whether it is overfunded or underfunded relative to the rest of the country. Explanation of the higher costs of services in London has variously attributed them to higher input prices (particularly for staffing and land), casemix complexity and deprivation. Taking the last hypothesised source first, there is sufficient evidence (discussed further in Chapter 3) to indicate that London scores highly on a number of key sociodemographic factors – including poverty, deprivation and social isolation – each of which has been found to be indicative of, or associated with, greater morbidity and mental health needs (Hirsch, 1988; Thornicroft, 1991; Glover et al, 1994; Carr-Hill et al, 1994). As outlined in Chapters 6 and 7, this is borne out by above-average admission rates, bed use and bed occupancy in the hospital sector and higher use of community and ambulatory services across London (MILMIS Group, 1995).

The higher labour costs in London were examined some years ago by the York Health Economics Consortium, which estimated that skilled labour costs were 22 per cent and unskilled labour 17 per cent higher in London than for England as a whole (Akehurst et al., 1991). In a more recent staffing survey of four local authorities, Bebbington and Kelly (1993) found higher pay, grading and appointment levels in two inner London Boroughs than in the other metropolitan districts. It has also been argued that resources are inefficiently used in London, in particular because patients stay longer in specialised hospital care than is necessary because of reductions or gaps in intermediate levels of support. Finally, there are grounds for suggesting that due to a combination of small catchment populations but high overheads (and morbidity), commissioning agencies in London may demonstrate greater diseconomies of small scale.

Previous research

The Centre for the Economics of Mental Health (CEMH) was previously funded under the King's Fund's *Fair Shares for London* Research Grants Scheme to examine the utilisation and costs of community health, hospital and some other services by people with mental health problems living in a variety of specialist residential accommodation settings (Knapp et al, 1995). In particular, the research focused on establishing, and then comparing, the level and composition of residential provision in and outside London, the associated costs of that provision, and the links between costs and the characteristics of residents, facilities and areas, which together enable the analysis of shifts in the balance and financing of care. At the level of summary sample descriptions and bi-variate tests, it was found that the costs of residential care packages (all settings) are 43 per cent higher in London than elsewhere; for hospital residents, the weekly differential is £187, for community residents it is £72 (1993/94 price levels).

These initial descriptive analyses were followed by an examination of the resource implications of variations in the characteristics of clients and facilities, the cost differences between facility types or sectors, the resident and cost differences between areas and the decomposition of the London cost differential into resident, price and technology components. The analyses led us to conclude that a substantial part of the difference between the London and non-London costs of accommodating people with mental health problems (about two-fifths of the overall difference) could be attributed to the *balance of care effect*, namely that relatively fewer people are accommodated in community residential accommodation rather than in hospital in London than in non-London districts. This is particularly because of a shortage of suitable community accommodation in the capital. The characteristics of individual residents with significant cost-raising implications, which together constitute what can be called a *needs effect*, account for a relatively small part of the inter-area difference. (In fact, non-London facilities accommodate a marginally more costly community care clientele than do London community residents, but London hospitals accommodate more costly inpatients.) The remaining difference is made up of the combined effects of *care technology and unit costs*, with the unit cost or input price effect apparently dominant. The decomposition of the 'London differential' is summarised in Figure 1.

Figure 1 Decomposing the London/non-London difference

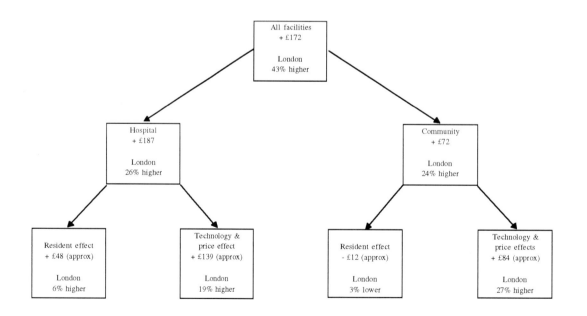

11.3 Methodology

The costing work reported here has drawn on a large number of data sources, necessitating a clear account of how these various sets of information were integrated into our overall methodological framework. The methodological principles, processes and (where necessary) assumptions described in this section of the report can be viewed as a preliminary set of guidelines for future use by commissioners or other interested parties in their own respective areas.

Costing principles

The broad perspective employed in the costing of mental health services is an economic one, such that in principle service costs are derived by reference to their marginal long-term opportunity costs. For example, the opportunity cost of an inpatient hospital bed is in principle to be based on established calculations of how those resources could be used in their best alternative use, such as a residential care place, an entirely different service within or outside mental health care or even the return on those resources that could be obtained through an interest-bearing bank account. In practice, however, derivation of costs in this way is elusive, and it is conventional to use short-term average costs as a reasonable proxy for long-run marginal costs (Beecham, 1995). There is widespread consensus in health economics as to the validity of these proxies in most circumstances. A further principle of cost evaluation is that the resource implications of *all* elements of a service should be considered, even though individual service planners may only be interested in the cost to their own agencies. Again, there are difficulties in realising this principle on pragmatic grounds; for instance, the full cost of a residential care place may include inputs from unpaid volunteer staff or financial contributions from clients over and above those of the managing agency. In costing the various service components of mental health care in London, we have taken as wide or comprehensive a perspective as time and effort would allow.

Unit cost data collection and calculation

Constructing a profile of the actual costs and resource implications of London's mental health services requires the combination of two sets of data, the first of which is information on current levels of service activity – the information used here was the data set already described in more detail in chapter 7 of this report. For each of the service components described – and this is the second set of data – an estimate of the cost associated with the provision of a unit of service provision is needed. The appropriate unit of analysis differs across the service components (for example, hospital inpatient beds are usually described in daily units, whereas residential places are more commonly described per week). For the purposes of comparison, each unit cost has been converted into an annual estimate.

London as an entity can be divided up in a number of different ways, for instance by borough, by health authority or by low/high Jarman score (Jarman, 1982). From a costing perspective, the most viable means of division is Inner/Outer London; accordingly, separate unit costs have been derived in order to reflect the differential costs of provision in these two areas. Where unit cost data are not specifically disaggregated for these two areas, adjustment factors for capital, revenue and overhead costs need to be established and applied to London-wide or national unit cost estimates. In this study, we have made adjustments for capital (based on surveys of tender prices; Building Cost Information Service, 1996) and staffing (area cost adjustments; Department of the Environment, 1996). Adjustment factors for non-staff revenue costs and overhead elements could not be calculated, but as these elements only represent approximately 25–30% of total unit costs, we are not substantially underestimating the differential costs of provision in Inner and Outer London.

Data used for the calculation of unit costs were obtained from a number of sources, including government statistics and returns, facility accounts, compilations of unit costs, individual research studies and published and unpublished reports on various specific services. The particular set of 'building blocks' and resulting best estimates of annual unit cost for hospital, residential and day care can be found in Table 1. For ease of reference, we briefly outline below the methods and sources used for the three main categories of service provision: hospital inpatient services; residential care facilities in the community; and day care/community mental health services.

Hospital inpatient services

Unit costs for acute and continuing care psychiatric inpatient care were derived on the basis of a sample of 25 acute and 19 continuing care psychiatric wards covered in a recent survey of residential care in eight district health authorities (described in Chisholm et al, 1997; and set out in Netten and Dennett, 1996). Capital estimates are based on average functional unit prices derived from the Building Cost Information Service (1996), and revenue costs were obtained from hospital accounts, broken down into salaries, supplies and services, and agency overheads. In this study, service activity data on continuing care wards have been merged with that on hostel ward provision. We have applied our unit cost estimate for continuing care wards (£48,929, Inner London; £46,047, Outer London) to this merged category, noting that this estimate falls close to the upper limit of the range (£35,000–£50,000) suggested in a recent report on 24-hour nursed care facilities (Department of Health, 1996c).

The annual estimate of £95,000 per bed for regional secure units is based on prices per bed for local health authority and Trust returns for the South Thames region (South Thames RHA, 1996). The local secure ward estimate is drawn from individual facility accounts as part of the North Thames reprovision study (Hallam et al, 1996).

Residential care

The primary source of costs data for 24-hour staffed hostels, day staffed hostels, and unstaffed hostels/group homes was a substantial survey of mental health residential care (Chisholm et al, 1997). Weekly establishment estimates are based on a London subsample of facilities, and are broken down into capital, salaries, running costs and overheads. Capital and salary components were adjusted to reflect the Inner/Outer differential as described above. These weekly estimates were then converted into annual unit costs.

Table 1 Derivation of unit costs: hospital, residential and day provision

Service component[1]	Unit of baseline measurement	Baseline unit cost (£, 1995/96)	Source (Ref.)	Range (sector means)	Adjustment factors[2]				Adjusted annual unit costs, London	
					Capital		Salaries			
					Inner	Outer	Inner	Outer	Inner	Outer
Regional Secure Unit	price per annum (S. Thames Region)	95,000	S. Thames returns	78,000–136,000	n/a	n/a	n/a	n/a	95,000	95,000
Local secure ward	per patient week (Outer London)	1,282.52	N. Thames study	n/a	1.06	1.00	1.10	1.00	72,442	66,871
Acute psychiatric ward	per patient day (London)	141.14	Unit Costs book	n/a	1.02	0.96	1.06	0.97	53,651	50,248
Continuing care ward/hostel ward	per patient day (London)	129.15	Unit Costs book	n/a	1.02	0.96	1.06	0.97	48,929	46,047
24 hour staffed hostel	per resident week (London)	399.72	Resid.l care study	(277.52 LA) (566.70 Vol)	1.02	0.96	1.06	0.97	21,748	20,305
Day staffed hostel	per resident week (London)	203.91	Resid.l care study	(155.82 LA) (216.84 Vol)	1.02	0.96	1.06	0.97	11,074	10,352
Unstaffed hostel/group home	per resident week (London)	167.39	Resid.l care study	(226.52 LA) (150.47 Vol)	1.02	0.96	1.06	0.97	9,021	8,495
Supportive housing	per resident week (Outer London)	140.19	N. Thames study	n/a	1.06	1.00	1.10	1.00	7,929	7,310
Day hospital[3]	per day (Outer Lon)	43.21	N. Thames study	n/a	1.06	1.00	1.10	1.00	11,539	10,586
Day care[3]	per day (London)	38.58	Unit Costs book	n/a	1.02	0.96	1.06	0.97	9,918	9,163

1 Service components as defined in PRiSM survey of Trusts and Local authorities
2 Adjustment factor for capital taken from BCIS (1996; adjustment factor for salaries taken from DoE (1996b)
3 Annual cost of day hospital/day centre attendance assumes 245 operational days per annum.

Day care and community mental health services

Day hospital estimates (£11,539, Inner; £10,568, Outer) are drawn from a single facility's accounts as part of the North Thames reprovision study (Beecham et al, 1997), and compare with an independent estimate of £15k-£20k per place for acute care for adults (Crilly and Robbins, 1996). Day centre cost estimates are based on the Unit Costs publication (Netten and Dennett, 1996), which coincide with the mean estimate for 8 units covered in the North Thames study (Beecham et al, 1997).

Two separate pieces of work informed the calculation of Community Mental Health Teams (CMHTs). Onyett et al (1995) describe the organisation and operation of CMHTs based on two national surveys, including the typical staffing composition of such teams. Median salaries for each type of worker represented in a typical team were multiplied by the proportion of that type of worker to produce a generic CMHT worker salary. Together with appropriate London multipliers (1.22; Akehurst et al, 1991) plus capital and staffing overheads, a unit cost of £41,504 per annum (or £27 per hour) is derived. The mean amount of face-to-face contact time for all these workers was 36 per cent, giving an estimate of £75 per hour of client contact (Netten and Dennett, 1996, pages 52 and 91). A further adjustment for differential labour and capital costs in Inner and Outer London gives estimates of £43,575 and £40,151 respectively.

The second piece of work was specifically commissioned to provide further evidence on this key service component. Two independent estimates of CMHT staffing, skill mix and associated costs were developed based on national averages and other indicators, as well as on the first-hand experience of two CMHSD consultants (Crilly and Robbins, 1996). CMHTs were assumed to undertake the following functions: screening, assessment, care programming, case management, monitoring and review; providing alternatives to inpatient treatment (i.e. home treatment and day treatment); primary liasion. Staffing levels exclude out of normal working hours crisis response (costed separately) and primary care workers (for people with less severe mental health problems).

Full time equivalent staffing levels per 100,000 population and unit cost estimates, together with an explanation of the basis of these estimates, can be found in Table 2. For a population of 100,000 with a standard profile of deprivation, it is estimated that a total of 37 w.t.e. posts are required, at a total annual cost of close to £1 million (including operational site overheads but excluding capital charges and corporate overheads). Once we have substituted the 10% estimate for site costs in this model with a fuller estimate of all operational, corporate and capital overheads (£6,544 per worker; Netten and Dennett, 1996) and included a regional multiplier for London, an alternative – and slightly lower – annual unit cost estimate of £36,201 per generic CMHT worker is reached. Estimates for Inner and Outer London are £38,010 and £35,024 respectively. For out of hours crisis cover, an estimated range of £20,000 – 40,000 per 100,000 population is calculated for the provision of 24-hour phone line and on-call rota services (it is assumed here that no additional staff are required).

Table 2 Derivation of unit costs: Community mental health teams (CMHTs)

Element[1]	WTE/100k population[2]		Source/assumptions	Unit cost[3]	Total cost[4]
	Low	**High**		**(£k)**	**(£k; Low)**
Consultant	2	3.3	Low = standard average; High = RCP guidelines	70	140
Other medical	1	2		30	30
CPN	8	13	Low = 1 CPN/12.5k popn; High = 1/7.5k	25	200
Support worker	8	-		12	96
Occupational therapist	2	5	No consensus; High assumes 1/20k popn	20	40
Psychologist	2	3	4.5/100k across all specialities; assume 66% on MH care	35	70
Admin & clerical	5	5	1 WTE per 5 professionals is assumed	12	60
Manager/coordinator	1	1		30	30
Social worker	8	8	No national figures available; Local studies suggest 1/12.5k	23	184
Total WTE staff[5]	**37**	**39.6**		-	**850**
Site costs @10%[5]			Operational overheads only: capital/corporate o'heads excluded		**85**
Total CMHT cost					**935**

1 Typically a CMHT comprises a psychiatrist, CPNs, social workers, with administrative support and input from occupational therapists and psychologists.
2 Staffing estimates are calculated on the assumption of a standard population and deprivation profile.
3 Includes salary on-costs but excludes non-pay on-costs/overheads.
4 Lower WTE estimates used as baseline for unit costs calculation, reflecting actual practice more than recommended guidelines.
5 See text for full unit cost estimation of generic CMHT worker, i.e. inclusive of capital and corporate overhead elements plus London multiplier.

Costing actual and predicted levels of service provision

Service activity and unit cost data were combined to reveal the current costs of provision (both per actual population and per 100,000 population in each borough) for a range of inpatient hospital (RSU, local secure ward) and residential care (hostel wards, 24-hour staffed/day/unstaffed hostels and group homes) service components for people with mental health problems. Hostel wards are taken to be a community-based residential service, following the recommendation of a recent report on this category of accommodation (NHS Executive, 1996d). Service activity data on day and community mental health service provision were not collected and therefore could not be costed on this basis (see next section). Service activity data on supportive housing and respite care places were incomplete, and have consequently been excluded from our descriptive analysis of costed actual provision (section 4.1).

Actual service provision for hospital and residential care, appropriately costed, was then compared to predicted numbers of places required in each of the boroughs and health authorities, using the Mental Illness Needs Index (MINI) developed by Glover et al (1994) . The version used was the revised version described in sections 7.5 and 7.6 of this report, which is intended to allow for the extremes of service use encountered in inner city areas. This MINI draws on original estimates of predicted hospital and residential places per 250,000 population produced by Strathdee and Thornicroft (1992) and Wing (1992), and was revised in the course of this study by the PRiSM team. (For a more detailed description of how the MINI was developed and utilised for the purpose of this study, see Chapter 7.) Where certain categories of community-based accommodation are merged (such as day- and unstaffed hostels), weighted average unit costs were used, based on the existing balance of service delivery. Since supported housing and respite care have been included in the latest MINI estimates of predicted places, we have incorporated available data into this comparative analysis in order to minimise underestimation of actual provision. These analyses allowed calculation of the resource or cost differential between actual and suggested levels of provision for these categories of accommodation, thereby providing an insight into the extent to which these key and cost-intensive services are under- or over-provided, and an estimate of the cost implications of that under/over provision in economic terms.

Scenario analysis of alternative service configurations

The preceding analyses do not provide an overall picture of mental health services. Other components, not covered by the PRiSM team's survey of actual provision or indeed in MINI estimates, include day care, either in hospital or community settings, a range of community care services (drop-in centres, sheltered workshops/employment schemes) and multidisciplinary sector teams (community mental health teams). Given the diversity of day and community service models and practices (in terms of caseload, volume and capacity), it was not possible to derive reliable estimates of locality-specific levels of provision.

In the absence of these estimates, these service elements were incorporated into our costing analysis by attaching unit cost estimates to a range of alternative service configurations. These alternative configurations are based on information from a number of sources, including the in-depth PRiSM survey of the spectrum of care in three London catchment areas (Camberwell, Ealing and Croydon) which is described in chapter 10, published literature on day care and CMHTs (e.g. Holloway et al, 1991; Onyett et al, 1995) and consultation with professionals. Clearly, these derived ranges remain indicative only, since they may not be representative of all London boroughs or authorities, and cannot reflect the wide diversity of alternative models of delivery. As such, we emphasise that this stage of the analysis is not an exercise in prescribing norms, but rather an attempt to provide a quantified estimate of the resource implications of alternative service configurations, which may form the basis for discussion and further development.

11.4 Results

Hospital inpatient and residential provision: actual costs

London boroughs

The total costs associated with actual levels of current hospital in-patient and residential care provision across all London boroughs amount to £312 million. Inner London boroughs consume £137 million, of which hospital services make up £78 million and residential care (including the category of hostel wards) £59 million, whilst costs in Outer London boroughs total £175 million, split between hospital service provision of £86 million and residential provision of £90 million (Figure 2).

Figure 2 In-patient hospital and residential care costs (Inner/Outer London boroughs)

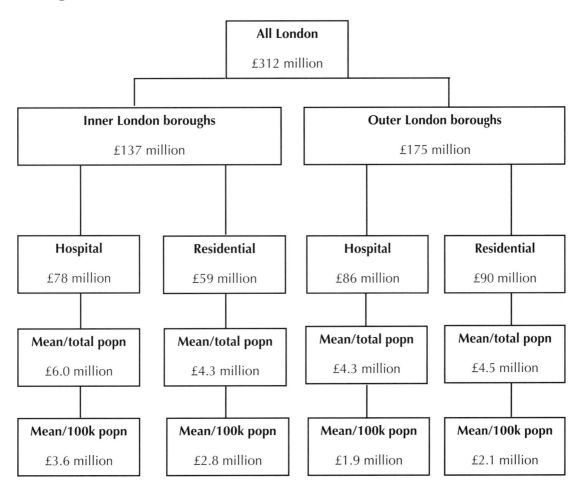

The mean cost for an Inner London borough is £6 million on in-patient hospital provision and £4.3 on residential care; for an Outer borough, the mean cost for inpatient hospital is £4.3 million and for residential provision £4.5 million. There is considerable variation in the total amount and make-up of costs between boroughs, as indicated in Charts 1 and 2. For instance, the costs of provision in the City of London amount to a little over £1/2 million, whilst costs in Lambeth approach £20 million.

When size of population is standardised in order to make inter-borough comparisons, there remain large variations in the costs of hospital in-patient and residential provision, as illustrated in Charts 3 and 4. City of London, with a population of 4129, has a very high level of provision on this basis, although it actually provides only 17 places. Of the Outer London boroughs, Brent stands out as the largest scale (and high cost) provider of services.

Chart 1 Total hospital and residential care costs
(Inner London boroughs: total = £137 million)

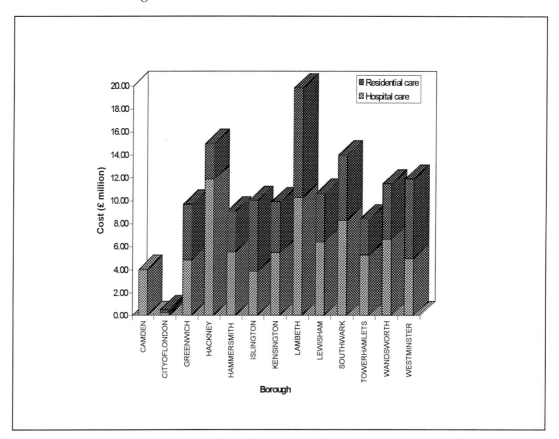

Chart 2 Total hospital and residential care costs
(Outer London boroughs: total = £175 million)

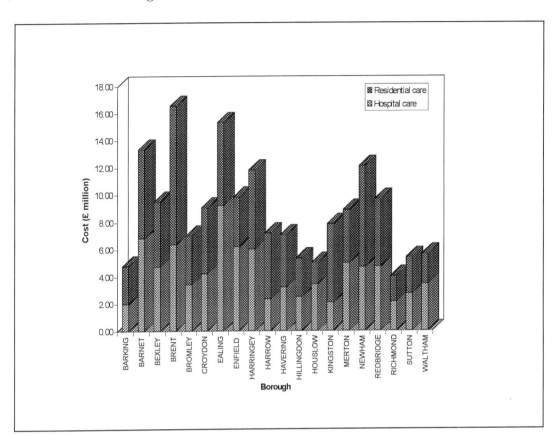

Chart 3 Hospital and residential care costs per 100k population
(Inner London boroughs)

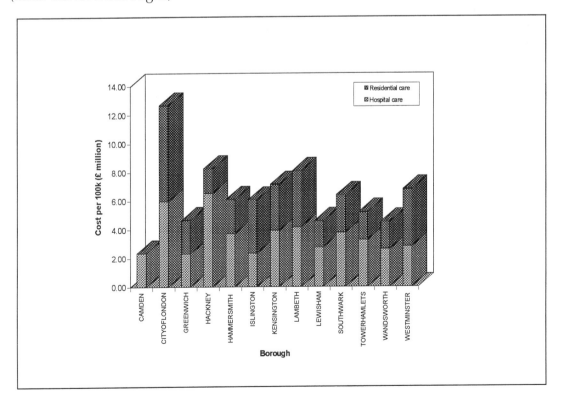

Chart 4 Hospital and residential care costs per 100k population
(Outer London boroughs)

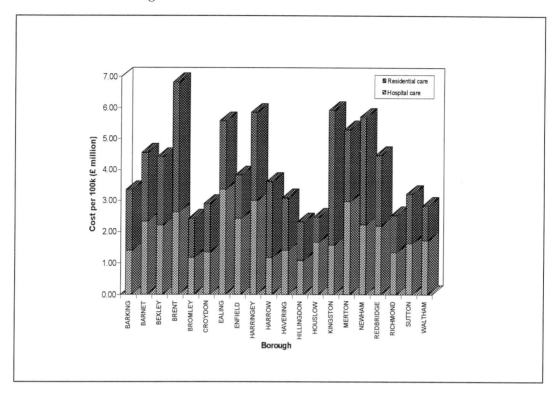

The mean costs (and ranges) per 100,000 population for Inner and Outer boroughs for each of the accommodation types surveyed can be found in Table 3. There is a consistent pattern between the Inner/Outer proportion of places and associated costs (43% Inner; 57% Outer); that is, Inner London boroughs contribute 43% towards the London-wide number of places and costs, even though the population of these boroughs (2.3 million) is only 35% of the total population. The mean number of total in-patient hospital beds and residential care places is 190 per 100,000 population for Inner boroughs (range 69-412), and 124 for Outer boroughs (66-216), at a cost of £6.4 million (range 3.3-12.7) and £4.0 million (2.3-6.8) respectively.

Table 3 Hospital and residential provision: places and costs (£k) per 100k population

Service component	Inner boroughs Mean (range)	Outer boroughs Mean (range)	Total Mean (range)
RSU			
- places	12 (4-23)	3 (0-11)	8 (0-23)
- cost	1,186 (339-2,206)	315 (0-1,071)	750 (0-2,206)
Local secure ward			
- places	7 (2-16)	3 (0-9)	5 (0-16)
- cost	500 (112-1,175)	221 (0-594)	360 (0-1,175)
Acute psych. ward			
- places	46 (31-66)	29 (19-49)	37 (19-66)
- cost	2,454 (1,688-3,551)	1,437 (934-2,450)	1,946 (934-3,551)
Total hospital beds			
- places	59 (40-98)	35 (21-57)	47 (21-98)
- cost	3,592 (2,323-6,542)	1,941 (1,085-3,356)	2,767 (1,085-6,542)
- % places	46%	54%	
- % costs	48%	52%	
Hostel wards			
- places	14 (1-33)	24 (0-65)	19 (0-65)
- cost	670 (72-1,626)	1028 (0-3,012)	849 (0-3,012)
24-hour staffed hostel			
- places	79 (13-266)	38 (12-240)	59 (12-266)
- cost	1,723 (293-5,794)	779 (240-1,757)	1,251 (240-5,794)
Day staffed hostel			
- places	20 (0-48)	7 (0-54)	14 (0-54)
- cost	220 (0-536)	75 (0-564)	148 (0-564)
Unstaff. hostel/grp home			
- places	19 (0-61)	19 (3-83)	19 (0-83)
- cost	170 (0-553)	158 (24-706)	164 (0-706)
Total residential places			
- places	131 (27-322)	89 (35-175)	110 (27-322)
- cost	2,777 (936-6,686)	2,111 (777-4,334)	2,444 (777-6,686)
- % places	41%	59%	
- % costs	38%	62%	
Total hospital/residential			
- places	190 (69-412)	124 (66-216)	157 (66-412)
- cost	6,370 (3,290-12,668)	4,052 (2,315-6,817)	5,211(2,315-12,668)
- % places / cost	43%	57%	

The relative balance or composition of services for Inner and Outer boroughs is shown in Chart 5. The main difference is the provision of hostel wards and 24-hour staffed hostels, with hostel wards making up 10% less of the overall cost in Inner London boroughs, compared to 6% more for 24-hour staffed hostels. Generally, however, there is a similar pattern of cost components for the two areas.

Chart 5 Hospital and residential care cost categories (% of total cost)

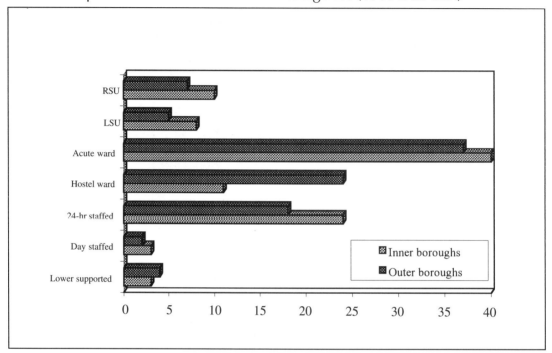

London health authorities

Service activity data across the various provider agencies were also ascribed to the 16 London health authorities. Chart 6 illustrates the total costs associated with inpatient hospital and residential care provision (£312 million across all London health authorities) for each authority, which range from £5-10 million in a number of the Outer London authorities to £35 million in East London and City and £44 million in Lambeth, Southwark and Lewisham. It is also evident from this chart that the costs of residential provision in a number of authorities are close to or actually exceed the costs of inpatient hospital provision.

Conversion into a standardised unit of population (100,000) allows variations in service volume to be observed, both in terms of beds/places provided and in terms of the costs of that provision (Chart 7). Hospital beds per 100,000 population averaged 40 (ranging between 21-63), at a cost of £2.3 million (range £1.1-3.9 million); mean provision of residential places was 100 (with a range of between 60-178) at a cost of £2.2 million (range £1.2-3.7 million). These figures indicate that there exists a threefold variation across London health authorities in the provision and cost of care, even after population size has been controlled for. The overall balance of costs across the range of hospital and residential facility types echoes the breakdown by boroughs found in Chart 5.

Chart 6 Hospital and residential care costs (£ million, by Health Authority)

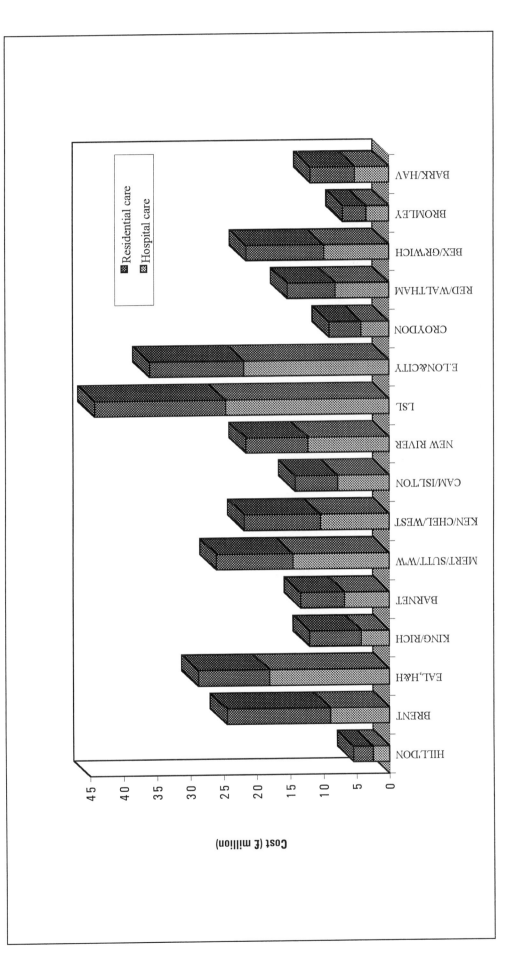

Chart 7 Hospital and residential care costs per 100k population (Health Authorities)

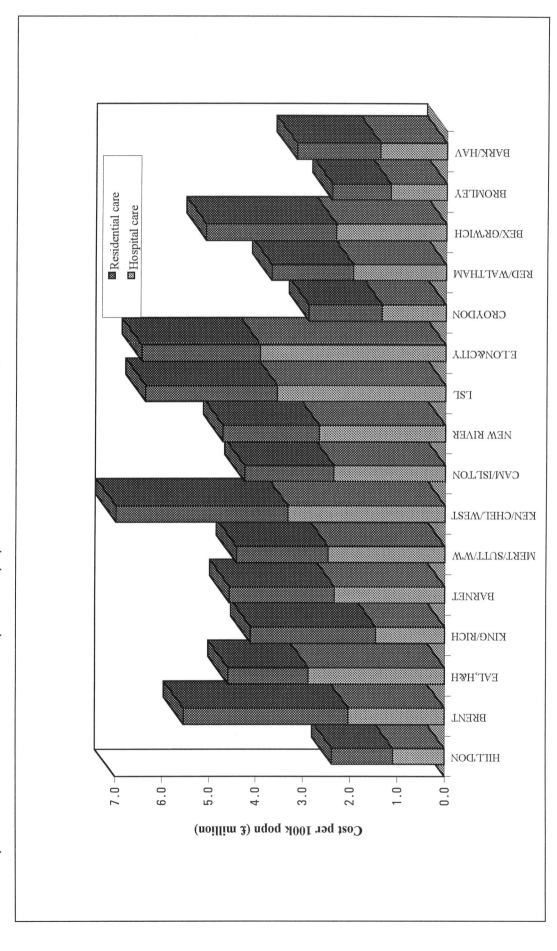
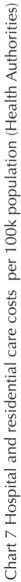

Hospital inpatient and residential provision: actual vs predicted costs

Actual service activity data and attendant costs were compared to deprivation-weighted and epidemiologically-based estimates of local service requirements. Charts 8 and 9 show the aggregated cost differentials between actual versus desirable levels of places for each London borough.

Chart 8 Cost differentials – Inner London boroughs
(actual minus predicted MINI estimates)

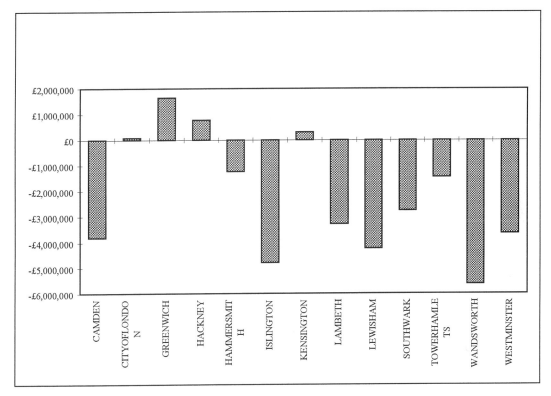

Chart 9 Cost differentials – Outer London boroughs
(actual versus predicted MINI estimates)

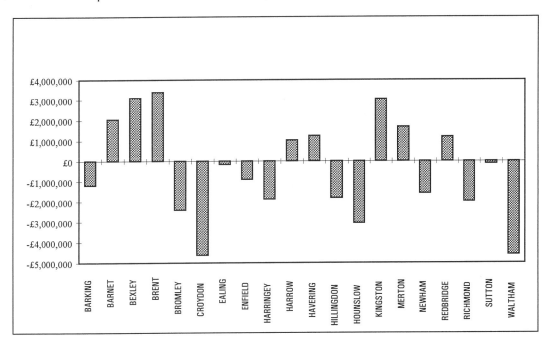

Chart 10 Cost differentials – Health authorities
(actual minus predicted MINI estimates)

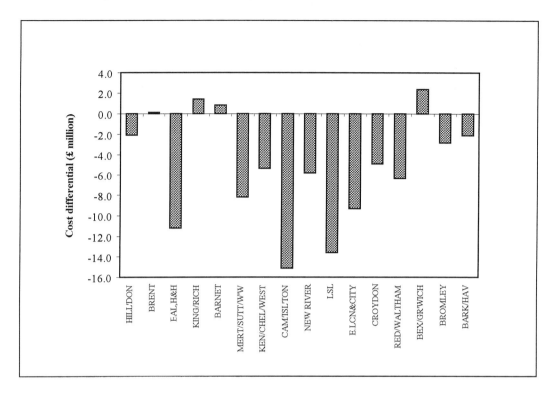

Chart 10 shows cost differentials by health authority. The general picture arising from this analysis is one of negative differentials, indicating under-provision of services (that is, the costs associated with actual provision are less than the costs associated with predicted service requirements). The extent of under-provision is particularly stark in the Inner London boroughs – 9 of the 13 boroughs have negative differentials, and 6 of these are in excess of £3 million per annum. The situation in Outer London boroughs is more varied, with 12 out of the 20 boroughs falling below the level at which actual and desired provision coincide. The negative differentials in certain boroughs, such as Croydon and Waltham, reach close to -£5 million, but in other boroughs – Bexley, Brent and Kingston – there is a positive differential in excess of £3 million. From the perspective of health authorities, 12 out of 16 have negative differentials, ranging from -£2-3 million (Hillingdon, Bromley, Barking and Havering) to more than -£10 million (Ealing, Hammersmith and Hounslow; Camden and Islington; Lambeth, Southwark and Lewisham).

The total predicted costs of hospital in-patient and residential provision across London amount to £391 million. This gives an overall, but overstated, difference of £79 million compared with actual costs. A more appropriate differential of £59 million is derived by separately calculating differentials for each category of accommodation in each borough, reflecting the fact that in many areas services are characterised by *mis*-provision rather than exclusively by under-provision.

There are a number of issues pertaining to these findings that deserve comment. Firstly, it is acknowledged that the deprivation-weighted index (MINI) to which the above estimates of required places have been attached has least predictive power in inner city areas, owing to the high degree of mobility, homelessness and population mix in these areas. This injects uncertainty into obtained results, but is likely to underestimate levels of need in London. Secondly, two important assumptions underlie the suggested targets: i) services should be community-based as far as possible, with community residential and day places taking the place of institutional care (Johnson et al, 1996); ii) there should be provision in all or most of the categories. The reality is of course very different, with certain groups of services absent or undersupplied, leading to greater or excessive demands being made on those services that are present, in particular long-established hospital services. This disparity between actual practice and ideal structures again suggests that the differentials observed can be interpreted not simply in terms of under/over-provision, but also in terms of overall mis-provision across the various service components. The relative imbalance of service categories is evident from Chart 11, which shows cost differentials by facility type for Inner and Outer London boroughs. Whilst the overall picture is clearly negative, indicating significant underprovision, there are certain service categories that appear to be overprovided, in particular nursed facilities/hostel wards in Outer London boroughs (+£24 million). The principal cost deficits relate to acute psychiatric inpatient provision (-£24 million across Inner boroughs, -£20 million across Outer boroughs) and 24-hour staffed hostels (Inner: -£14 million; Outer: -£10 million).

Chart 11 Cost differentials by facility type (Inner and Outer London boroughs)

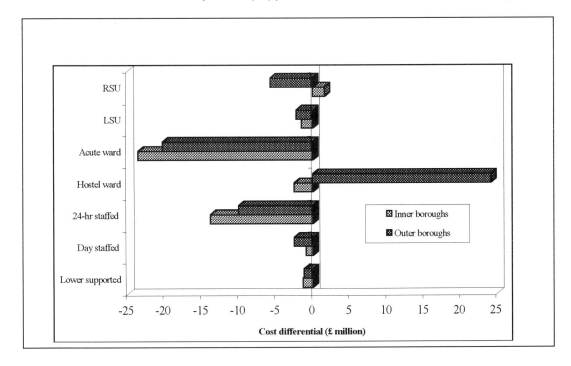

Resource implications of alternative service configurations

In attempting to quantify the resource implications of service provision over and above in-patient hospital and residential care, a series of range estimates (both for provision per 100,000 population and the annual cost of a unit of provision) were derived for day hospital and day care services, sheltered employment/work schemes, and community mental health teams. Derived estimates of service provision were largely drawn from the PRiSM spectrum of care survey in three London catchment areas (Camberwell, Ealing and Croydon). These range estimates, together with an indication of their sources, are summarised in Table 4. The uncertainty and width of these range estimates has already been emphasised, and is a direct consequence of the shortage of available

Table 4 Full service configurations: range estimates of service provision and unit costs (Inner and Outer London boroughs)

Service component	Unit of measurement	Unit cost range (£ p.a., 1995/96)		Indicative range of provision per 100k popn	Primary source(s)	Total cost (£k p.a., 1995/96) per 100k population	
		Inner	Outer			Inner	Outer
CMHTs[1]							
normal working hours	Generic CMHT worker	38,010 – 43,575	35,024 – 40,151	25 – 37	PRiSM 3 area survey Crilly and Robbins (1996)	950 – 1,612	875 – 1,485
out of hours crisis cover	Cost per 100k	20,000 – 40,000	20,000 – 40,000	-	Crilly and Robbins (1996)	20 – 40	20 – 40
Day hospital	Place(s)	11,539	10,586	50 – 100	PRiSM 3 area survey (Chapter 10)	577 – 1,154	529 – 1059
Day care centre	Place(s)	9,918	9,163	40 – 80	PRiSM 3 area survey; Holloway (1991)	397 – 793	367 – 733
Supported housing/flats	Place(s)	7929	7310	10 – 20	PRiSM 3 area survey	79 – 158	73 – 146
Employment schemes	Place(s)	2,500 – 6,500 (National estimates)[2]		50 – 70	PRiSM 3 area survey	125 – 455	125 – 455

1 See text for description of CMHT functions assumed and derivation of generic CMHT worker unit costs.
2 Net expenditure per place, based on seven schemes, including Industrial Therapy Unit, vocational rehabilitation, and clubhouse settings (Schneider, 1996).

and reliable data on local levels of current provision of these services. For instance, we have estimated that the annual cost of providing comprehensive CMHT support to a population of 100,000 is between £950,000 and £1.6 million in Inner London boroughs, and between £875,000 and £1.5 million in Outer London boroughs.

These estimates are (deliberately) wide, but can nevertheless provide data that may be useful, particularly to mental health planners and purchasers. The conversion of the above CMHT estimates to the total population of London, for instance, leads to estimates of £60-100 million.

On the basis of these estimates, a series of scenarios were developed. These scenarios indicate the cost consequences of a number of alternative service configurations under different sets of assumptions. The principal variables in these analyses are unit costs (high and low estimates of the costs of a generic CMHT worker, out of hours cover, and employment schemes); levels of provision (low and high estimates, reflecting levels currently found in certain London boroughs (low) versus levels that might be expected to be found); and interchangability of services (high and low estimates of levels of overlapping service functions, in particular day hospital, day centre and community mental health team support).

The resource implications of eight alternative scenarios are given in Table 5. Each scenario shows the predicted additional costs of providing differential levels of supported housing, employment schemes, day hospital/centre places and CMHT support (that is, those key service components *not* covered by the PRiSM survey of borough-by-borough activity).

The total costs of these services per annum for all London boroughs range from £136 million (scenario 3) to £268 million (scenario 8), which represent between 43% and 85% add-ons to the previously calculated total costs of £312 million for in-patient hospital and residential care provision only. On the basis of these add-ons, it is estimated that the full resource consequences of all service activity across London are a minimum of £443 million and a maximum of £573 million per annum, with a median of close to £500 million. Expressed as a proportion of this combined total of all costed service activity, the additional day and community care elements modelled here account for between 30% and 46% of total cost.

Finally, we altered the existing balance of provision across London in order to observe the cost consequences of (hypothetical) shifts in the locus of care. In view of the current debate on the under-provision of 24-hour staffed residential facilities, we first imputed an increase of 10% to the number of 24-hour nursed and other staffed hostel places. The costs associated with this increase are £12.9 million (£5.5 million in Inner London boroughs, £7.4 million in Outer London boroughs). By way of illustration, this is equivalent to 250 (or 9.5% of) acute psychiatric beds. At a wider level, if all in-patient hospital categories (RSU, local secure, acute) are reduced by 10% (291 beds across London), this would reduce costs in this sector by an estimated £16.7 million. These costs are equivalent to the provision of 744 residential places. Alternatively, 291 residential places could be provided for £10.2 million less than their current cost within the hospital sector.

Table 5 Full service configurations: alternative scenarios (London wide)

Scenario[1]	Configurations	Additional cost (£k)		Add-on[2] %	% of total cost[3]
		Total popn	**per 100k popn**		
1	Low support.housing/ employ schemes, high day, low CMHT	197,582	2,967	63%	39%
2	Low support.housing/ employ schemes, low day, high CMHT	179,294	2,692	57%	36%
3	Low support.housing/ employ schemes, low day, low CMHT	136,147	2,045	43%	30%
4	Low support.housing/ employ schemes, high day, high CMHT	240,729	3,615	77%	43%
5	High support.housing/ employ schemes, high day, low CMHT	224,567	3,372	72%	42%
6	High support.housing/ employ schemes, low day, high CMHT	206,279	3,098	66%	40%
7	High support.housing/ employ schemes, low day, low CMHT	163,279	2,450	52%	34%
8	High support.housing/ employ schemes, high day, high CMHT	267,715	4,020	85%	46%

1   All scenarios incorporate differential levels of supportive housing, employment schemes, day hospital/centre places and CMHT cover.
2   Proportional add-on to hospital in-patient and residential care costs(£317 million).
3   Proportion of total costs (all service categories)

Clearly these analyses can be no more than illustrative, since no account is being taken of the myriad of factors that may influence the ability to effect such changes, including the characteristics of clients, levels of unmet need and the organisation/historical development of local services. However, they do provide a rudimentary indication of the relative size of resource flows that follow from changes to the balance of provision. A fuller account and treatment of these issues in the context of a recent survey of residential care can be found in Knapp et al. (1997), who concluded that whilst the costs of inpatient hospital treatment for inappropriately placed patients greatly exceeded the costs of community-based care, further reduction of hospital beds is not the panacea for an appropriate balance of mental health. Rather, service providers and purchasers should focus on developing community-based care (including increased provision of 24-hour nursed beds) by ensuring that resources released through earlier closure programmes have been redeployed for their intended use and by accessing additional pump-priming and/or bridging resources.

11.5 Summary and conclusions

This research study set out i) to establish the cost implications of existing mental health service provision in London, ii) to compare these derived costs with the costs associated with predicted service requirements, and iii) to explore (where possible) the efficiency with which resources are being utilised in different localities in the capital.

The costs of mental health service provision

With respect to the first of these intentions, we have been able to complement the work undertaken by the PRiSM team by attaching (annual) unit cost estimates to the current activity levels of a range of in-patient hospital and residential care services. The total costs associated with the provision of these services is over £300 million, of which 43% is accounted for by the 13 Inner London boroughs (with 35% of the total London population), and 57 % by the 20 Outer London boroughs (see Figure 2 for an overview). We also find, as expected, considerable variation in the balance of provision and consequent resource flows, even after population size has been standardised (Charts 1-7). Although unable to indicate relative efficiency or cost-effectiveness, these descriptive costs data provide an up-to-date overview of the resource implications of current levels of mental health hospital and residential provision in London.

Actual versus predicted costs of provision

Comparison of these estimates of actual service costs with the costs of desirable service levels (based on MINI estimates) was expected to reveal any differential that might exist in London, thereby providing an insight into the extent to which services are under- or over-provided. The results of our analyses based on the revised version of the MINI described in chapter 7 predominantly suggest *under-* rather than over-provision, particularly in relation to acute inpatient wards and 24-hour staffed hostels. Across all categories of accommodation, the implied deficit in some Inner London boroughs is £4-5 million per annum and in some health authorities localities is as much as £10 million or more (Charts 8-11). The total negative differential across London is estimated to be as much as £59 million.

Analysis of full service configurations

Our capacity to realise the third of our study aims – to explore the efficiency of resource use – has been hampered by a shortage of normative data on expected levels of provision for a number of key service categories, and a lack of evidence upon which to indicate the likely trade-offs or substitutions that would be required to move from potentially inefficient models of current service delivery to more efficient modes of practice. The House of Commons Health Select Committee (1994) recommended that the Department of Health issue instructions on minimum acceptable levels of provision for the following categories of mental health services: 24-hour staffed community houses; day staffed residential care; day centre and day hospital places; provision of community-based multi-disciplinary teams. In a similar vein, the Audit Commission (1994a) recommended that purchasers should review the balance of expenditure on hospital and community resources and should investigate the scope for the possible substitution of some hospital care with community alternatives, including both 24-hour staffed accommodation and less intensively staffed provision.

Whilst there have certain developments in this respect – including recent publications on 24-hour nursed beds, the spectrum of care and auditing the care programme approach (Department of Health, 1996a, 1996c, NHS Executive, 1996c) – there remains a lack of clearly defined guidelines on recommended *levels* of service provision, particularly for day and community mental health care. From an economic perspective, and despite the difficulties of doing so, such a baseline is needed in order to systematically (as opposed to hypothetically) examine the key issue of service efficiency. The development of programme-budgeting in mental health would similarly benefit from specification of the service levels to be attached to service functions.

In the absence of official recommendations, a series of range estimates (per 100,000 population) were derived for possible levels and costs of day and community mental health care provision (Table 4). These estimates were then combined in a number of different configurations. The total London-wide cost of these services (CMHT support, day hospital/centre places, employment schemes and supported housing) ranged from £136 million to £267 million, representing between 43% and 85% add-ons to the total costs of £312 million derived for in-patient hospital and residential care (Table 5). As a proportion of the totality of costs for all service categories, the additional components modelled in our analyses account for between 30% and 46%. In short, the cost implications of providing a comprehensive range of services under a range of alternative scenarios appear to be very considerable. Examination of the extent to which local services in London are providing this full range of services was precluded by the absence of service activity data for day and community mental health services.

Changes to the balance of provision

In view of the considerable resource implications of providing a comprehensive range and sufficient volume of services, we altered the existing pattern of provision in order to observe the cost consequences of such potential changes. For example, increased provision of hostel wards/24-hour staffed residential facilities by 10% carries an additional cost of £5.5 million in Inner London boroughs, £7.4 million in Outer London boroughs. These costs equate, again for example, to 102 acute in-patient psychiatric beds in Inner London boroughs (9.8% of beds), or 148 (or 9% of) beds in Outer London boroughs. At a wider level, if all in-patient hospital categories (RSU, local secure, acute) are reduced by 10% (291 beds across London), this would reduce costs in this sector by an estimated £16.7 million. These costs are equivalent to the provision of 744 residential places. Alternatively, 291 residential places could be provided for £10.2 million less than their current cost within the hospital sector. These analyses are clearly illustrative only, since no account is being taken of the characteristics of clients, levels of unmet need and the organisation/historical development of local services.

Chapter 12

The obstacles to and the opportunities for the development of mental health services in London: the perceptions of managers

Edward Peck, Helen Smith, Ingrid Barker and Gregor Henderson

Introduction

The study described in this chapter aimed to obtain descriptive data about the management of London's mental health service alongside an account of the concepts, behaviours and perceptions of the people responsible for managing the service system. It is only through understanding the nature of the interface between the system and those responsible for managing it that solutions to the systems pathologies, described both below and elsewhere in this book, can effectively be tackled. Simply introducing particular interventions, such as increased funding or a new policy requirement, will not necessarily lead to improvements in services unless the impact of these interventions is understood in terms of management capacity and capability to act on these changes and their likely response to them.

Methodology

The use of structured questionnaires is well known from the literature on qualitative research methods (e.g. Fontana and Frey, 1994) and this approach was used in this study to collect organisational and personal information. Analysis of participant narratives was chosen as the primary method for obtaining data on perceptions and views. This method produces a rich source of data from which to identify common underlying phenomena influencing the management of mental health care; explore un/common decision making processes and map the range of contributory elements that influenced service management and, in turn, service delivery. It was hoped that this would produce a 'shared rhetoric' (Lewis, 1995) about London's mental health services.

All transcripts were indexed for systematic charting using the 'Frameworks' approach to qualitative data analysis (Ritchie and Spenser, 1994). The generative strategies emerged through expert analysis of the data from researchers experienced in both mental health systems and management theories.

The authors devised, piloted and conducted a structured interview with fifty-seven managers in London identified by their organisations as the most senior manager explicitly responsible for mental health services. The sample consisted of mental health purchasers in HAs (13) and managers responsible for mental health services in NHS trusts (21) and in Social Services Departments (23). The interviews were conducted by the authors. The interviews lasted around one-and-a half hours. Tables 1 and 2 present the sample size and composition.

The structured questionnaire was a combination of closed questions and open questions. The responses to the questionnaires were placed on a database (in Microsoft Access). The answers to open questions were placed on the database as open text, the interviewers then allocated all open text to a series of categories devised on the basis of the content of that open text. The analysis of the data derived from the database was undertaken by the four interviewers together. Pilot interviews, including pilot narrative recordings, were conducted with four managers in London by the four interviewers working in pairs. These interviews were used to refine the questionnaire, ensure the effectiveness of the narrative dictation, and to develop a reliable approach between the interviewers.

As senior managers, it was assumed that participants would be confident using dictaphones, and they were asked to dictate, in the presence of the interviewer, an uninterrupted narrative of recent personal experience in developing a local mental health project. In order to stimulate the thoughts of participants, an introductory letter suggested some broad categories within which they may wish to construct their narrative. These categories were: the nature/origins/sources of the change/innovation; the drivers for the change; obstacles; and lessons learnt for the future. The majority of participants (50) were comfortable with this approach and dictated narratives lasting on average around twenty minutes. Subsequently, these narratives were transcribed for analysis.

The four interviewers agreed a coding framework for the document analysis based upon notes made during the dictation of the narrative. This framework contained thirteen themes in three areas (see Table 3). The analysis examined the transcripts for the presence of the theme, recorded its presence and selected quotations which illustrated the point being made. In addition, the analysis recorded the subject addressed in the narrative and any topics lying outside the themes or categories, and not covered in the questionnaire, which were of crucial importance to the participants. The authors shared the outcome of this analysis and looked to establish points of similarity and dissimilarity between participants from different agencies.

Table 1 Size of the sample

Narratives recorded:	50	64.10%
Completed questionnaires:	57	73.08%
Total possible sample:	78	100.00%

Table 2 Composition of the sample

Nature of Agency	Total possible sample	Actual sample	Percentage of possible sample represented
Health Authorities	16	13	81.25%
Social Services	33	23	69.70%
trusts	29	21	72.41%

Table 3 Coding frame for the narrative transcripts

Content	Process	Context
Overall resource level declining	Organisational culture and approaches to development	Capacity and power
Complexity of financial rules relating to PFI	Political complexion of LAs (including public opinion)	Issues relating to non-MH and Community trusts
Problems of CMHTs	User involvement	Organisational geographical boundaries
Problems with CPA/care management	Role of product champions	GP Fundholders pressure: dual agenda
		Role animosity

Analysis of and Commentary on the Structured Questionnaire

This section presents data from the analysis of the structured questionnaire and a commentary on that data. Each table reproduces the question. On occasions, the analysis compares data from two questions and these figures reproduce both questions. The tables are grouped into broad subject headings.

The Person and the Post

Table 4 What is the agency that you work for?

Nature of Agency	Count	Percentage
Health Authority	13	22.81%
Social Services	23	40.35%
Combined Trust	13	22.81%
Community MH Trust	3	5.26%
MH Trust	5	8.77%

The sample reflects the fact that there are more combined trusts (providing acute, community, and mental health services) than community/mental health trusts and mental health trusts in London. This fact distinguishes London from many other UK cities and may have implications for the seniority and job stability of the officers responsible for mental health services within London trusts. The large number of social services departments is unique to London amongst cities in the UK. It is presumed that this feature may make collaborative working between agencies, which is a central theme of recent policy (e.g. HMSO, 1995), more difficult to achieve.

Table 5 How long have you been employed by this agency?

Months in Organisation	Count	Percentage
0 to 6	2	3.51%
7 to 12	5	8.77%
13 to 24	8	14.04%
25 to 36	3	5.26%
37 to 60	14	24.56%
61 +	25	43.86%

This table indicates a high level of organisational stability amongst managers, with almost 75% having been in their current organisation for more than two years, and 44% for five years or more.

Table 6 How long have you been in your current post?

Months in Post	Count	Percentage
0 to 6	7	12.28%
7 to 12	11	19.30%
13 to 24	15	26.32%
25 to 36	10	17.54%
37 to 60	10	17.54%
61 +	4	7.02%

This table is important. If it is assumed that it takes at least 12 months to become effective in a new job, then almost one third of managers (32%) are still in that initial 12 month phase. Well over 50% have been in post for less than two years. This represents significant job instability amongst the most senior managers responsible for mental health services in London. Further analysis shows no significant bias in this distribution between agencies.

Table 7 How long have you worked in mental health in total?

Years in MH (aggregate)	Count	Percentage
2 up to 3	2	3.51%
3 up to 5	7	12.28%
5 up to 10	15	26.32%
11 or over	33	57.89%

This figure demonstrates the very substantial experience of mental health services possessed by managers in London, with only 4% having less than three years experience in aggregate during their career. This finding is partially explained by examination of Table 11, which shows that almost 75% of managers come from practitioner backgrounds.

Table 8 How long have you worked in mental health continuously?

Years in MH (continuously)	Count	Percentage
less than 1	5	8.77%
1 up to 2	1	1.75%
2 up to 3	5	8.77%
3 up to 5	10	17.54%
5 up to 10	14	24.56%
11 or over	22	38.60%

This table shows that over 75% of managers have been working continuously in mental health for over three years and well over 50% for more than 5 years. This concentration on mental health, presumably again a product of managers' practitioner backgrounds, suggests an excellent knowledge of mental health services.

Table 9 How many people are there between you and Chief Executive/Director?

No. between Interviewee and CE/Director	Count	Percentage
-1	7	12.28%
0	13	22.81%
1	28	49.12%
2	7	12.28%
3	1	1.75%
4	1	1.75%

This figure shows that 12% of the participants were the chief officer of their organisations, and that 22% were the immediate subordinates of the chief officer. In just over one third of the sample, therefore, the most senior manager responsible for mental health services could be expected to be a member of the board/senior management team of the organisation. However, in almost two thirds of the sample this is not the case. Given the policy priority being given to mental health services, and the complexity of the issues perceived to be faced by mental health services in London (see Tables 40 and 41), this is an important finding.

Table 10 Analysis of number of people between interviewee and Chief Executive/ Director by agency

No. Between Interviewee & CE/Director	Nature of Agency	Count	Percentage
-1	Combined Trust	2	3.51%
	MH Trust	5	8.77%
0	Health Authority	2	3.51%
	Social Services	3	5.26%
	Combined Trust	6	10.53%
	Community MH Trust	2	3.51%
1	Health Authority	7	12.28%
	Social Services	15	26.32%
	Combined Trust	5	8.77%
	Community MH Trust	1	1.75%
2	Health Authority	4	7.02%
	Social Services	3	5.26%
3	Social Services	1	1.75%
4	Social Services	1	1.75%

In trusts, the most senior manager is the chief executive, and the community/mental health trusts show similar seniority for the mental health manager. It is the combined trusts that do not, in the majority of cases, have the most senior manager responsible for mental health services reporting directly to the senior officer in the organisation. Most health authorities are in a similar position, with a small number having a junior manager responsible for mental health. The overwhelming majority of social services departments do not have the most senior mental health manager reporting directly to the director. This is a worrying result, not only because of the likely consequences of the lack of seniority of many managers responsible for mental health, but also because of the disparity of seniority that may be present between officers charged with working in partnership to develop services.

Table 11 What is your professional background?

Professional Background	Count	Percentage
Medical	4	7.02%
Manager	10	17.54%
Nurse	13	22.81%
Occupational Therapist	1	1.75%
Other	2	3.51%
Private Sector	2	3.51%
Psychologist	2	3.51%
Social Worker	22	38.60%
Voluntary Sector	1	1.75%

This table presents one of the most striking findings of the research: almost 70% of the managers come from a practitioner background. All but one of the social services managers is a social worker. Further analysis reveals that five of the ten managers, the two private sector people, the two others (researcher and librarian) and the voluntary sector person are working in the health authorities. Only three of the health authority managers are from a practitioner background (two public health doctors and one nurse). The majority of the trust managers have a nursing qualification. This data suggests that the managers in the three agencies exhorted by policy to work together come to that collaboration with very different experiences and expectations, and that there is little interchange of staff between those agencies (particularly social workers and nurses into health authorities and anyone into or out of social services). In particular, the understanding of the clinical experience of patients in the health domain is restricted to the trusts; this may explain why trust managers' voice frustration with the health authorities (see next section). However, the managerial orientation of the health authority managers may explain their frustration with their partners in trusts.

Table 12 What qualifications do you possess?

Qualification	Count	Percentage of total questionnaires
1st Degree	44	77.19%
Management qualifications	26	45.61%
MBA	9	15.79%
Professional qualifications	39	68.42%

This table shows a broadly well educated set of managers, with significant professional qualifications. However, less than half possess a management qualification of any description (from Certificate of Management to Masters in Business Administration). This suggests that over half of the managers may possess little or no training in the complexities of the management of change that they are grappling with. It is a worrying, and perhaps, significant result, which may indicate that practitioners are being inadequately prepared for their managerial role.

Table 13 Gender

Gender	Count	Percentage
Female	25	43.86%
Male	32	56.14%

Table 14 How would you describe your ethnic origin?

Ethnic Origin	Count	Percentage
African Sub-continent	1	1.75%
Indian	1	1.75%
White, British	47	82.46%
White, Irish	4	7.02%
White, Other	4	7.02%

A worrying, if perhaps unsurprising finding is that managers do not reflect the ethnic mix of their city.

Table 15 How much of your time is given to mental health?

% Time in a Week Given to MH	Count	Percentage
11 to 20	1	1.75%
21 to 30	5	8.77%
31 to 40	3	5.26%
41 to 50	2	3.51%
51 to 60	2	3.51%
61 to 70	5	8.77%
71 to 80	7	12.28%
81 to 90	9	15.79%
91 to 100	23	40.35%

This table shows that only just over 50% of the sample estimate giving over 80% of their time to mental health.

Table 16 Analysis by agency of amount of interviewees' time given to mental health

Nature of Agency	% Time in a Week Given to MH	Count
Health Authority	21 to 30	2
	41 to 50	1
	51 to 60	2
	71 to 80	2
	81 to 90	2
	91 to 100	4
Social Services	11 to 20	1
	21 to 30	2
	31 to 40	2
	41 to 50	1
	61 to 70	3
	71 to 80	1
	81 to 90	3
	91 to 100	10
Combined Trust	21 to 30	1
	31 to 40	1
	61 to 70	2
	71 to 80	3
	81 to 90	3
	91 to 100	3
Community MH Trust	71 to 80	1
	91 to 100	2
MH Trust	81 to 90	1
	91 to 100	4

Looked at in more detail, the data reveals that amongst trusts, it is the mental health and community/mental health trust managers that give most time to mental health. Less than half of the managers in combined trusts commit 80% of their time to mental health; so not only are they more junior but they are also more likely to have non-mental health responsibilities.

Work Context

Table 17 How many management re-structurings have there been in the last three years (since April 1993) which have involved the most senior manager responsible for mental health in a change of roles/ responsibilities/position in hierarchy?

Number of Restructurings	Count	Percentage
0	10	17.54%
1	20	35.09%
2	12	21.05%
3	14	24.56%
4	1	1.75%

All but ten of the organisations have restructured since April 1993. It is possible to predict significant turnover, loss of attention to task and fracturing of relationships during and after such restructurings. This table may suggest a significant cause of slow progress in developing mental health services in many parts of London.

Table 18 Analysis by agency of the number of management re-structurings in the last three years

Nature of Agency	Number of Restructurings	Count
Health Authority	0	1
	1	4
	2	4
	3	3
	4	1
Social Services	0	6
	1	7
	2	3
	3	7
Combined Trust	0	3
	1	7
	2	1
	3	2
Community MH Trust	1	1
	2	1
	3	1
MH Trust	1	1
	2	3
	3	1

This table shows that social services are most prone to repeated restructurings, otherwise there is no bias in the distribution.

Table 19 How secure do you feel in your current post?

Secure in post?	Count	Percentage
Completely	6	10.53%
Very	14	24.56%
Reasonably	20	35.09%
Not very	11	19.30%
Not at all	4	7.02%
Unsure	2	3.51%

Given the number of restructurings, it is perhaps not surprising that over 25% of the sample felt not very or not at all secure in their position. Over one third felt only reasonably secure. This is an important finding if it is presumed that lack of security inhibits performance, in particular in the creation and sustenance of confiding and confident inter-agency relationships.

Table 20 How long do you anticipate staying in your present position?

Plan to Stay?	Count	Percentage
0 to 6	4	7.02%
7 to 12	13	22.81%
13 to 24	13	22.81%
25 to 36	7	12.28%
37 to 60	6	10.53%
61 +	3	5.26%
unsure	11	19.30%

Over 25% of the sample do not expect to be in their present post in twelve months time. This response suggests that the historical instability presented in Table 6 is set to continue. Furthermore, almost 20% do not know how long they will be in their present post, indicating a lack of career planning or uncertainty in their future beyond their control (or both).

Table 21 How well prepared do you feel for your current mental health responsibility?

Preparedness for Current Responsibility	Count	Percentage
Very	23	40.35%
Sufficiently	28	49.12%
Insufficiently	5	8.77%
Poorly	1	1.75%

There is a need to be alert to bias in this response, but almost 90% of participants feel prepared for their responsibilities. This seems to suggest a high level of personal confidence amongst managers, despite the complexities and obstacles identified by the participants, and the widespread concern about the quality and quantity of mental health services in London.

Table 22 What would make you feel more prepared for your current mental health responsibility?

Factor mentioned	Count	Type of training	Count
More training	14	Current issues training	8
More time to prepare themselves	13	Management training	4
To see other services	2	Commissioning training	2
Total number of responses to this half of question	33		

and/or why do you feel so well prepared for your current mental health responsibility?

Factor mentioned	Count
Experience in mental health	28
Clinical background	7
Good inter-agency relationships	5
Thorough training	3
Total number of responses to this half of question	35

NB: It is not valid to express these figures in percentage form, as a number of interviewees expressed more than one reason.

Notwithstanding the apparently high level of personal confidence, well over 50% of participants felt that they would benefit from more preparation, in particular, training and time to prepare. The reasons that respondents gave for feeling well-prepared overwhelmingly relate to experience, presumably clinical experience, or clinical background, in mental health services This is perhaps not surprising in the light of Table 11. However, it assumes that experience, in particular clinical experience, in mental health services, is sufficient of itself to prepare people for the managerial challenge. Managers are not stating that their skills in the management of change or their understanding of the impact of policy on practice have prepared them for their current responsibilities. Given that less than 50% possess any management qualification, there must be a serious concern that many of the managers may lack skills relating, for instance, to the management of change, and that many do not know what they do not know. Only 4 out of 33 replied that they felt that they required management training.

Table 23 Who are your key (agency-title) partners outside your agency?

Agency	No. of mentions	Agency	No. of mentions
Carers	3	Private sector	1
GPs	8	Probation	4
GP Fundholders	1	Social Services	33
Health Authority	39	trusts	38
Housing	13	User groups	16
Police	6	Voluntary	32
Prison	1	Sector	

Of the 13 Health Authority representatives:	13 mentioned Social Services, 11 mentioned trusts.
Of the 23 Social Services representatives:	23 mentioned trusts, 22 mentioned Health Authorities.
Of the 21 Trust representatives:	19 mentioned Social Services, 17 mentioned Health Authorities.

NB: There was no limitation to the number of agencies each interviewee might name.

It is striking that the managers from the three agencies participating in the study recognised each other as key partners, and also recognised the voluntary sector. The message of the DoH concerning partnerships (e.g. Department of Health, 1995a) is having an impact. Beyond that, however, only user groups and housing have any significant presence in the partnerships. Despite the policy emphasis on a primary care-led NHS, GPs do not figure strongly, and despite the policy emphasis on MDOs, police, prison and probation hardly figure at all. This may suggest either a significant time-lag between policy dissemination and response from the field or a lack of congruence between the policy priorities of the DoH and those of managers responsible for their implementation, or both.

Table 24 How often do you meet with these partners collectively?

Frequency of Collective Meetings	Count	Percentage
weekly	1	1.92%
monthly	21	40.38%
every 6 weeks	14	26.92%
quarterly	8	15.38%
annually	1	1.92%
regularly	2	3.85%
unstructured	1	1.92%
never	3	5.77%
don't know	1	1.92%
Total	**52**	**100.00%**

Over 80% of the participants met their partners at regular meetings, mostly monthly, and over 50% of the sample said that their partners rarely missed the regular meetings.

Table 25 What degree of trust do you have in your key partners?

Trust in Key Partners	Count	Percentage
2 (low trust)	1	3.85%
4	3	11.54%
5	6	23.08%
6	4	15.38%
7	1	3.85%
8	10	38.46%
9 (high trust)	1	3.85%
	26 (45.61% of sample)	100.00%

Participants could respond to this question overall or they could differentiate between partners. This table shows that the managers in the sample split into two camps: around 45% have high trust (8/9) in their partner agencies whereas almost 40% have low trust (2,3,4,5). Further analysis reveals that of the participants in the sample that differentiated between managers, those participants rated health authorities as being the most trustworthy, except where there was very low trust. Partners had less polarised views about social services and trusts. Impressionistic as it is, this response demonstrates that in many localities there is a lack of trust that must inhibit service development.

Table 26 How well prepared do you think your lead partners are?

Preparedness of Lead Partners (All)	Count
Very	5
Sufficiently	15
Insufficiently	3

Preparedness of Lead Partners (HAs)	Count
Very	2
Sufficiently	6
Insufficiently	2
Poorly	5
Preparedness of Lead Partners (Social Services)	**Count**
Very	6
Sufficiently	3
Insufficiently	2
Poorly	1
Preparedness of Lead Partners (trusts)	**Count**
Very	4
Sufficiently	9
Insufficiently	2
Poorly	3

The interviewees responded to this question either by referring to all their lead partners, or separating out individual agencies. For this reason, this analysis is presented in the form of tally marks for each registered answer. Respondents were keen to differentiate between partners. Participants from all of the three agencies gave examples of the other agencies being insufficiently or poorly prepared; however, Health Authorities were more often cited as being insufficiently or poorly prepared than social services or trusts. This lack of perceived preparedness may be related to the views of practitioners about having to deal with non-practitioners.

Table 27 In what areas are your partners unprepared?

Type of difficulty	Count	Percentage
Relationships	11	19.30%
Personality	11	19.30%
Capacity	8	14.04%
Capability	22	38.60%
Other	3	5.26%
Don't know	2	3.51%

Table 27 is revealing. It suggests that over one third of participants think that their partners lack the capability to perform their role, a much larger percentage than think that they lack capacity. Furthermore, almost 20% of respondents specified one particular aspect of capability, i.e. the capability to create and sustain inter-agency relationships. These responses, when compared with those in Table 21 which sought to establish how well prepared respondents believed themselves to be, suggest an element of 'I'm OK, you're not OK'. Similarly in Table 22, participants were not suggesting that they felt that they needed help in creating and sustaining relationships. In this case, it is possible that training might assist. It is striking that in almost 20% of cases, respondents felt that partners did not have the right personality to create and sustain relationships. In such cases, presumably training would not assist; this response may be symptomatic of considerable personal animosity between players.

Table 28 What are the implications of current organisational boundaries for joint working?

Response	Count	Percentage of total questionnaires
Positive	19	33.33%
Negative	42	73.68%

This table confirms that the current geographical boundaries used by the agencies are perceived as having negative implications for the development of mental health services in London.

Policy Direction

Table 29 What are the influences that shape the policy priorities of your agency (focus on three) ?

Influence	Count
Local pressures	40
National Initiatives	36
Finance	26
Needs Assessment	14
Health Authority priorities	8
Local Incidents	7
User Views	4
Hospital Closure	3
Ethnicity	1
GP pressure	1
Learning of the staff	1

NB: These figures may not be expressed as percentages as each interviewee mentioned a number of influences.

Overall, national initiatives, money and local pressures are the major influences on the policy priorities of the three agencies. The significant impact of national initiatives may initially appear reassuring for the DoH, but it puts a responsibility on policy makers and performance managers within the DoH to frame and disseminate policy in a fashion which assists the relationships of the agencies in the field; the mental health scene is apparently very sensitive to the interventions of the centre. At the same time, money, or the lack of it, for service development and the reduction of resources to sustain current services (in particular in social services) appear to be major constraints.

This focus on national initiatives, money and local pressures suggests that two sets of significant voices (users and practitioners) are not currently influential on the policy of local agencies. In the case of users, this will be a continuation of tradition. However, the apparent lack of influence over policy exercised by practitioners may be a major change from tradition, especially for psychiatrists. In these circumstances, it would not be surprising to find that practitioners are responding less than enthusiastically to policy that they may have played a reduced role in formulating.

Table 30 Which three national policy interventions have had the most impact on your work and priorities over the last five years (focus on three)?

National policy	Count
CPA	60
NHS & Com. Care Act	19
Financial Incentives	13
MDOs	13
Health of the Nation	10
Hospital Closures	5
Primary Care-led NHS	3
Continuing Care Guidance	3
MH Task Force	2
Audit Commission	2
Malone Review	2
The Children's Act	1

While CPA is represented as a single category in Table 30, the respondents expanded this definition into two sub-categories: 'CPA/CM integration' and 'CPA & discharge'.
NB These responses cannot be expressed as percentages as each interviewee could specify up to three interventions.

The most important policy initiative of the past five years is the care programme approach and associated innovations (i.e. supervised discharge, integration with care management). This very specific piece of policy, perhaps better viewed as a national *operational* policy, is mentioned 60 times by respondents. Unlike their HA and trust colleagues, social services departments make reference also to the NHS and Community Care Act. This may signal an important difference between the approach of the health agencies and social services to the CPA. For social services, care management (of which the CPA is a specialist category) represents a major change to their role and function which has had significant implications for organisational structure and practitioner culture. Health, on the other hand, has tended to graft the CPA onto an practitioner culture largely untouched by the NHS and Community Care Act; in that sense it has had a very narrow focus. This difference may be a cause of significant tension between health and social services, and between managers and practitioners within health. This tension within health may be felt particularly by the managers from a practitioner background struggling to implement the CPA and achieve integration with care management without the active support of practitioners, in particular some psychiatrists (see next section).

Respondents were asked to rate the significance of three interventions, two of which were NHS Executive interventions (the Mental Health Task Force and the 'Malone Review'), and were mentioned by a small number of respondents spontaneously (see Table Thirty), and one inquiry report into an incident involving a mental health service user (publication of the Clunis Inquiry Report – Ritchie et al, 1994).

Table 31 Mental Health Task Force – significant or not?

MH Task Force Significance	Count
Significant	20
Not significant	33
Don't know	4

Clunis Inquiry – significant or not?

Clunis Significance	Count
Significant	47
Not significant	8
Don't know	2

'Malone Review' – significant or not?

Malone Significance	Count
Significant	28
Not significant	24
Don't know	5

In respect of the Mental Health Task Force London Project, health authorities were more likely to rate it as significant than either social services or trusts. The report of the inquiry into the care of Christopher Clunis was seen as significant by an overwhelming majority of the sample. The 'Malone review' was again perceived as significant by health authorities, less so by trusts and by only 50% of the social services departments.

Table 32 What was the meaning that you ascribed to:

Mental Health Task Force

Meaning mentioned	Count
Political motives	11
Raising the profile of mental health	7
Prompted by public concern	2
Other	29
Total number of responses	49

Clunis Inquiry Report

Meaning mentioned	Count
Joint working & co-ordination of care	20
Establishment of a blame culture through accountability	15
Furtherance of CPA	4
Risk assessment	4
Other	14
Total number of responses	57

Malone Review

Meaning mentioned	Count
Furtherance of CPA	13
Health Authorities 'being told to get their act together'	12
Political Motives	10
Challenge Fund money	3
Other	10
Total number of responses	48

In the meaning ascribed to the Mental Health Task Force and the 'Malone review', there is evidence of attribution of political motives to national initiatives by around 25% of the sample. It was clear to the interviewers that this attribution was pejorative and may indicate a significant strand of cynicism amongst the managers responsible for achieving change. Over 25% cite the establishment of a 'blame culture' within mental health services as the meaning that they ascribed to the Clunis Report. Such a culture is not conducive to creative practice and may account for the apparent reluctance of psychiatrists to operate multi-agency procedures which impinge on traditional patterns of clinical decision-making and accountability.

Local Agendas

Table 33 What are your current priorities for implementation?

Priority	Count
CMHTs	31
CPA development	15
Bed management	10
Financial priorities	9
Crisis services	8
Joint working	8
Hospital closure	7
Day care	7
Ethnic issues	5
Links with GPs	4
Child & Adolescent services	3
Mentally Disordered Offenders	3
Out-of-hours services	3

NB: It is not possible to express these figures as percentages, as each interviewee gave a list of priorities.

This table presents current priorities in July 1996. It is striking that over 50% of the sample have CMHTs as a *current* priority for implementation. CMHTs have been emerging as a model of practice (although a very inconsistent model of practice) since the mid-1980s (see Peck 1994). In 'Building Bridges' (Department of Health, 1995a) it was assumed that localities possessed CMHTs as the method of integrating health and social care (and the CPA/care management), and the October 1995 performance management checklist for health authorities contained CMHTs as one of the eight components, although the creation of CMHTs has never been explicit DoH policy. The delay in the full implementation of CMHTs (the policy vehicle for service integration) in London requires explanation. Firstly, it may suggest that there is a significant time-lag between early innovations and mainstream service developments. It is reasonable to assume that implementation of particular policy requirements will take longer than policy-makers may wish, especially where specific policy initiatives are issued: without explicit reference to the local strategy and practice context into which they are to be incorporated; without guidance on the process of establishment; and without targeted resources. Secondly, the slow development of CMHTs in London may suggest either further evidence of the limitations of inter-agency service development or further evidence of practitioner resistance to change (or both).

Table 34 Would you say your work is driven more by long term/strategic or short term/fire-fighting objectives?

Long Term or Short Term	Count	Percentage
Long term/strategic	18	31.58%
Short term/fire-fighting	16	28.07%
Balance	19	33.33%
Don't know	4	7.02%

This table suggests that although local policies and priorities are influenced by national initiatives, over 25% of the sample see short-term, firefighting objectives as taking priority, with a similar number seeing the long-term and short-term as in balance.

Table 35 Are acute admission beds an issue?

Acute Admission Beds an Issue	Count	Percentage
yes	51	89.47%
no	6	10.53%

and for which client group?

Client Group	Count	Percentage
Adult general	38	74.51%
Mentally Disordered Offenders	2	3.92%
Substance abusers	2	3.92%
Elderly	1	1.96%
Men	1	1.96%
New long stay	1	1.96%
Don't know	6	11.76%

Admission beds are an issue for almost 90% of the sample. However, less than 20% of managers mentioned bed management amongst their current priorities (see Table 33), nor would creating more beds be a priority if more resources became available (see Table 37).

Table 36 What is the issue for acute admission beds?

Issue	Count
Not enough beds	32
Discharge arrangements	10
Clinical practice on admission	7
Lack of alternatives to hospital admission	3
ECR issues	3
Inadequate housing	2

NB: It is not possible to express these figures as percentages as interviewees could state more than one issue.

This table shows that well over 50% of the 90% in Table 35 thought that the issue was a lack of beds. Less than 50% mentioned other problems, and only around 5% made reference to a lack of alternatives to admission, although work reported elsewhere in this book (Chapter 8) found them to be largely absent. Over 25%, however, cited problems relating to practice on admission and discharge arrangements.

Table 37 What would be your priority if you were given 10% more resources tomorrow?

Priority	Count
CMHTs	18
Staff	10
Housing	9
Crisis services	8
Bed management	5
Out-of-hours services	3
Mentally Disordered Offenders	2
Day care	2
Ethnic issues	1

NB: It is not possible to express these figures as percentages, as there was no limit on the number of priorities the respondents might mention.

This table shows that almost 33% of managers in the sample would invest in CMHTs, suggesting that they believe that the delay in creating CMHTs is at least in part a resource problem. In contrast, no manager would spend money on the CPA, suggesting that the delay in implementation and integration with care management is not a resource problem, and neither is joint working. Managers may also believe that effective CMHTs would reduce pressure on adult acute admission beds. Only two managers would spend the money directly on providing more adult acute admission beds, a surprising finding in the light of Table 36, the other three who cited bed management would invest elsewhere in the system to relieve pressure on admission beds. However, only one manager, in apparent contravention of recent guidance (Department of Health, 1996c), and in the context of the problems caused by the lack of such provision identified in this book would explicitly invest in 24 hour nursed beds. However, nine managers would invest in housing, and eleven would invest in crisis or out of hours services, all of which might be predicted to reduce the pressure on acute beds.

Managers in the sample overwhelmingly recognise that adult acute admission beds are an issue, and they largely believe that there are not enough beds, a message they presumably hear regularly from practitioners. Nonetheless, creating more beds is neither an agency priority for HAs, trusts and social services, nor is it a personal priority for managers in the event of increased resources. This apparent paradox may be explained by a number of factors: firstly, CMHTs and crisis/out of hours responses appeared in the NHS Executive performance management checklist in October 1995 and are perceived as a high agency and personal priority; secondly, creating more beds may be seen as addressing the effect not the cause; thirdly, that cause is perceived to a be lack of alternatives to admission or options for discharge.

In fact, and in contrast to Table 33, managers showed a striking variety of personal priorities for investment, often completely unconnected with the agency priorities. This disparity suggests that managers may not believe that the agenda set by national initiatives contains the issues of most pressing local importance.

Obstacles and Opportunities

Table 38 What are the three major obstacles that you have encountered in the development of mental health services?

Nature of obstacles	Count
Financial	28
Joint Working	22
Managerial	16
Clinicians	14
GPs	11
Change	7
Recruitment	4
Personal	4

NB: It is not possible to express these figures as percentages, as there was no limit to the number of priorities respondents might mention.

The most significant obstacle was financial; a more detailed review of the responses show a concern both about maintaining current levels of resource (especially social services') and locating new resources for service development. Perhaps managers will always want more money, but there is a consistency about the response to this question and elsewhere which suggests that it is a genuine obstacle, a conclusion borne out elsewhere in this book, although it is important to recognise that some responses in this category are as much to do with financial mechanisms as adequacy of budgets (e.g. GP Fundholding, approach of Finance Directors, separation of health and social services budgets).

Problems around joint working are cited by well over a third of the sample; this is clearly a source for concern as it is an obstacle which is capable of being overcome. It is not mentioned by a majority of the sample, and the same number of respondents saw it as an opportunity (see Table 39) as saw it as an obstacle. This impression that the problem is resolvable is supported by the frequency of comments referring to culture, although it is important to record the frequency of comments referring to structure.

Over 25% of the sample mention obstacles relating to management. The most consistent problem appears to be capacity, although there are some strong comments relating to the capability of colleagues. There would appear to be some support for an integrated management structure between health and social services.

Almost 25% saw the attitude of clinicians, or to be more specific consultant psychiatrists, as an obstacle. Almost 20% had a similar view about GPs, in particular Fundholders. Both responses suggest a worrying split between managers and clinicians within the health domain.

Table 39 What are the opportunities?

Opportunity	Count
Joint working	22
Finance	18
Staff	14
Focus on mental health	11
CMHTs	9
Users	8
CPA	4
Voluntary Sector	3
Training	2

NB: It is not possible to express these figures as percentages, as each respondent mentioned several opportunities.

It is encouraging to note that, in relation to joint working there are exactly the same number of the sample citing it as an opportunity as an obstacle. Similarly, almost 33% see finance as an opportunity, especially the additional local resources being invested in response to the perceived crisis in the system and the national funding initiatives (e.g. MISG). It is also important to recognise that almost 25% see staff as an opportunity, in particular clinical staff and including consultant psychiatrists. It is interesting that although 31 respondents have CMHTs as a priority for implementation, only 9 saw them as an opportunity.

Table 40 Do you think any of the issues you have covered are unique to London, and if so what are they?

London Issues	Count	Percentage
Yes	22	38.60%
Matter of degree	19	33.33%
No	15	26.32%
Don't know	1	1.75%

and chart of all issues mentioned by those answering 'yes' or 'matter of degree'

London issues	Count
Transient population	14
Ethnic diversity	8
Bed pressure	8
Intensified problems	6
Recruitment	6
Deprivation	5
Morbidity	5
Underfunding	3
MDOs	2

NB: There was no limit to the number of issues each respondent might mention.

Table 41 Do you think that the issues covered are unique to mental health? If so which?

Mental Health Issues	Count	Percentage
Yes	41	71.93%
Matter of degree	9	15.79%
No	6	10.53%
Don't know	1	1.75%

and chart of all issues mentioned by those answering 'yes' or 'matter of degree'

Mental Health Issue	Count
Public unpopularity	14
Need for joint working	13
Media unpopularity	8
Bed pressure	3
Underfunding	3
Defensive clinical practice	3
MDOs	2
Users uncooperative	2

NB: There was no limit to the number of issues each respondent might mention.

It is worth considering these tables together. Almost 75% of the sample believed that some of the issues facing mental health services in London were unique to London either because of their nature or because of their degree. Almost 75% of the sample believed that the issues facing mental health services were unique to mental health because of their nature. Furthermore, respondents produced a wide range of such issues in response to each question.

Analysis of and Commentary on the Narrative Transcriptions

The analysis of the narratives is supported by quotations, with the organisational origin of the manager being quoted in brackets. On occasions the quotations have been edited either to protect the anonymity of the manager or to remove the circumlocution inevitable in taped accounts. Table 42 identifies how often each theme was mentioned and by whom. The commentary which follows does not exactly match the themes identified in the table, as much of the content of each theme overlapped, or was mutually reinforcing.

Table 42 Number of times particular themes emerged in the transcripts

(Total number of transcripts)	Trusts (18)	Health Authorities (11)	Social Services (22)
CONTEXT			
Power and Capacity	5	7	14
Organisational boundaries	7	4	8
Issues relating to GP fundholders	6	2	4
Role animosity	7	2	11
CONTENT			
Declining resources	7	4	8
Financial complexity	3	3	2
CMHTs	7	3	13
CPA/care management	1	2	11
PROCESS			
Service development	8	6	12
Political influences of LAs	4	3	7
User-led issues	4	4	7
Product champions	6	2	5
Single/combined Trust	1	0	0

Declining Resources and Decreasing Capacity

Unsurprisingly, the issue of declining resources was raised by many interviewees, the effects of which were spread throughout the service system and not just felt in financial terms, for instance in staff turnover: *'another crucial factor is the loss of expertise of experienced staff that is created by this sort of major change. Certainly, we are feeling that we've lost experienced staff, particularly in relation to nursing, but also in other areas, particularly administration. These were people that have gained tremendous experience over a long period of time, and there's not replacement people for them out there who are readily available ... And so therefore I think the resource issue's not one just about money, but is certainly around available skills as well'* (Trust).

Many health authorities, in particular, seem simply to have insufficient people working on mental health issues to make any real impact upon local services. Health authorities are thus, more than ever, reliant on trusts to operationalise joint working with social services. This lack of management capacity is felt acutely in combined trusts where the perception of the interviewees was that mental health services has borne the brunt of the required reduction in management costs and some interviewees have seen a commensurate reduction in the status of their position.

Many services saw declining resources as having a clear impact on service development: *'The second thing was no additional resources, so you were trying to actually implement this process, which has very far reaching effects on practice and culture and inter-relationships, without having an infrastructure to support that'* (SSD). The wider effects were a large number of re-structurings, often to reduce costs, resulting in increased organisational instability: *'I've had to apply for my job three times, including getting the job in the first place. There are any number of people in exactly that same position. I just happened to be the one who's always stayed around. The Trust has reorganised internally twice, to my knowledge, and there have been sort of subtle shifts and changes of responsibility on top of that. The local authority have reorganised at least twice, and again there have been subtle changes that I haven't necessarily been aware of'* (HA). *'The biggest single obstacle to change is the fact that I've had to work with eight changes of lead responsibility within the Trust during the course of three and a half years'* (SSD).

The effect of 'down-sizing' has been to cast an ever more focused spotlight on joint working between those individuals who are in positions of seniority: *'Now, when the management structures of the health authority, the Trust and social services are getting smaller and smaller and there are two or even four personalities that don't get on with one another, it's really difficult'* (HA).

Problems imposed by Organisational Boundaries

Reinforcing findings from elsewhere, the lack of co-terminosity appears to be causing widespread problems in London. The problems of matching locality teams/CMHTs to GP practices has caused significant inter-agency difficulties, particularly with social services colleagues, who have put considerable effort (with health colleagues) in achieving co-terminosity of operational team boundaries. *'Social services won't wear any changes in boundaries to match GPs – it will be the demise of the locality teams'* (SSD). There have also been some idiosyncratic influences on boundary issues: *'Over the last 3-4 years, we've made some progress in reshaping boundaries...however, we have still ended up with some discrepancies. For example, we have a Professor who wanted a morbid patch which is less than half the size of the others. So all the other disciplines have had to carve up their resources to meet that sized patch'* (Trust). *'They* [the Trust] *started from a position of wanting each sector to be different, because they wanted to research them! Which was fine for them, but not really for us or the local population'* (HA).

Problems with CMHTs

A large number of the transcripts were about CMHTs. The problems of reducing management capacity are matched, in some areas, by problems in finding managers with adequate experience and management skills. *'We struggled through getting team managers of the calibre that we really wanted...'* (Trust). Some trusts have actively tackled this problem:

> *'We have restructured managerially to give some more dedicated support to the development of the CMHTs. At the time I came in, whilst the service had developed a huge amount, we had not looked at the management structure and what that should look like to reflect a much bigger service and a much more complex service. I created a dedicated project management post for a year to help with the development of the CMHTs. It's given the CMHT managers somebody who they feel is their person to give them some dedicated support and time, and who's not been from a clinical background, so they haven't had some of the clinical support they might have liked, but have been able to complement their clinical skills by providing some business support skills, and helping them with some elements of the job that they didn't feel comfortable with'* (Trust).

Nevertheless, problems with – and for – CMHT managers are well documented (e.g. Onyett, Standen and Peck, in press) and are unlikely to be easily resolved. There is no identified primary professional background for this job and no recognised training associated with the post. Team managers may have to be clinicians to gain sufficient credibility with the majority of team members – but this may cause conflicting loyalties with the provider management they are there to represent and, of course, with social services colleagues who may feel their interests are not being fully represented. '*In fact we have a mixture of local authority and health service personnel in those positions* [CMHT managers]. *However, it is our experience that it's more successful where health service personnel lead it, and that, of course, doesn't help*' (Trust).

Many agencies had faced major difficulties in finding suitable premises for their teams. '...*capital was the biggest stumbling block* [to the development of CMHTs]. *Without capital it was almost impossible for us to make a move. We only have half the revenue costs now to run* [the CMHT base] *so we may have to think very hard, possibly make some staff redundant as a result, just to pay for the base*' (Trust). '*There've been lots of problems about the building, which seems to me extremely expensive*' (HA)

Some services have found creative ways round the potential professional dislocation felt by workers in the shift to a team base. However, the experiences for many professionals within teams remains an unhappy one:

> '*To begin with, I felt: 'Look, we've really got to go with health into these CMHTs." You know: sit in the same place, the same building, rub shoulders, [then] people will share things, information will be exchanged. I pushed very hard for that to happen. I then got much closer to our social workers who were in the team and it emerged that actually they were in one room and they barely ever spoke to anybody. They only ever came together when they had their team meeting. The thing that frustrated them was that there was ... all this mirroring of meetings. They had ... the CMHT meetings, their own team meetings, the business meetings, and then they had to meet with their own managers, there were just all these masses of different meetings ... It felt like relationships weren't anywhere near as good as was being painted, so ... they said they wanted to come out of the CMHTs. They felt that ... we could meet with the teams without people having to sit together. So we honoured that wish*' (SSD).

Social services, in particular, voiced concerns about the implications for their workers of moving into teams: '*Social workers perceived moving to CMHTs, at worst, as the HA being imperialist and snaffling up one of our (area) teams*' (SSD). Some agencies had set up pilot CMHTs, although this did not necessarily alleviate the problems of future teams. For some, a pilot project was in danger of stalling the whole development process. '*It [CMHT] is seen as a kind of problem child. Which is not good, if that's really the way we're thinking of going in the future. If this is a pilot project, people are going to be fed up with it before it's even got out of the pram*' (SSD). Although having a pilot did quickly highlight local problems. '*There were no policies or procedures agreed between social services and health as to how this team would operate. In hindsight, we probably went into implementation before we'd actually done the planning and that created a number of different problems around the staff that were assimilated, certainly from social services' perspective, who were not, I don't think, particularly prepared as to what they were going into, what kind of animal this was, and what the expectations were'* (SSD).

A striking omission in all but a very small number of transcripts was of any clear definition of what CMHTs were there to *do*. The development of the service was described as an end in itself, without any clear sense coming across in the transcripts as to what was the function of the teams and what was their role within a comprehensive mental health service. This may have led, in part, to the role animosity and confusion which still characterises these services and it is notable that those interviewees who did cite successful CMHTs, described them in terms of their function and what the teams would seek to achieve for service users. Despite all this, whatever their problems, CMHTs are clearly felt by many to represent an improvement in services. *'Reassuringly, some of those staff who've made the transition [to CMHTs] when asked would they go back to the old way of working, wouldn't touch it with a bargepole. I think we've got one of the best services in the country'* (Trust).

CPA/Care Management

Eleven social services interviewees discussed the CPA/CM in their narratives, yet it was only mentioned by 1 Trust and 2 HA interviewees – from the transcripts alone, it did not appear to be as pressing an issue for health services. Those agencies that did talk about the CPA/care management often noted positive effects: *'The mechanisms force us to work together, like CPA and care management. I feel quite optimistic about that. We've got a long way to go, but anything that can force us to be talking ...'* (SSD). There was a fair degree of support for integration of the CPA and care management, although the practical difficulties of integration loomed large: *'Management should have spent more time dealing with concrete issues rather than theoretical issues. It is quite easy to gain theoretical assent as being a good idea. There has been a lot written and discussed about who is in the care programme approach and care management and desirability of working together and training needs and development needs etc. etc. The things that have been difficult are when health staff stated that social services can't use the car park or decisions about whether social workers are sitting at their desk as a part of a multi-disciplinary team or sit dispersed amongst health colleagues at integrated desks as part of a multi-disciplinary team'* (SSD).

The following quote from an outer London SSD, summarises the feelings of many social services interviewees:

1 *The Trust was required by [the] HA as purchasers to implement CPA, and did not involve social services at an early stage. Now, I think that's partly because they had their own changes to cope with, but also because we were pretty poor on mental health anyway. So you've got two insular organisations trying to actually look at implementing something that required considerable joint working.*

2 *The second thing was no additional resources, so you were trying to actually implement this process, which has very far reaching effects on practice and culture and inter-relationships, without having an infrastructure to support that. Eventually, we put joint finance alongside it on a time limited project. That project has now stopped, and I would argue that we still haven't got the implementation right or complete, so [there are still] inadequate resources.*

3 *The third thing is it was owned by everyone as a good thing, but small powerful groups within the conglomeration of people involved with mental health services were saying it is a good thing publicly, but not subscribing to it in terms of their own professional practice. In some instances it was a complete professional group, and in some instances it was individuals. Any process imposed without having due time to actually think through how you are going to take people with you, is almost sure to fail.*

4 *The other problem has been that if you have two ostensibly separate systems (CPA and care management) it's extremely difficult to get them to court each other and subsequently come into some sort of partnership. That remains a problem.*

The overall feeling seemed to be that, given that the CPA and care management were imposed, with inadequate recognition of implementation costs, insufficient lead-in time and a possible conflict of interest between the national versus local agenda, it is hardly surprising that the culture shift required to make it work properly has not happened.

Animosity between professional groups and agencies

Discussion of the CPA and care management prompted many interviewees to describe significant problems working with psychiatrists. Social services in particular, are frustrated at spending a substantial amount of time developing operational policies, particularly in relation to patient care, then finding this overturned by one consultant, or a small number of consultants, who carry on implementing traditional clinical ways of working. This is a particular problem in developing integrated CPA/CM procedures, (some psychiatrists, for example, will not accept a single assessment). '*... towards the end of the time during which the working party was completing its task there was a new appointment [...] of a lead clinician. Unfortunately the lead clinician was clear that he was not in favour of amalgamated assessments in any form and felt that everything should be separate. This caused tremendous upset between the two authorities. The current position is that the whole project can best be described as being on hold, as the lead clinician would seem to be in a position where his views can supersede those of the steering group, the working party, the health purchasers, although the local authority is not willing to accept the position*' (SSD).

Part of the problems is that: '*the obstacles to change* [vis-à-vis psychiatrists] *are around tradition. We need to develop a management of change package for a particularly intractable group who see themselves as the leaders but take no responsibility. We have actually managed to make the case for more psychiatrists, but, on a bad day, I'm not sure that was so clever*' (Trust). As a profession, psychiatrists need to be fully involved in the changes facing mental health services; the findings from the transcripts indicate that this may require a more formal framework of accountability for psychiatrists which extends to individual professionals. The problems highlighted in working with psychiatrists did extend to other professional groups. National polices may be profoundly threatening to professional status in a way which has, hitherto, not been explored.

Alongside this professional animosity, went animosity between agencies which, between trusts and social services, often lay in the nature of their approaches. Trusts are driven by clinical imperatives, surviving in the market place and, in the main, take a non-strategic/pragmatic approach to providing services. Social services are driven by political imperatives and a procedural approach, most strongly characterised by child protection work, but also in evidence in their approach to mental health care. There was also evidence of the parochialism of trusts being challenged in the move away from a hospital base: '[The trust] *didn't appreciate the complexities of funding around community services. They assumed that if they moved to the community and set up these things then social services would simply go along with them and set up their arrangements alongside and around, without actually having the discussions with social services first to find out what they were prepared to do. A part of the trust's learning curve around moving to the community has to be around realising that they have to work with other people quite closely'* (HA).

The animosity between trusts and HAs often centred around confusion as to who is responsible for what within the service system, leading to real issues of territoriality. The confusion over strategic versus operational responsibilities is, perhaps, most clearly highlighted in the CPA, where HAs are responsible for ensuring the policy is in place, yet trusts are responsible for setting the structure in place and individual professionals for its implementation.

Service Development

This theme was reflected, of course, throughout all the transcripts, given the nature of what interviewees were asked to discuss. However, there were specific issues in relation to service development which warrant further comment.

Agencies rarely lacked service plans. *'A number of reviews had been carried out; in fact when we counted them, a health service colleague and I, we came to a total of eight different reviews that had been carried out by both sides, both health and social services. Different managers at different times ... they'd been carried out, come to a conclusion, and filed away'* (SSD). There was recognition of the need to take a 'whole system' approach, although the process of how the three statutory agencies arrive at a comprehensive map of services to guide service developments was not once mentioned. However, once a strategy had been developed many agencies had problems in successfully implementing the plans. There was little evidence of a systematic organisational approach to this issue – many senior managers did not know how to engage their own or other agencies in implementation, so they did it themselves, or trusted to a few individuals to push the process through. This often failed, leaving patchy implementation.

The theme of the strategy not being needs-led emerged throughout the interviews. *'The health authority's strategy that was adopted was not a needs-led strategy, and it changed several times en route ...'* (HA). *'My concern at the moment is that we're not looking at real need assessments, we're not developing the services based on real need assessment. They're all on epidemiology, national trends, rather than on what's happening locally, rather than looking at: "What do we have? How many homes do we have locally? What's the actual utilisation of the services? What's the homeless position like here?" I think we need to emphasise the importance of real needs assessment with our purchasers, and do joint needs assessment, and get somebody in to come and do it properly, and then base the service development on that'* (SSD).

Professional investment in the status quo was a significant barrier to the implementation of service plans which many agencies had not overcome. *'It seems to me that there is a sensible way forward about developing a comprehensive, seamless needs-led mental health service. I think I made the mistake of assuming that everybody agreed with that. Again I knew it, or perhaps under-estimated it, and that's underestimating the power of vested professional interests ...'* (SSD). This effect of professional power to inhibit service development was forcibly expressed by some interviewees. *The whole idea that there may be a different way of doing things is ... is alien, I think, to a lot of people. Some of the debates I've had with staff about some of the changes, you'll get them to a stage of accepting needs assessments, and you say to people: "What do you actually want? What would make your life better?" And they'll say: "Well, yeah, that's fine for people who are physically disabled, but you can't apply it to mentally ill people. We're the professionals; we know best."'* (SSD).

However, the influence of service users, particularly on HAs, is growing: *'A lot of it* [pressure for change] *came from service users, and it was the express wishes of service users, who were expressing their dissatisfaction with our service that was based on hospital beds'* (HA); *'The nature and origin of the change is, in its initial form, the demand by mental health service users for a more responsive service: one that was more responsive than what they saw as simply 'get admitted to hospital or don't'* (HA).

Perhaps one of the most useful lessons for agencies to learn in relation to service development is the inter-dependence of the statutory agencies in successfully bringing about change: *'The problems have mainly stemmed from a lack of communication and not getting all agencies on board right from the start. I suppose ... we've learnt from that, I mean we wouldn't do it that way again. It's been a springboard in many ways for us to get much closer co-operation with, particularly with Housing, so the problems have brought benefits. And I think the trust will have learnt a lot of lessons from that as well: primarily that they do have to talk to others in advance of deciding what they're going to do! Which is, I think, is a real culture shock for them'* (HA).

Table 43 Table showing the major stories of the transcripts

Trusts	Health Authorities	Social Services
6 – CMHTs	1 – reprovision	11 – CMHTs
1 – A&E Triage	1 – accommodation	1 – setting up a duty team
1 – employment	1 – secure provision	3 – crisis service
2 – reprovision	1 – crisis response	4 – CPA/care management
1 – acute bed pressure	4 – CMHTs	1 – day services review
1 – joint purchasing of a service		1 – accommodation
1 – high dependency unit		2 – assertive outreach team
1 – primary care link worker		
1 – care management		
1 – medical recruitment		
1 – attention to hospitalisation		

Major Themes from Both Sources of Data

There are a number of themes which emerge from both the questionnaires and the transcripts. It should be stressed that, as far as possible, they are summarised in this section from the perspective of participants (and do not necessarily represent the views of the authors on these issues).

The apparent lack of management capacity

There appears to be a lack of capacity to create and sustain local, comprehensive mental health services in London. Social services departments, health authorities and trusts are all under financial pressure which leads to a reduction in management capacity, health agencies are additionally experiencing explicit targets for management cost which are further reducing capacity. This financial pressure is one influence on the regularity of restructurings. The lack of capacity leads to managers combining operational and strategic responsibilities with priority inevitably being given to the reactive and short-term rather than the proactive and long-term. This problem is exacerbated in those organisations which have never possessed sufficient and/or senior mental health management (e.g. combined trusts). In these circumstances, it is increasingly difficult to identify managers to work on project management or to support (or become) product champions for change.

The apparent organisational and personal instability

There appears to be significant organisational and job instability in the management of mental health services in London. This instability results in frequent changes in those managers responsible for the creation and sustenance of services which, in turn, produces problems in developing relationships within and between agencies.

The apparent cultural obstacles to joint working

There appear to be significant cultural problems which act as impediments in many localities to effective joint working between managers in social services, health authorities and trusts. In brief, managers come from different professional backgrounds, with long experience of mental health practice from different perspectives, working for agencies with different pressures and aspirations, and different forms of internal and external accountability.

The apparent impact of policy-making and performance management

There appear to be problems arising from the way in which policy is made and disseminated. The health aspect of mental health policy in the DoH is made by expert clinicians and focuses increasingly on the what (CPA, Spectrum of Care, 24 hour nursed beds). However, it says little or nothing about the how, that is, the process by which change is achieved in a complex service system. Given the sensitivity of health managers to the content of national initiatives (either policy or performance), the absence of guidance or support relating to the process of change is a significant issue.

The apparent problems of accountability of consultant clinical staff

There appear to be problems with the accountability of consultant clinical staff for their agreement to and compliance with local agreements between agencies which seek to implement national policy. This problem is apparent despite the preponderance of managers who are, or were, practitioners. The reluctance of some consultants to conform, even when they have been involved in the formulation of agreements, is perhaps a consequence of the perceived threat to their autonomy in the changes to practice in mental health services.

The apparent problems of managing in a service of public and political concern

There appear to be problems with managing in a service which has been the subject of so much public and political debate. This has two implications: the first is the political aspect of policy making and performance management being perhaps more emphasised than local priorities and clinical discretion; the second is the practical aspect of managing staff who perceive themselves to be vulnerable to blame for what they perceive to be service deficiencies.

Chapter 13

Interpreting the evidence: conclusions and possible solutions

Sonia Johnson & Graham Thornicroft

13.1 Introduction

This chapter summarises the main evidence on Londoners' mental health needs, on the condition of the city's mental health services, and on gaps between need and provision. Each major area of service provision is discussed in turn, and suggestions are made for possible solutions to the difficulties identified. We draw on proposals made by all contributors to the book.

13.2 Information

A significant obstacle to rational planning of comprehensive local strategies in many areas is the lack of interpretable and accurate information. The care system has become more complex since the introduction of the internal market, and with it the task of assessing what provision is really available to a local population. Important difficulties are:

- Lack of standard formats and of categories of services and of client groups for recording service provision across different agencies.
- Lack of co-ordinated systems for monitoring services within a catchment area across all statutory and independent sector agencies, and for making this information readily accessible.
- Lack of information about what provision is actually available locally at any given time – information about places occupied does not indicate what options there are for making new placements.
- Lack of procedures for regularly up-dating data collection about catchment area services and thus establishing trends over time.
- Lack of detailed information about the level of support which facilities can provide and the client groups for which they are suitable.
- A frequent absence of information on place of origin of clients in residential services, so that, particularly for voluntary sector facilities with wide catchment areas, it is uncertain how far they are providing for the local population and how far increasing local needs by importing patients into the catchment area.
- There is no regular system of data collection across London as a whole.

Possible solutions

Co-ordinated data collection across health service, local authority and voluntary sectors within each catchment area would facilitate rational planning at a local level. A single multi-agency group should collate and disseminate all relevant information within an area, avoiding wasteful parallel procedures. Such a process could helpfully take place at the level of a Health Authority or a Borough. The development of standardised formats for recording service provision by all agencies would make data comparable and interpretable, and should include clearly defined categories for service types and for client groups.

The difficulties encountered in data collection and service assessment in this report also indicate the need to assess not only numbers of places currently in use, but also current service availability, including delays experienced and needs for service provision which cannot be met. As well as devising systems for local monitoring, London as a whole needs a system for regular collection and collation of data, allowing continuing monitoring of the state of the city's services and their ability to meet the population's needs.

13.3 Londoners' needs and the resources available to meet them

There is very strong evidence both from epidemiological studies and from service utilisation that the mental health needs of Londoners are at an extreme in the national range. Levels of social deprivation, unemployment, social isolation and homelessness in London are at the top end of the national spectrum. These factors are associated not only with a greater prevalence of morbidity, but also with greater disability and disadvantage among the mentally ill in London compared with elsewhere in the country. The large ethnic minority and refugee populations also have specific service needs. Demand for in-patient services for young males is especially high.

Even though London purchasers currently appear to be spending relatively high proportions of their budgets on mental health services, many London services appear to be falling below reasonable minimum standards in the extent to which they can meet these extreme needs. In many of the chapters of this book, evidence has been presented which strongly suggests the conclusion that mental health services in London are substantially underfunded. Despite this, while preparing the book, we have been aware of proposals to reduce funding for mental health services in many London boroughs. We therefore need to address the wider issue of how resources are allocated to health authorities. This issue is the subject of a very detailed recent House of Commons Health Select Committee report, 'Allocation of Resources to Health Authorities' (House of Commons, 1996). The current arrangement is that the proposals of the University of York Consortium, produced in 1994, have been implemented by weighting 64% of funds allocated to health authorities by their acute services formula and 12% by their mental illness formula, with the remaining 24% of total funds allocated unweighted. The decision to weight the three components of the funding formula in this way has very important consequences for the total amount of allocation to each health authority. An examination of these consequences was published in 1995 by the University of York Consortium (Peacock and Smith, 1995). This report shows the consequences for funding two health authorities for all health services of using different possible funding formulae: the previous basis (the square root of the standard mortality ratio of those aged under 75), the York Acute Prediction Model, the York Mental Illness Model, the current NHS Executive formula, and the 'full' York Needs formulae. The total amount of funding allocated to City and Hackney, for example, would be 3.93% greater if the entire allocation were based upon the York Needs formulae, rather than on the current NHS Executive formulae. Conversely, the amount allocated to mid Surrey on the basis of the York formula would be 5.26% less than under the current arrangement.

Possible solutions

Resources: In view of the very high levels of need and the evidence that London providers are struggling to meet them within existing resources, the adequacy of current resources for London should be reassessed, and the implication for inner city areas of current national capitation formulae should be reconsidered. We agree with the conclusions of the Health Select Committee that 'the current situation in which some 24% of hospital and community health services expenditure is unweighted for need is unsatisfactory'. The considerable pressures currently experienced by mental health services throughout London, particularly in inner city boroughs, might be alleviated at least in part by a revision of the funding formulae in the direction of the full proposals made by the University of York.

For several of the groups who are highly represented in London, further research is required in order to reach an understanding of the group's needs and of ways of meeting them:

Young people: Many existing services were developed for the generation first discharged in large numbers from the asylum, a generation now approaching old age. However, the younger generation of patients now predominating in London have not experienced long term institutionalisation and have different needs and expectations in areas such as work and housing. This generation's needs and preferences need to be investigated and appropriate service models piloted and evaluated.

For young men in particular, the rising demand for in-patient services is a major cause for concern. Reasons are not well understood, but may include rising unemployment, increasing substance abuse, clinicians' concern about risk of violence, or alienation from community psychiatric services, especially among young men from ethnic minority groups. The causes of this rise in admission need to be investigated and ways sought of engaging young men more effectively in community services.

Ethnic minorities: A greater understanding is needed of the needs of members of ethnic minorities, and of the most acceptable and effective ways of providing services for them. This applies especially to refugees, to people with milder mental health problems, and to groups such as the Chinese and Black African communities, who are a significant presence in London, but are not highly represented enough to have attracted much specific research or service provision.

User and carer perspectives: Future assessments of needs for services in London should fully represent the perspectives of service users and carers.

13.4 Acute beds

There is overwhelming evidence that a crisis exists in acute bed provision in psychiatric wards in Inner London, with many Outer London services also experiencing considerable pressure. Bed occupancy is excessive and wards are accessible only to be the most severely disturbed. This is despite higher levels of acute bed provision in Inner London than elsewhere in the country. Expenditure on extra-contractual referrals (ECRs) is diverting large quantities of resources away from local services. The rate of 'new long stay' patients, who occupy beds on acute admission wards for periods in excess of six months, is also higher than elsewhere in the country, reducing the numbers of beds actually available for acute admissions.

Possible solutions

Acute beds are only one component in the system of care, and should not be considered in isolation from other elements whose availability is likely to have substantial effects on acute bed occupancy. In particular, more high support residential facilities (including facilities with 24 hour nursing care) need to be made available for placement of the most disabled patients who currently remain for unnecessarily long periods on the in-patient ward. As yet it is uncertain how far intensively staffed residential care or intensive 24 hour community services may be effective in preventing admission, and research on these questions in an inner city setting may be needed. The threshold for admission currently seems to be high in London, so that only very intensive services of a kind not generally available in the city at present seem likely to be potential substitutes for admission. In some parts of London, some extra acute beds may be needed to alleviate current pressures on staff and patients, and to reduce expenditure on extra-contractual referrals to the private sector.

13.5 Residential care

Although expenditure on residential services is high in relation to national levels, shortages of a range of community residential facilities are experienced in many catchment areas. As discussed above, some 'new long term' patients who would otherwise remain inappropriately in acute beds are likely to require facilities with 24 hour cover provided by nurses. There is also evidence that placements are often not well matched with the support needs of patients, and many more highly staffed facilities may be occupied by older, long term residents who no longer need this level of support, but for whom the facilities have become a permanent home. Many longer-established facilities may be unacceptable to younger people who are unwilling to share rooms or live among older patients.

Possible solutions

Provision of residential care in each catchment area should be reviewed in detail, with a particular view to ensuring that places are currently available in facilities with a wide range of levels of support, including 24 hour cover by nurses, and in facilities which younger people and people from ethnic minority groups find acceptable. For those who do not require 24 hour care, the supported tenancies being developed in some areas of London promise to be a very useful model. Permanent tenancies with varying levels of support according to current need allow flexibility, may be more acceptable to younger people, and provide patients with permanent tenancies, which they can continue to hold when support is no longer needed and has been withdrawn. Delays before placement vary widely through the capital, and minimum standards should be agreed and implemented for acceptable waits for assessment and for appropriate residential care. We suggest that an acceptable level of service would be placement of all patients in appropriate accommodation within a month.

13.6 Community teams

An organisational infra-structure has been established in most places for community-based services through sectorisation and the development of integrated multidisciplinary teams. However, in many areas premises in the community within sectors (such as community mental health centres) are not yet available. The intensity of the home treatment which such teams can provide is still very limited, and is not generally comparable with care delivered by research-based model services. There are shortages of CPNs in many areas. There are very wide differences between the level of community support available in different parts of the city, fluctuations which do not appear to correspond in any way to need. Practices vary on how sector boundaries are defined (whether by social services catchment areas or general practice lists) and whether separate rehabilitation services are maintained: there is little evidence of policy guidance available to inform decisions of this sort about which community team model to adopt.

Possible solutions

Where teams are currently based at sites which are not within or very close to the sectors they serve, the provision of more local community premises should be considered. Currently the speed of response and intensity of service available from teams in different areas varies very widely. Minimum standards should be set for these, and ways found of implementing them throughout the city. We suggest as an acceptable minimum standard that it should be possible for acutely ill or relapsing patients to be visited at least once per working day when required, that initial contact should be available within 24 hours, and that longer term allocation to a CPN or social worker caseload should take place within two weeks. The effectiveness of different community mental health team models should be investigated and guidance developed on these questions.

13.7 Day care and employment

Shortages of long term day care are experienced in some areas of London, and the health service seems to be a major provider of such services, at least in some areas. It is uncertain how far this is an appropriate role for services in which many of the staff are trained mental health professionals. Employment services appear to be very underdeveloped in most of London, and there is little variety in the schemes offered. This is despite evidence that many users and carers give a very high priority to employment services, and that they have beneficial effects on patients' outcome. Day care, employment and activity services have not been central in the mental health policy, research or public discussion of the 1990s, and this seems to be reflected in a patchy and limited service.

For acute day care, there are some acute day hospitals in Outer London which are able to respond quickly enough to emergencies for it to be realistic to expect them to prevent some admissions, but in Inner London, most of the existing day hospitals seem to have long delays for admission, so that they are unlikely to be capable of fulfilling such a function. However, it is not established whether acute day hospitals would in any case be an appropriate placement for many of the very severely disturbed individuals currently admitted to London's wards.

Possible solutions

Within each catchment area, current levels of provision of day care and employment scheme should be reviewed, with the aim of ensuring that such placements are available to all severely mentally ill patients who appear likely to benefit from them. The needs and preferences of service users in relation to long term day care and work schemes and the degree to which existing services meet these should be investigated. Schemes which help patients find open market employment and give them intensive support in retaining such jobs constitute a promising form of care which has so far been implemented and evaluated little in London.

13.8 Ethnic minorities

How to provide appropriate services for ethnic minorities is one of the central questions facing London's mental health services, particularly in view of the city's great ethnic diversity, and of the evidence that members at least of some minorities are unlikely to reach the services by voluntary routes, but at an increased risk of reaching them by compulsory means. Some voluntary sector services for specific groups have been developed, but their contribution is likely to remain significant but very circumscribed, as they are generally providing just one or two service components to a single minority group. Most service provision to most members of ethnic minorities is likely to continue to be from the generic services rather than from specific services, and strong concerns have been expressed that such services do not engage and meet the needs of members of minority groups.

Possible solutions

A central focus in service development for members of ethnic minority groups should be on how to make the **whole** mental health care system culturally sensitive and accessible to local ethnic minorities, and on provision of training in cross-cultural working for all mental health staff, regardless of their ethnic origin or work setting. Such initiatives to make the generic services culturally sensitive and accessible to local ethnic minorities should be based on widespread consultation both with service users from ethnic minorities and with other members of their communities. Research should be commissioned into the effectiveness of these initiatives. There is a particular need to examine the working of the Mental Health Act in relation to ethnic minorities, and introduction of legal representation and of advocates at an earlier stage in its implementation should be considered.

13.9 The homeless

There are large concentrations of homeless people in London, and very high rates of psychiatric disorder have been demonstrated among them. Many are unlikely to receive care unless specific intensive outreach services actively seek to engage them. Current barriers to effective provision include the effects of rigidly implemented catchment areas, problems registering with GPs, the inability of services to address multiple needs simultaneously (e.g. for physical and for mental health problems), and a tendency for homeless people to give a higher priority to basic needs such as housing and food than to health care.

Possible solutions

Difficulties in allocating responsibility for homeless patients may be overcome by provision of multidisciplinary teams with clear responsibility for assessing and meeting the needs of the homeless mentally ill in each health district with a homeless population. The foundations for comprehensive provision of this type have been laid in the development of five specialist teams for the homeless mentally ill established in three Thames Regions under the homeless mentally ill initiative. These multidisciplinary teams should take the lead in gathering local information on the extent of homelessness, and in establishing links between local agencies. Primary care agencies should also be closely involved for planning for the local homeless, and examination is need of the implications of fundholding for primary care of the homeless. Housing associations and special needs housing require good support and joint initiatives involving this sector should be encouraged, especially for longer-term move-on accommodation.

13.10 Services for mentally disordered offenders

Demand for in-patient secure facilities from inner London districts is at the extreme end of the national spectrum, with figures in some areas as much as ten times the national average. The demand on budgets is considerable. Community support by trained staff and highly supported residential care is in limited supply for individuals discharged from secure facilities. Problems with staff recruitment and retention make it more difficult to provide adequate services. Whilst some development has taken place of services for identification and diversion into the mental health system of mentally disordered offenders appearing in magistrates' courts, psychiatric services in prisons remain very variable in intensity and quality.

Possible solutions

A review of funding formulae should take place, to consider whether London's extreme needs for secure services are adequately taken into account, particularly in inner city areas. Sources of funding for community residential care for those discharged from secure hospital care should also be re-examined.

Attention is needed to training of staff in a range of community agencies in assessment of risk and management of mentally disordered offenders, and to finding ways of making working conditions and environments in London seem more attractive to staff. Research should be commissioned into the extent and adequacy of current psychiatric provision in London prisons.

13.11 Provision for carers

Provision of family interventions and of services supporting carers is very patchy, with some areas of London reporting that no such interventions can be provided locally. This is despite the proven clinical effectiveness of family interventions in psychosis and the fact that care in the community risks imposing a substantial burden on informal carers if they are not adequately supported.

Possible solutions

Services need to actively seek to give families the opportunity to be directly involved in the care of their mentally ill relatives, and, with patients' consent, fully aware of it. Specific services supporting carers, including carers' groups and respite care, should be available throughout the city, as should the family interventions which have proven efficacy for people with psychotic illnesses and their relatives.

13.12 Advocacy services

Advocacy services are becoming available in most areas, but the funding is often still precarious, and little information is available about the precise activities and outcomes.

Possible solutions

Research should be commissioned into the nature and effectiveness of advocacy services currently provided, and whether users find them helpful. Where there is evidence that advocacy services are found helpful by users and carers, their funding should be placed on a more secure long-term footing.

13.13 Services for older people

Inner London has high rates relative to other cities of admission for people between 65 and 75, but low rates for people over 75. The models of care used in community services for the elderly are highly variable across the city – in a few areas, innovative multidisciplinary models of home care have been developed, but in other areas the extensive support often required to maintain the elderly mentally ill at home does not seem to be fully available. With regard to residential care, there are again some impressive innovative models, but levels of provision in London are generally low, with less increase in private sector provision having taken place in London than elsewhere in the country in the last decade. This appears to be resulting in placement of substantial numbers of the elderly mentally ill in nursing homes outside London, which may result in isolation from existing social networks.

Possible solutions

Home care services for the elderly could be improved by development of the role of 'trained' carers (employed by the health service) to assist in the practical, day to day support of the elderly mentally ill at home, by the expansion of the use of intensive home care management, and by further development of multidisciplinary community teams. Where residential placements are needed, these should be available close to people's current homes.

13.14 Child and adolescent services

In London, rates of children being in local authority care ('looked after') or on child protection registers, are high compared with national figures. This is likely to be associated with considerable demands for child and adolescent services. Increased numbers of young people among the homeless, rising numbers of refugee children, and increasing rates of crime, substance misuse and suicide among children and adolescents are all likely to put pressure on London's services. Shortages of permanent social work staff, withdrawal of social workers in some services, and the demise of a single central educational authority for London appear to have increased demands for provision by the health services. Despite policy guidance advocating joint service planning, inter-agency working between child psychiatric services, paediatrics, social services and educational authorities remains fragmented and poorly co-ordinated, probably more so in London than elsewhere in the country.

Possible solutions

A categorisation of children with mental health problems should be agreed across health, education, social services and youth justice, so that databases can be developed providing standardised information about these children and adolescents. Overlaps and fragmentation of care for children with mental health problems need to be investigated in order to improve joint planning and commissioning between health, social services and education authorities. Staffing levels and spending on child and adolescent services are low in an international context, and their adequacy should be reviewed. Perverse incentives for in-patient treatment should be removed by adequate resourcing of mental health services in the community and cost-shunting between agencies. The effects of a primary care led NHS on strategic planning for child mental health services should be examined. Training of primary care staff in detection and treatment of child mental health problems should be reviewed, and in particular health visitors should be trained in behaviour modification and parent management techniques. All primary care staff including general practitioners should be trained in child protection in joint multi-professional training involving social services, education and local specialist child mental health problems.

13.15 Substance misuse

A high proportion of the nation's drug users are concentrated in London. Substance misuse services have expanded considerably over the last two decades, but recently have not kept pace with the rise in rates of substance misuse disorders. This is reflected in substantial waiting times for services in many areas. There has been a shift from specialist in-patient care to community services, and expansion particularly in the voluntary sector, but co-ordination between agencies and between areas often remains poor. Drug misuse in prisons is a substantial problem which has not been well addressed, nor have the needs of the homeless for substance abuse treatment. People with dual diagnosis of substance misuse and psychosis are a group who are present in considerable numbers in London and overlap substantially with the homeless mentally ill and mentally disordered offenders. As yet, most services do not appear to have established strategies for managing this group, and, in particular, for providing them with integrated care for psychosis and substance misuse.

Possible solutions

Rapid access services with minimal waiting times need to become available, as recommended in recent policy guidance. Better mechanisms need to be developed both for local co-ordination between health service, social services, voluntary sector agencies, police and probation services, and for co-ordination of services on a pan-London basis. Service models need to be developed and evaluated to meet the needs of adolescents and young people involved in substance misuse, dual diagnosis patients, the homeless and prisoners with substance misuse problems.

13.16 Liaison psychiatric services

Liaison services remain under-developed in London, despite substantial evidence that such services are beneficial to patients in acute hospital settings, and few services currently anticipate much growth.

Possible solutions

Clear guidelines should be agreed for adequate levels of liaison psychiatry provision, and these should be implemented and supported by a specific budget in all general hospitals.

13.17 Services for HIV/AIDS-related mental health problems

HIV infection and related mental health problems are again highly concentrated in London, which has almost 70% of the cases reported so far in the UK. There has been considerable service development for HIV infection and AIDS, including some specific psychiatric services, but for the first time, funding levels have fallen in 1996/7. Services for HIV-associated dementia remain patchy.

Psychiatric populations are potentially a group at risk of HIV infection. Mental health specialists also have a potential role in developing strategies to help the small group of individuals who have considerable difficulties in reducing their risk behaviours.

Possible solutions

New cases of HIV infection continue to occur, and patients with symptomatic disease live longer, with increased risk of having psychiatric and social difficulties: reduction in resources available for mental health services for HIV thus seems inadvisable. Better assessment of service needs and co-ordination of provision are needed for individuals with HIV associated dementia. Among psychiatric populations, the prevalence of HIV infection needs to be monitored over the next few years, and education strategies implemented for both patients and staff.

13.18 Mental health services in primary care

London's primary care services have been found to be of generally poorer quality than those elsewhere in the country, although excellent innovative services have been established in a few practices. GPs appear often to lack fundamental skills and knowledge in management of mental health problems, distribution of mental health professionals in primary care is patchy, and use of case registers and practice protocols are not widespread.

Possible solutions

Training of primary care staff needs to become a high priority, with a focus on developing the detection and management skills of general practitioners and practice nurses. Availability of counsellors and psychologists in primary care is currently very patchy, and ways should be found of making this more equitable. Case registers and practice protocols are aspects of good practice which should be generally adopted.

Community mental health teams should consider ways of increasing integration with primary care services – this may include aligning boundaries to general practice populations, developing shared care registers, and establishing clinics by psychologists and psychiatrists in larger practices.

13.19 Management of services

The management structures of London's mental health services appear to be characterised by high levels of organisational and job instability, and problems in joint working with other agencies and also with medical colleagues. Obstacles continue to hinder the full implementation of community mental health teams. In many parts of London, there is also evidence of a lack of management capacity and capability to manage change in a highly complex service system.

Possible solutions

Managers need to be provided with adequate training, support and guidance in policy implementation, comprehensive service planning and the management of change. The impact on morale and staff effectiveness of repeated organisational restructurings need to be considered. Ways need to be found of improving inter-agency joint working and communication.

13.20 Staff

Recently, there has been growing evidence of a recruitment crisis for mental health professionals of all disciplines in London, and there is evidence that levels of staff 'burnout' are high. Pressure on services and the stresses associated with caseloads on which a high proportion of patients are severely disabled and disadvantaged may contribute to staff stress, as may anxieties aroused by the recent public and media concern about violent acts perpetrated by the severely mentally ill.

Possible solutions

A major review should be carried out of the causes of difficulty in recruiting and retaining staff, and of ways of improving working conditions and attracting adequate numbers of appropriately qualified staff to work in the capital. Procedures for maximising the safety of staff dealing with those severely ill patients who may become violent should be developed as soon as possible.

References

Abas, M. et al. (1996) Depression and anxiety among older people in the UK: screening unmet need and the provision of appropriate services. *International Journal of Geriatric Psychiatry*, **11**, 377–382.

Abas, M. and Silverman, M. (1996) Community care of the elderly, some problems viewed from one inner city area. *Psychiatric Bulletin*, **20**, 169–171.

Abrahams, C. and Mungall, R. (1992) *Runaways:Exploding the Myths*. London, NCH.

Abrams, F. and Ashton, K. (1995) Are Britain's school children more trouble than they used to be? *Independent*, 15th June, pp. 12–13.

Acharyya, S. et al. (1989) Nafsiyat: a psychotherapy centre for ethnic minorities. *Psychiatric Bulletin* **13**(7), 358–360.

Adam, S. (1991) What the government should do. *British Medical Journal*, **302**, 1120–1123.

Advisory Council on the Misuse of Drugs (1982) *Treatment and Rehabilitation*. Department of Health and Social Security, London.

Advisory Council on the Misuse of Drugs (1993) *AIDS and Drug Misuse Update*. London, HMSO.

Ahmad, W. (1993) Making black people sick: race ideology and health research. In W.I.U. Ahmad (ed.), *Race and Health in Contemporary Britain*. Buckingham, Open University Press.

Ahmad, W. (1996) Family obligations and social change amongst the Asian community. In W. Ahmad & K. Atkin (eds), *Race and Community Care*. Buckingham, Open University Press.

Ahmad, W. & Atkin, K. eds (1996) *Race and Community Care*. Buckingham, Open University Press.

Ahmed, R. (1995) Services for Asian communities. In C. Harding, *Not just black and white: an information pack about mental health services for people from Black communities*. London, Good Practices in Mental Health.

Akehurst, R., Hutton, J. & Dixon, R. (1991) *Review of higher costs of health care provision in inner London and a consideration of implications for competitiveness: final report*. York Health Economics Consortium, University of York.

Alberti, K. (1995) Local research ethics committees. *British Medical Journal*, **311**, 639–640.

Anderson, J., Dayson, D., Wils, W., Gooch, C., Margolius, O., O'Driscoll, C. & Leff, J. (1993) The TAPS Project 13, Clinical and social outcomes of long stay psychiatric patients after one year in the community. *British Journal of Psychiatry*, **162** (Supplement 19), 45–46.

Arie, T. (1970) The first year of the Goodmayes psychiatric service for old people. *Lancet*, **ii**, 1175–1182.

Armstrong, E. (1996) Local guidelines in primary care – health promotion by practice nurses. Conference on Prevention of mental illness and mental health promotion in primary care, 12–15 July, Kensington Town Hall, London, Department of Health.

Association of Directors of Social Services and the Royal College of Psychiatrists (1995) Joint statement on an integrated mental health service for children and adolescents. ADSS Secretariat of The Royal College of Psychiatrists, 17 Belgrave Square, London SW1X 8PG.

Atkin, K. & Rollings, J. (1993) *Community Care in Multi-Racial Britain. A critical review of the literature*. London, HMSO.

Atkin, K. (1996) An opportunity for change: voluntary sector provision in a mixed economy of care. In W. Ahmad & K. Atkin (eds), *Race and Community Care*. Buckingham, Open University Press.

Atri, J. et al. (1996) Fair shares in health care? Ethnic and socio-economic influences on recording of preventive care in selected inner London general practices. *British Medical Journal*, **312**, 614–617.

Audini, B., Marks, I.M., Lawrence, R.E. et al. (1994) Home based versus outpatient/inpatient care for people with serious mental illness. Phase II of a controlled study. *British Journal of Psychiatry*, **165**, 204–208.

Audit Commission (1994a) *Finding a Place. A review of mental health services for adults*. London, HMSO.

Audit Commission (1994b) *Seen but not Heard. Coordinating local health and social services for children in need*. London, HMSO.

Audit Commission. (1996a) *Fundholding Facts. A digest of information about practice with the scheme during the first five years*. London, HMSO.

Audit Commission. (1996b) *What the Doctor Ordered. A study of GP fundholders in England and Wales*. London, HMSO.

Bachrach, L.L. (1984) Young adult chronic patients, an analytic review of the literature. *Hospital and Community Psychiatry*, **33**, 189–197.

Bagley, C. (1971) The social aetiology of schizophrenia in immigrant groups. *International Journal of Social Psychiatry*, **17**, 292–304.

Bal (1984) *The Symptomatology of Mental Illness amongst Asians in the West Midlands*. BA Dissertation. Department of Economics and Social Sciences, Wolverhampton Polytechnic.

Balabil, S. & Dolan, B. (1992) A cross-cultural evaluation of expectations about psychological counselling. *British Journal of Medical Psychology*, **65**, 305–308.

Balarajan, R. (1996) Health trends ethnicity and variations in the nation's health. *Health Trends* **27**(4), 114–119.

Balarajan, R., Raleigh, V. & Yuen, P. (1991) Hospital care among ethnic minorities in Britain. *Health Trends* **23**(3), 237–239.

Balarajan, R. & Raleigh, V.S. (1992) The ethnic populations of England and Wales: the 1991 census. *Health Trends* **24**(4), 113–115.

Ball, C.J. (1993) The rise and fall of the day hospital: The future of day care in old age psychiatry. *Psychiatric Bulletin*, **17**, 427–428.

Banerjee, S., Lindesay, J. & Murphy, E. (1993) Psychogeriatricians and general practitioners, a national survey. *Psychiatric Bulletin*, **17**, 592–594.

Banerjee, S. et al. (1994) *Deaths of detained patients. A review of reports to the mental health act commission*. London, Mental Health Foundation.

Banerjee, S., O'Neill-Byrne, K., Exworthy, T. & Parrott, J. (1995) The Belmarsh Scheme. A prospective study of the transfer of mentally disordered remand prisoners from prison to psychiatric units. *British Journal of Psychiatry*, **166**, 802–805.

Bardsley, M. & Hamm, J. (1995) *The Health of Londoners Project. London's Health, Key Facts and Figures*. Health of Londoners Discussion Paper No. 1. Public Health Directorate, East London and City Health Authority.

Bebbington, A.C. & Kelly, A. (1993) *Area differences in labour costs of personal social services.* Discussion Paper 898, Personal Social Services Research Unit, University of Kent at Canterbury.

Bebbington, A.C. & Darton, R.A. (1995) *The supply of long-stay facilities for elderly people in London.* PSSRU Discussion Paper 1139/3, University of Kent.

Bebbington, P. et al. (1981) Psychiatric disorders in selected immigrant groups in Camberwell. *Social Psychiatry*, **16**, 43–51.

Bebbington, P.E., Feeny, S.T., Flannigan, C.B., Glover, G.R., Lewis, S.W. & Wing, J.K. (1994) Inner London Collaborative Audit of Admissions in two Health Districts. *2. Ethnicity and Use of the Mental Health Act. British Journal of Psychiatry*, **165**, 743–749.

Beecham, J., Cambridge, P., Hallam, A. & Knapp, M. (1993) The costs of domus care. *International Journal of Geriatric Psychiatry*, **10**, 827–832.

Beecham, J.K. (1995) Collecting and estimating costs. In M.R.J. Knapp (ed.), *The Economic Evaluation of Mental Health Care*. Aldershot, Ashgate.

Beecham, J.K., Hallam, A. and Knapp, M.R.J. (1997) Costing care in hospital and in the community. In J. Leff (ed.), *Community Care: Illusion or Reality?* Chichester, John Wiley & Son.

Bcliappa, J. (1991) *Illness or Distress. Alternative models of mental health.* London, Confederation of Indian Organisations.

Benjamin, M. (1985) *Juvenile Prostitution: a portrait of the life.* Toronto, Min. of Comm. & Soc. Serv.

Bennet, F.J. (1995) Qualitative and quantitative methods: in depth or rapid assessment? *Social Sciences and Medicine*, **40**(12), 1589–1590.

Bentley et al. (1988) Rapid ethnographic assessment: applications in diarrhoea management program. *Social Sciences and Medicine*, **27**(1), 107–116.

Benzeval, M., Judge, K. & Solomon, M. (1992) *The Health Status of Londoners: a comparative perspective.* Working Paper No.1, King's Fund London Acute Services Initiative, London.

Berrington, A. (1994) Marriage and family formation among white and ethnic minority populations in Britain. *Ethnic and Racial Studies*, **17**(3), 517–546.

Bhopal (1986) The inter-relationship of folk, traditional and western medicine within an Asian community in Britain. *Social Sciences and Medicine*, **22**(1), 99–105.

Bhopal, R. & White, M. (1993) Health promotion for ethnic minorities: past, present and future. In W.I.U. Ahmad (ed.), *Race and Health in Contemporary Britain*. Buckingham, Open University Press.

Bhugra, D. et al. (1992) Homelessness and Mental Illness. Working Party Report. London, Royal College of Psychiatrists.

Bhugra, D. (1993) Unemployment, poverty and homelessness. In D. Bhugra & J. Leff (eds), *Principles of Social Psychiatry*. Oxford, Blackwell.

Bhugra, D., Bridges, K. & Thompson, C. (1995) *Caring for a Community*. Royal College of Psychiatrists Council Report CR 36. London, Gaskell.

Bhugra, D. & Bhui, K. (1996) Cross-cultural assessments. *Advances in Psychiatric Treatment* (in press).

Bhugra, D. et al. (1996a) Attempted suicide in West London I: rates across ethnic groups. Manuscript submitted.

Bhugra, D. et al. (1996b) Attempted suicide in West London: a case control study of South Asian women. Manuscript submitted.

Bhugra, D. et al. (1996c) Setting up psychiatric services: cross-cultural issues. *International Journal of Social Psychiatry* (in press).

Bhugra, D., Bhamra, J. & Taylor, P. (1996d) A survey of drop-in services for the homeless. *International Journal of Social Psychiatry* (in press).

Bhui, K. (1994) Somatic symptoms in Asian patients. MSc thesis, UMDS, University of London.

Bhui, K. et al. (1993) Asian inpatients in a district psychiatric unit: an examination to presenting features and routes into care. *International Journal of Social Psychiatry*, **39**, 208–220.

Bhui, K., Christie, Y. & Bhugra, D. (1995a) The essential elements of culturally sensitive psychiatric services. *International Journal of Social Psychiatry*, **41**, 342–356.

Bhui, K. et al. (1995b) Developing culturally sensitive community psychiatric services. *British Journal of Health Care Management*, **1**(16), 817–822.

Bhui, K. et al. (1996) Ethnicity and remanded mentally disordered offenders. Preliminary findings. Paper in preparation for submission.

Bhui, K. (1996a) The language of compliance: health policy for the severely mentally ill. *International Journal of Social Psychiatry* (in press).

Bhui, K. (1996b) Checklist: addressing the needs of minority ethnic groups. In *Effectively managing mental health service development*. London, The Sainsbury Centre for Mental Health.

Bindman, J., Johnson, S., Wright, S., Szmukler, G., Bebbington, P., Kuipers, E. & Thornicroft, G. (1996) Integration between primary and secondary services in the care of the severely mentally ill: patients' and GPs' views. Accepted by *British Journal of Psychiatry*.

Bines, W. (1994) *The health of single homeless people.* University of York.

Black health workers and patients group (1983) Psychiatry and the corporate state. *Race & Class*, **25**, 49–64.

BMA (1995) Multicultural Health Care. Current practice and future policy in medical education. London, British Medical Association.

Boardman, A.P. (1987) The General Health Questionnaire and the detection of emotional disorder by general practitioners. *British Journal of Psychiatry*, **151**, 373–381.

Bond, T. (1991) HIV Counselling: Report on National Survey and Consultation 1990. British Association for Counselling and Department of Health Joint Project.

Bonnerjea, L. (1990) *Leaving care in London.* London Boroughs Children's Regional Planning Committee.

Boyle, S. & Smaje, C. (1992) *Acute health services in London: an analysis.* Working Paper No.2, King's Fund London Acute Services Initiative, London.

Bowden, P. (1978) Men remanded into custody for medical reports, the selection for treatment. *British Journal of Psychiatry*, **132**, 320–331.

Bowden, P. (1990) Mentally disordered offenders. In R. Bluglass & P. Bowden (eds), *Principles and Practice of Forensic Psychiatry*. Edinburgh, Churchill Livingstone.

Bradley, C., Marchall, M. & Gath, D. (1995) Why do so few patients appeal against detention under section 2 of the mental health act? *British Medical Journal*, **310**, 364–367.

Breakey, W., Fischer, P., Kramer, M. et al. (1989) Health and health problems of homeless men and women in Baltimore. *Journal of the American Medical Association,* **262**, 1352–1357.

Brewin, C. (1980) Explaining the lower rates of psychiatric treatment among Asian immigrants to the United Kingdom. *Journal of Social Psychiatry,* **15**, 17–19.

Brixton Circle Project (1992) *Annual report of the Brixton Circle Project.* London.

Brown, P., Challis, D. & von Abendorff, R. (1996) The work of a community mental health team for the elderly. Referrals, caseloads, contact history and outcomes. *International Journal of Geriatric Psychiatry*, **11**,29–39.

Building Cost Information Service (1996) *Surveys of Tender Prices.* Kingston-upon-Thames, The Royal Institution of Chartered Engineers.

Bulmer, M. (1996) The ethnic question in the 1991 Census of population. In D. Coleman & J. Salt (eds), *Ethnicity in the 1991 Census, Vol 1: Demographic characteristics of the ethnic minority populations.* OPCS. London, HMSO.

Burke, A. (1986) Racism, prejudice and mental illness. In J.L. Cox (ed.), *Transcultural Psychiatry.* London, Croom Helm.

Burke, A. (1984) Racism and psychiatric disturbance among West Indians in Britain. *International Journal of Social Psychiatry,* **30**, 50–68.

Burney, E. & Pearson, G. (1995) Mentally Disordered Offenders: finding a focus for diversion. *The Howard Journal,* **34**(4), 291–313.

Burti, L. & Tansella, M. (1995) Acute home-based and community psychiatry. In M. Phelan, G. Strathdee and G. Thornicroft (eds), *Emergency Mental Health Services in the Community.* Cambridge, Cambridge University Press.

Buszewicz, M. & Phelan, M. (1994) Schizophrenia and the environment. *British Journal of Hospital Medicine*, **52**, 149–154.

Callan, A. (1996) Schizophrenia in Afro-Caribbean immigrants. *Journal of the Royal Society of Medicine*, **89**, 253–256.

Camden Health and Race Group et al. (1992) *A changing health services in Camden and Islington to meet the needs of Black and other minority communities.* Report on a conference held on 8th October, Bloomsbury and Islington Health Authority & Commission for Racial Equality.

Cantwell, R. & Harrison, G. (1996) Substance misuse in the severely mentally ill. *Advances in Psychiatric Treatment*, **2**, 117–124.

Carr-Hill, R.A., Hardman, G., Martin, S., Peacock, S., Sheldon, T.A. & Smith, P. (1994) *A formula for distributing NHS revenues based on small area use of hospital beds.* University of York, Centre for Health Economics.

Carr-Hill, R.A. et al. (1996) Socio-economic determinants of rates of consultation in general practice. *British Medical Journal*, **312**, 1008–1013.

Castle, D., Scott, K., Wesseley, S. & Murray, R. (1993) Does social deprivation during gestation and early life predispose to later schizophrenia? *Social Psychiatry and Psychiatric Epidemiology,* **28**, 1–4.

Carter, D., Drake, M. Liltler, T. et al. (1989) *The faces of homelessness in London.* Guildford, University of Surrey.

Catalan, J., Riccio, M. & Thompson, C. (1989) HIV disease and psychiatric practice. *Psychiatric Bulletin*, **13**, 316–332.

Catalan, J. (1993) *HIV infection and mental health care: implications for services*. World Health Organisation, European Office, Copenhagen.

Catalan, J. Burgess, A. & Klimes, I. (1995a) *The Psychological Medicine of HIV Infection*. Oxford Medical Publications, Oxford, Oxford University Press.

Catalan, J., Meadows, J., Baldeweg, T. (1995b) *Epidemiology of HIV-associated dementia in London 1991–1994*. London, Department of Health.

CDR (1996a) AIDS and HIV-1 infection in the UK, monthly report. *Communicable Disease Report*, **6**, 25–28.

CDR (1996b) The incidence and prevalence of AIDS and other severe HIV disease in England and Wales for 1995 to 1999, projections using data to the end of 1994. *Communicable Disease Report*, **6**, R1–R24.

Chandra, J. (1996) Role and models of purchasing health for black and minority ethnic populations. In *Locating the goalposts. Health promotion and purchasing for black and minority ethnic health*. London, Health Education Authority.

Cherrett, M. (1996) *Diversion at the police station*. Report to the Metropolitan Police (unpublished).

Chinese Mental Health Association (1995) *Annual report for the year 1994/5*. London.

Chisholm, D., Knapp, M.R.J., Beecham, J.K., Astin, J., Audini, B. & Lelliott, P. (1997) The mental health residential care study: The costs of provision. *Journal of Mental Health* (in press).

Christie Y. (1995) Overview. In C. Harding (ed.), *Not just black and white: an information pack about mental health services for people from Black communities*. London, Good Practices in Mental Health

Clement, S. and Stockwell, T. (1988) *Community Alcohol Teams*. Report to the Department of Health.

Clinical Standards Advisory Group Committee on Schizophrenia (1995) *Schizophrenia, Volume 2, Protocol for Assessing Services for People with Severe Mental Illness* (2nd Version). London, HMSO.

Cochrane, R. & Stopes-Roe, M. (1981) Psychological symptom levels in Indian immigrants to England. A comparison with native English. *Psychological Medicine*, **11**, 319–327.

Cochrane, D., Conroy, M. & Lewis, R. (1994) *A Profile of London's Mental Health Services. A Report for the Mental Health Task Force London Project*. Conrane Consulting.

Cochrane, R. et al. (1977) Mental illness in immigrant groups to England and Wales: an analysis of mental hospital admissions, 1971. *Social Psychiatry*, **22**, 181–191.

Cochrane, R. et al. (1989) Mental hospital admission rates of immigrants to England: a comparison of the 1971 and 1981 data. *Social Psychiatry and Psychiatric Epidemiology*, **24**, 2–11.

Cochrane, R. et al. (1996) Ethnicity and patterns of alcohol consumption. In *Ethnicity: an agenda for mental health*. London, Gaskell (in press).

Cochrane, R. & Sashidharan, S.P. (1996) Mental health and ethnic minorities: a review of the literature and service implications. In *Ethnicity and Health: reviews of literature and guidance for purchasers in the areas of cardiovascular disease, mental health and haemoglobinopathies*. CRD Report 5. NHS Centre for reviews and dissemination social policy research unit. University of York.

Cohen, C. and Crane, M. (1996) Old and homeless in London and New York City: a cross-national comparison. In D. Bhugra (ed.), *Homelessness and Mental Health*. Cambridge, Cambridge University Press.

Coid, J. (1988) Mentally abnormal prisoners on remand. I. rejected or accepted by the NHS? *British Medical Journal*, **296**, 1779–1784.

Cole, E. et al. (1995) Pathways to care for patients with a first episode of psychosis. A comparison of ethnic groups. *British Journal of Psychiatry*, **167**, 770–776.

Cole, T. (1986) *Residential Special Education*. Milton Keynes, Open University Press.

Collighan, G., Macdonald, A., Herzberg, J., Philpot, M. & Lindesay, J. (1993) An evaluation of the multidisciplinary approach to psychiatric diagnosis in elderly people. *British Medical Journal*, **306**, 821–824.

Confidential Inquiry into Homicides and Suicides by mentally ill people (1994) *A preliminary report on homicide*. London, Royal College of Psychiatrists.

Confidential Inquiry into Homicides and Suicides by mentally ill people (1996) *Report of the Confidential Inquiry*. London, Royal College of Psychiatrists.

Conway, A., Hale, A. & Melzer, D. (1994) The outcome of targeting community mental health services, evidence from the West Lambeth schizophrenia cohort. *British Medical Journal*, **308**, 627–630.

Cooke, D.J. (1992) Reconviction following referral to a forensic clinic: the criminal justice outcome of diversion. *Medicine, Science and Law*, **32**, 325–330.

Cooper, B. (1991) Principles of service provision in old age psychiatry. In R. Jacoby & C. Oppenheimer (eds), *Psychiatry in the Elderly*. Oxford, Oxford University Press.

Corney, R. (1996) Links between mental health professionals and general practices in England and Wales: the impact of fundholding. *British Journal of General Practice*, **46**, 221–224.

Court, S.D.M. (1976) *Fit for the Future: The Report of the Committee on Child Health Services* ('The Court Report'). London, HMSO.

Craig, T. (1995) *The Homeless Mentally Ill Initiative: An evaluation of four clinical teams*. London, Department of Health.

Craig, T. & Timms, P. (1992) Out of the wards and onto the streets? *Journal of Mental Health*, **1**, 265–275.

Craig, T., Bayliss, E., Klein, O., Manning, P. & Reader, L. (1995) *The homeless mentally ill*. London, Department of Health.

Crane, M. (1993) *Elderly homeless people sleeping on the streets in inner London*. London, Age Concern.

Crane, M. (1994) The mental health problems of elderly people living on London's streets. *International Journal of Geriatric Psychiatry*, **9**, 87–95.

CRASH (1995) *Winter shelters provided in London*. London, CRASH.

Crawford, A., Plant, M.A., Kreitman, N. & Latcham, R.W. (1987) Unemployment and drinking behaviour: Some data from a general population survey of alcohol use. *British Journal of Addiction*, **82**, 1007–1016.

Crilly, T. & Robbins, J. (1996) *Community Mental Health Teams*. London, Centre for Mental Health Services Development.

Crisis (1995) Central London Street Monitor. May 25. *Homeless Network*, London.

Cunningham, D. (1983) *Overview of psychiatric services in London health districts*. Paper presented for King's Fund Conference, Issues for London DHAs: the development of psychiatric services.

CVS Consultants and Prince Evans Solicitors (1995) *Caring for Citizens – A review of the fixed points and realistic choices in the financial rules surrounding the implementation of community mental health services*. A report for the Centre for Mental Health Services Development and the Audit Commission. Available from CMHSD.

Dauncey, K., Giggs, J., Baker, K. & Harrison, G. (1993) Schizophrenia in Nottingham: lifelong residential mobility of a cohort. *British Journal of Psychiatry*, **163**, 613–619.

Davidge, M., Elias, S., Jayes, B., Wood, K. & Yates, J. (1993) *Survey of English Mental Illness Hostels, Prepared for the Mental Health Task Force*. Health Services Management Centre, University of Birmingham.

Davies, S., Thornicroft, G., Leese, M., Higginbotham, A. & Phelan, M. (1996) Ethnic differences in risk of compulsory admission among representative cases of psychosis in London. *British Medical Journal*, **312**, 533–537.

Dayson, D. (1993) The TAPS Project 12, Crime, vagrancy, death and readmission of the long-term mentally ill during their first year of local reprovision. *British Journal of Psychiatry*, **162** (Supplement 19), 40–44.

Dean, C., Phillips, J., Gadd, E., Joseph, M. & England, S. (1993) Comparison of community-based service with hospital-based service for people with acute severe psychiatric illness. *British Medical Journal*, **307**, 473–476.

Dean, G. et al. (1981) First admissions of native born and immigrants to psychiatric hospitals in South East England, 1976. *British Journal of Psychiatry*, **139**, 596–12.

Dell, S., Robertson, G., James, K., Grounds, A. (1993) Remands and Psychiatric Assessments in Holloway Prison I, The Psychotic population. *British Journal of Psychiatry*, **163**, 634–640.

Dening, T. (1993) Community psychiatry of old age, a UK perspective. *International Journal of Geriatric Psychiatry*, **7**, 757–766.

Department for Education (1993) *A new deal for out of school pupils*. Press Release 126/93.

Department of Education (1994) *Pupils with Problems*. London, HMSO.

Department of the Environment (1996a) *The Next Challenge*. London, Department of the Environment.

Department of the Environment (1996b) *Standard Spending Assessments 1996/97: Guide to methodology*.

Department of Health (1989a) *Caring for People. Community care in the next decade and beyond*. London, HMSO.

Department of Health (1989b) *Working for Patients. The National Health Service Review*. London, HMSO.

Department of Health (1990) *The Care Programme Approach for People with a Mental Illness referred to Specialist Psychiatric Services. Joint Health/Social Services Circular HC(90)23/LASSL(90)11*. London, HMSO.

Department of Health (1991) *Children in Care of Local Authorities, year ending 31st March 1988*. Government Statistical Office, England.

Department of Health (1992a) *The Health of the Nation. A strategy for health in England*. London, HMSO.

Department of Health (1992b) *Report of the Inquiry into London's Health Service, Medical Education and Research* ('The Tomlinson Report'). London, HMSO.

Department of Health (1993a) *Caring for People. Information Pack for the Voluntary and Private Sectors.* London, HMSO.

Department of Health (1993b) *On the State of the Public Health 1992.* London, HMSO.

Department of Health (1993c) *Making London Better.* Department of Health Health Publication Unit, Lancashire.

Department of Health (1993d) *Public Health Common Data Set, 1992.* Surrey Institute of Public Health, University of Surrey.

Department of Health (1994a) *Priorities for Action. A Report by the Mental Health Task Force. London Project.* London, HMSO.

Department of Health (1994b) *Assessment of Needs for Mentally Disordered Offenders in response to NHS(M)E EL(93)68.* Unpublished.

Department of Health (1994c) *The Health of the Nation. Key Area Handbook Mental Illness* 2nd Edition. London, HMSO.

Department of Health (1994d) *Local systems of support: A framework for purchasing for people with severe mental health problems. A report by the Mental Health Taskforce and the NHS Executive.* London, HMSO.

Department of Health (1995a) *Building Bridges: A guide to arrangements for inter-agency working for the care and protection of severely mentally ill people.* London, HMSO.

Department of Health (1995b) *Mental Health Task Force London Project. Follow-up report.* London, NHS Executive.

Department of Health (1995c) *NHS responsibilities for meeting continuing health care needs, HSG(95)8.* London, HMSO.

Department of Health (1995d) *Children Looked after by Local Authorities, 14th October 1991 to 31st March 1993.* Government Statistical Office, England.

Department of Health (1995e) *Annual Reports of Area Child Protection Committees 1993/94.* Department of Health ACPCs Series 1995. Report No. 1.

Department of Health (1995f) *Children Accommodated in Secure Units, Year ending 31 March 1995.* Government Statistical Office, England.

Department of Health (1995g) *Child Protection, Messages from Research.* London, HMSO.

Department of Health (1995h) *NHS Day Care Facilities in England.* London, HMSO.

Department of Health (1996a) *The Spectrum of Care: Local Services for People with Mental Health Problems.* Leeds, NHS Executive.

Department of Health (1996b) *Mental Health in England.* London, Government Statistical Service.

Department of Health (1996c) *24 hour nursed care for people with severe and enduring mental illness.* Leeds, NHS Executive.

Department of Health and Home Office (1991) *Review of Health and Social Services for Mentally Disordered Offenders and Others Requiring Similar Services* ('The Reed Report'). The Reports of the Service Advisory Groups, an Overview. London, Department of Health.

Department of Health and Home Office (1992) *Review of Services for Mentally Disordered Offenders. Report of the Staffing and Training Advisory Group.*

Department of Health and Home Office (1994) *Report of the Department of Health and Home Office Working Group on Psychopathic Disorder.*

Department of Health and Office of Population Censuses and Surveys (1992) *The Government's Expenditure Plans 1993–94 to 1995–96.* London, HMSO.

Department of Health and Social Security (1970) *Psychogeriatric assessment unit, HM(70)11.* London, HMSO.

Department of Health and Social Security (1971) *Hospital Services for the Mentally Ill, HM(71)97.* London, HMSO.

Department of Health and Social Security (1972) *Services for mental disorder related to old age, HM(72)71.* London, HMSO.

Department of Health and Social Security (1974) *Report on Security in NHS Hospitals* ('The Glancy Report'). London, HMSO.

Department of Health and Social Security (1975) *Better Services for the Mentally Ill.* London, HMSO.

Department of Health and Social Security (1980) *Organisational and Management Problems of Mental Illness Hospitals. Report on a Working Group.* London, HMSO.

Department of Health and Social Security (1985) *Government Response to the Second Report from the Social Services Committee, 1984–85 Session.* London, HMSO.

Department of Health and Social Security and Welsh Office (1975) *The Census of Residential Accommodation, 1970. II. Accommodation for the Mentally Ill and for the Mentally Handicapped.* London, DHSS.

Department of Health and Welsh Office (1983) *Mental Health Act 1983 Code of Practice. Published pursuant to Section 118 of the Act.* London, HMSO.

Donaldson, L.J. & Hill, P.M. (1991) The domiciliary consultation service: Time to take stock. *British Medical Journal*, **302**, 449–451.

Donnan, S. (1996) Epidemiology and health services research in 1996. *Journal of Epidemiology and Community Health*, **30**, 113.

Drake, R.E., Becker, D.R., Biesanz, J.C., Torrey, W.C., McHugo, G.J. & Wyzik, P.F. (1994) Rehabilitative Day Treatment vs. Supported Employment, 1.Vocational Outcomes. *Community Mental Health Journal*, **30**, 519–531.

Doyle, Y. et al. (1994) Coping with disabilities: the perspective of young adults from different ethnic backgrounds in Inner London. *Social Sciences and Medicine*, **38**(11), 1491–1498.

Doyle, Y. (1995) Disability use of independent living fund in SE London and users' views about the system of cash for care. *Journal of Epidemiology and Community Health*, **49**(1), 43–47.

Eaton,W.W. (1974) Residence, social class and schizophrenia. *Journal of Health and Social Behaviour*, **15**, 289–299.

Eaton,W.W. (1985) Epidemiology of schizophrenia. *Epidemiological Reviews*, **7**, 105–126.

El-Kabir, D. & Ramsden, S. (1996) Primary health care of the single homeless. In D. Bhugra (ed.), *Homelessness and Mental Health*. Cambridge, Cambridge University Press.

Ernst, E. (1995) Complementary medicine: common misconceptions. *Journal of the Royal Society of Medicine*, **88**, 244–247.

Exworthy, T. & Parrott, J. (1994) Evaluation of a diversion from custody scheme at magistrates' courts. *Journal of Forensic Psychiatry*, **4**(3), 497–505.

Fahy, T.A. (1989) The police as a referral agency for psychiatric emergencies – a review. *Medicine, Science and the Law*, **29**, 315–322.

Faris, R. & Dunham, H. (1939) *Mental Disorders in Urban Areas*. Chicago, University of Chicago Press.

Fasey, C. (1994) The day hospital in old age psychiatry: the case against. *International Journal of Geriatric Psychiatry*, **9**, 519–523.

Faulkner, A., Field, V. & Lindesay, J. (1992) Who is Providing What? Information about UK Residential Care Provision for People with Mental Health Problems. Research and Development for Psychiatry; 134–138 Borough High Street, London SE1 1LB.

Fernando, S. (1988) *Race, Culture & Psychiatry*. London, Routledge.

Fernando, S. (1992) Roots of racism in psychiatry. *Open Mind*, **59**, 10–11.

Fernando, S. (1995) Culture, race and mental health: an historical approach. In C. Harding (ed.), *Not just black and white: an information pack about mental health services for people from Black communities*. London, Good Practices in Mental Health.

Fernando, S. (1996) *Mental Health in Multi-ethnic Society*. London, Routledge.

Fisher, N., Turner, S., Pugh, R. & Taylor, C. (1994) Estimating numbers of homeless people and the homeless mentally ill. *British Medical Journal*, **308**, 207–230.

Flannigan, C.B., Glover, G.R., Feeney, F.T., Wing, J.K., Bebbington, P.E. & Lewis, F.W. (1994a) Inner London Collaborative Audit of Met Admissions in two Health Districts. 1. Introduction, Methods and Preliminary Findings. *British Journal of Psychiatry*, **165**, 734–742.

Flannigan, C.B., Glover, G.R., Wing, J.K., Lewis, F.W., Bebbington, P.E. & Feeney, F.T. (1994b) Inner London Collaborative Audit of Admissions in two Health Districts. 3. Reasons for Admission. *British Journal of Psychiatry*, **165**, 750–759.

Fontana, A. & Frey, J. (1994) Interviewing: the art of science. In N. Denzin & Y. Lincoln (eds), *Handbook of Qualitative Research*, London, Sage.

Ford, R. & Sathyamoorthy, G. (1996) Team Games. *Health Service Journal*, 27 June, 32–33.

Fox, R. (1996) What do patients want from medical research? *Journal of the Royal Society of Medicine*, **89**(6), 301–302.

Francis, J. (1994) No more excuses. *Community Care*, 16–22 June, 21–23.

Frankel, S. et al. (1991) Lay epidemiology and the rationality of responses to health education. *British Journal of General Practice*, **41**, 428–430.

Frese, M. & Mohr, G. (1987) Prolonged unemployment and depression in older workers: a longitudinal study of intervening variables. *Social Science and Medicine*, **25**, 173–178.

Fullard, E., Fowler, G. & Gray, M. (1987) Promoting prevention in primary care: controlled trial of low technology, low cost approach. *British Medical Journal*, **294**, 1080–1082.

Furnham, A. & Li, Y. (1993) The psychological adjustment of the Chinese community in Britain: a study of two generations. *British Journal of Psychiatry*, **162**, 9–13.

Furnham, A. & Shiekh, S. (1993) Gender, generational and social support correlates of mental health in Asian immigrants. *International Journal of Social Psychiatry*, **39**, 22–33.

Gammell, H., Ndahiro, A., Nicholas, M. & Windsor, J. (1993) *Refugees (Political asylum seekers) Service Provision and Access to the NHS. A study by the College of Health for Newham Health Authority and Newham Healthcare.*

Gath, C. & Higginson, I. (1995) *Report of the Mental Health Census. A point prevalence study. Joint project to identify people with severe and enduring mental health problems in Kensington and Chelsea and Westminster.* Department of Public Health, Kensington and Chelsea and Westminster Health Commissioning Agency.

General Medical Council (1993) *HIV infection and AIDS, the Ethical Considerations.* London, GMC.

Gillam, S., Jarman, B., White, P. & Law, R. (1989) Ethnic differences in consultation rates in urban general practice. *British Medical Journal*, **289**, 953–957.

Glover, G.R. (1989) The pattern of psychiatric admissions of Caribbean-born immigrants in London. *Social Psychiatry & Psychiatric Epidemiology*, **24**, 49–56.

Glover, G.R. (1996) Mental Illness Needs Index (MINI). In G. Thornicroft & G. Strathdee (eds), *Commissioning Mental Health Services.* London, HMSO.

Glover, G.R., Robin, E., Emami, J. & Arabscheibani, G.R. (1996) *A needs index for mental health.* (Submitted).

Goldberg, D. (1996) Cultural aspects of mental disorder in primary care. In *Ethnicity: An Agenda for Mental Health.* London, Gaskell (in press).

Goldberg, D. & Huxley, P. (1980) *Mental illness in the community.* London, Tavistock.

Goldberg, D. & Huxley, P. (1992) *Common Mental Disorders.* London, Routledge.

Goldberg, D., Mann, A., Pilgrim, D. et al. (1996a) *Developing a strategy for a primary care focus for mental health services.* Institute of Psychiatry and the Department of General Practice, UMDS, London.

Goldberg, D., Sharpe, D., Nanayakkara, K. (Goldberg et al., 1996b) The field trial of the mental disorders section of ICD10 designed for primary care. *Family Practice*, **12**, 466–473.

Good, B.J. & Good, M.D. (1981) The meaning of symptoms: a cultural hermeneutic model for clinical practice. In L. Eisenberg & A. Kleinman (eds), *The Relevance of Social Science for Medicine.* Dordrecht, D. Reidal.

Gorst-Unsworth, C. (1992) Adaptation after torture: some thoughts on the long term effects of surviving a repressive regime. *Medicine and War*, **8**, 164–168.

Graham, P. (1996) The thirty year contribution of research in child mental health to public policy and clinical practice in the UK. In J. Brannen & B. Bernstein (in press).

Grant, C. & Deane, J. (1995) *Brixton Refugee Health Project, Factors which influence uptake and provision of primary health services for refugees.* London, Brixton Challenge.

Gray, P. (1996) Voluntary organisations. In *Ethnicity: An Agenda for Mental Health.* London, Gaskell (in press).

Green, A.E. (1994) *The geography of poverty and wealth.* The Institute of Employment Research. University of Warwick.

Greenwood, A. (1993) Ethnic minorities mental health: the case for a specialist unit. *Ethnic Minorities Current Awareness Bulletin*, **4**(2): i–iii.

Greve, J., Page, D. & Greve, S. (1971) *Homelessness in London*. Edinburgh, Scottish Academic Press.

Guite, H., Beveney, P. & Field, V. (1995) *The 1994 mental health bed crisis*. Report to Lambeth, Southwark and Lewisham Health Commission and the Department of Health Mental Health Task Force.

Guite, H., Curtis, S., Banerjee, S. & Parrott, J. Diversion from courts and prisons to psychiatric in-patient care in an inner city district (unpublished).

Gunaratnam, Y. (1994) *Health & Race. A starting point for managers on improving services for black populations*. London, King's Fund.

Gunn, J., Maden, T. & Swinton, M. (1990) *Mentally disordered prisoners. A report commissioned and published by the Home Office*. (Revised 1991).

Gunn, J., Maden, A. & Swinton, M. (1991) Treatment needs of prisoners with psychiatric disorders. *British Medical Journal*, **303**, 338–340.

Gunn, J. & Taylor, P. (1993) *Clinical, Legal and Ethical Issues*. Oxford: Butterworth Heinemann.

Gupta, S. (1991) Psychosis in migrants from the Indian sub-continent. A preliminary study on the use of psychiatric services. *British Journal of Psychiatry*, **159**, 222–225.

Gupta, K., Coupland, L. & Fottrell, E. (1996) A two-year review of an 'open access' multidisciplinary community psychiatric service for the elderly. *International Journal of Geriatric Psychiatry*, **11**, 795–800.

Hadley, T. et al. (1996) Mental health policy and its problems in the UK: déjà vu. *Current Opinion in Psychiatry*, **9**, 105–108.

Hall, D. & Hill, P. (1994) Community child health services. In A. Stevens & J. Raftery (eds), *Health Care Needs Assessment*. Oxford, Radcliffe Medical Press.

Hallam, A. (1996) Costs and outcomes for people with special psychiatric needs. *Mental Health Research Review*, **3**, 10–13.

Handysides, S. (1993) Helping people with dementia feel at home. *British Medical Journal*, **306**, 1115–1117.

Harrison, G., Owens, D., Holton, A., Neilson, D. & Boot, D. (1988) A prospective study of severe mental disorder in Afro-Caribbean patients. *Psychological Medicine*, **18**, 643–657.

Harrison, J., Barrow, S. & Creed, F. (1995) Social deprivation and psychiatric admission rates among different diagnostic groups. *British Journal of Psychiatry*, **167**, 456–462.

Harvey, C., Pantelis, C., Taylor, J., McCabe, P., Lefevre, K., Campbell, P. & Hirsch, S. (1996) The Camden Schizophrenia Surveys, II. High Prevalence of Schizophrenia in an Inner London Borough and its relationship to socio-demographic factors. *British Journal of Psychiatry*, **168**, 418–426.

Harvey, C. (1996) The Camden Schizophrenia Surveys, I. The psychiatric, behavioural and social characteristics of the severely mentally ill in Inner London. *British Journal of Psychiatry*, **168**, 410–417.

Health Action for Homeless People (1994) *North Thames and South Thames RHA Homeless Figures*. London, Health Action for Homeless People.

Health Advisory Service (1982) *The rising tide: developing services for mental illness in old age*. London, Health Advisory Service.

Health Advisory Service (1986) *Bridges over Troubled Waters. A Report from the NHS Health Advisory Service on Services for Disturbed Adolescents*. London, HMSO.

Health Advisory Service (1994) *Comprehensive Mental Health Services*. Sutton, NHS Health Advisory Service.

Health Advisory Service (1995) *Together We Stand: the Commissioning, Role and Management of Child and Adolescent Mental Health Services*. London, HMSO.

Health Education Authority (1994) *Health and Lifestyles: Black and Minority Ethnic Groups in England*. London, HEA.

Health Education Authority (1996) *Locating The Goalposts. Health Promotion And Purchasing For Black And Minority Ethnic Health*. London, HEA.

Helman, C. (1990) *Culture, Health And Illness*. Oxford, Butterworth Heinemann.

Hendessi, M. (1994) *From here to equality. CHCS, race and ethnicity*. London, Greater London Association of Community Health Councils.

Herridge, C. (1989) Treatment of psychotic patients in prison. *Psychiatric Bulletin*, **13**, 200–201.

Herzberg, J. (1987) No fixed abode. *British Journal of Psychiatry*, **150**, 621–627.

Higginson, I., Mallandain, I., Butters, E. & Wilkins, S. (1995) *What services are needed to care for people with HIV/AIDS encephalopathy in North Thames? Estimates of need and the views of clients, carers and professionals*. Health Services Research Unit, London School of Hygiene and Tropical Medicine, London.

Hill, P. (1996) Child and adolescent psychiatry, a new century. In J. Harris-Hendriks & M. Black (eds), *Child and Adolescent Psychiatry: a new century*. Royal College of Psychiatrists Occasional Paper 33.

Hinton, T. (1992) *Health and homelessness in Hackney*. London, The Medical Campaign Project.

Hinton, T. (1994) *Battling through the barriers*. London, Health Action for Homeless people and CELFHSA.

Hirsch, S. (1988) *Psychiatric beds and resources: Factors influencing bed use and service planning*. London, Gaskell (Royal College of Psychiatrists).

HM Prison Service (1996) *Prison Health: Report from the Director of Health Care*.

Hoge, M.A., Davidson, L., Hill, W.L., Turner, V.E. & Ameli, R. (1992) The promise of partial hospitalization, a reassessment. *Hospital and Community Psychiatry*, **43**, 345–354.

Hollander, D., Powell, R.B. & Tobiansky, R.I. (1996) Bed occupancy in psychiatric units in Greater London is 113%. (Letter). *British Medical Journal*, **313**,166.

Holloway, F. et al. (1991) Day care in an inner city: I. Characteristics of attenders. *British Journal of Psychiatry*, **158**, 805–810.

Home Office (1990) *Provision for mentally disordered offenders*. London (Circular 66/90).

Home Office and Department of Health and Social Security (1974) *Interim Report of the Committee on Abnormal Offenders* ('The Butler Report'). London, HMSO.

Home Office, Department of Health, Department of Education and Science and Welsh Office (1991) *Working Together under the Children Act, 1989, A guide to arrangements for inter-agency co-operation for the protection of children from abuse*. London, HMSO.

Home Office Statistical Bulletin (1995a) *Statistics of Drug Addicts and the Development of Drug Services in England*. University of London, Birkbeck College.

Home Office Statistical Bulletin (1995b) Asylum Statistics. Issue 15/95. Home Office Research and Statistics Department, 50 Queen Ann's Gate, London SW1 9AT.

Hotopf, M. et al. (1995) Are ethical committees reliable? *Journal of the Royal Society of Medicine*, **88**, 31–33.

Hoult, J. & Reynolds, I. (1984) Schizophrenia: a comparative trial of community orientated and hospital orientated psychiatric care. *Acta Psychiatrica Scandinavica*, **69**, 359–372.

House, A. & Hodgson, G. (1994) Estimating needs and meeting demands. In S. Benjamin, A. House & P. Jenkins (eds), *Liaison Psychiatry: Defining Needs and Planing Services*. London, Gaskell.

House of Commons (1959) *The Mental Health Act 1959*. London, HMSO.

House of Commons (1970) *Local Authority Social Services Bill*. London, HMSO.

House of Commons (1990) *National Health Service and Community Care Act*. London, HMSO.

House of Commons Health Select Committee (1993) *Community Care, Funding From April 1993*. London, HMSO.

House of Commons Health Select Committee (1994a) *Better off in the Community? The care of people who are seriously mentally ill*. London, HMSO.

House of Commons Health Select Committee (1994b) *Memorandum from the Department of Health on Public Expenditure on Health and Personal Social Services*. London, HMSO.

House of Commons Health Select Committee (1996) *Allocation of resources to health authorities*. London, HMSO.

Howard, R. (1994) Day hospitals: The case in favour. *International Journal of Geriatric Psychiatry*, **9**, 525–529.

Huby, G. et al. (1989) General medical practice in a multi-cultural and multi-racial environment: report from a multi-disciplinary casework seminar. *Health Trends*, **21**, 36–89.

Huka, G. (1995) Needs assessment and civil liberties. In *Mental Health in Black and Minority Ethnic people. Time for action*. London, The Mental Health Foundation.

Hudson, D., James, D. & Harlow, P. (1995) *Psychiatric Court Liaison to Central London. A report on the service at Horseferry Road magistrates' court March 1994–March 1995*. Riverside Forensic Services.

Hughes, T., Garralda, M.E. & Tylee, A. (1994) *Child Mental Health Problems. A Booklet on Child Psychiatry Problems for General Practitioners*. London, St Mary's.

Huka, G. (1995) Services for African and Caribbean Communitites. In C. Harding (ed.), *Not just black and white: an information pack about mental health services for people from Black communities*. London, Good Practices in Mental Health.

Ineichen, B. (1990) The mental health of Asians in Britain. *British Medical Journal*, **300**, 1669–1670.

Inhorn, M. (1995) Medical Anthropology and Epidemiology: divergence and convergence. *Social Science and Medicine*, **40**(3), 285–290.

Ismail, K. (1996) Planning services for black women. In K. Abel, M. Buszewicz, S. Davison, S. Johnson, and E. Staples (eds), *Planning Community Mental Health Services for Women*. London, Routledge.

Jacob, K. Bhugra, D. & Mann, A.H. et al. (1996) *The use of the general practitioner by Indian females with psychiatric morbidity: recognition of the disorder and the role of social and cultural factors in help seeking. Brief report of preliminary findings.* Submitted for publication (Section of Epidemiology and General Practice, Department of Psychiatry, Institute of Psychiatry, London).

Jacobs, A. (1995) Services for refugee communities. In C. Harding (ed.), *Not just black and white: an information pack about mental health services for people from Black communities.* London, Good Practices in Mental Health.

Jahoda, M. (1979) The impact of unemployment in the 1930s and the 1970s. *Bulletin of the British Psychological Society,* **32,** 309–314.

James, D.V. & Hamilton, L.W. (1991) The Clerkenwell scheme, assessing efficacy and cost of a psychiatric liaison service to a magistrate's court. *British Medical Journal,* **303,**282–285.

Jamdagni, L. (1996) *Purchasing for Black populations.* London, King's Fund.

Janes, C., Stall, R. & Gifford, S. (1986) *Anthropology and Epidemiology.* Dordrecht, D Reidal.

Jarman, B. (1983) Identification of underprivileged areas. *British Medical Journal,* **286,** 1705–1709.

Jarman, B. (1984) Underprivileged areas, validation and distribution of scores. *British Medical Journal,* **289,** 1587–1592.

Jarman, B. (1988) Identification of under-privileged areas, *British Medical Journal,* **296,** 1705–1709.

Jarman, B. and Hirsch, S. (1992) Statistical models to predict district psychiatric morbidity. In G. Thornicroft, C. Brewin & J.K. Wing (eds), *Measuring Mental Health Needs.* Royal College of Psychiatrists, Gaskell Press.

Jarman, B., Hirsch, S, White, P. & Driscoll, R. (1992) Predicting psychiatric admission rates. *British Medical Journal,* **304,**1146–1151.

Jennings, S. (1996) The process of partnership. In *Creating Solutions. Developing alternatives in Black mental health.* London, King's Fund.

Jezzard, R. (1996) A perspective on the future of child and adolescent mental health services. In *Child and Adolescent Psychiatry, a New Century.* London, Department of Health.

Johnson, S. & Thornicroft, G. (1993) The Sectorisation of Psychiatry in England & Wales. *Social Psychiatry & Psychiatric Epidemiology,* **28,** 45–47.

Johnson, S. & Thornicroft, G. (1995) Emergency psychiatric services in England and Wales. *British Medical Journal,* **311,** 287–288.

Johnson, S., Thornicroft, G., Phelan, M. & Slade, M. (1996) Assessing needs for mental health services. In G. Thornicroft and M. Tansella (eds), *Mental Health Outcome Measures.* Heidelberg, Springer.

Jolley, D.J. (1995) The first year of the Goodmayes Psychiatric service for old people. Commentary. *International Journal of Geriatric Psychiatry,* **10,** 930–932.

Jones, G. & Berry, M. (1986) Regional secure units: the emerging picture. In G. Edwards (ed.), *Current Issues in Clinical Psychology* IV. London, Plenum Press.

Jones, R. (1995) Why do qualitative research? *British Medical Journal,* **311,** 2.

Joseph, P. & Potter, M. (1993) Diversion from custody. I. Psychiatric assessment at the magistrate's court. *British Journal of Psychiatry,* **162,** 325–330.

Juss, S. (1993) *Immigration, Nationality and Citizenship.* London, Mansell.

Juss, S. (1995) The constitution and Sikhs in Britain. *Brigham Young University Law Review*. No 2. J Reuben Clark Law School, Utah, USA.

Kammerling, R.M. & O'Connor, S. (1993) Unemployment rate as a predictor of psychiatric admission. *British Medical Journal*, **307**, 1536–1539.

Karmi, G. (1992a) Refugee Health Requires a Comprehensive Strategy. *British Medical Journal*, **305**(25), 206–207.

Karmi, G. (1992b) *Refugees and the National Health Service*. London, NW and NE Thames Regional Health Authorities.

Kasper, J.A., Steinwachs, D.M. & Skinner, E.A. (1993) Family perspectives on the service needs of people with serious and persistent mental illness, Part II, Needs for assistance and needs that go unmet. *Innovations and Research*, **1**, 21–33.

Katschnig, H. & Konieczna, T. (1990) Innovative approaches to delivery of mental health services in Europe. In I.M. Marks, & R.A. Scott (eds), *Mental Health Care Delivery*. Cambridge, Cambridge University Press.

Katschnig, H. (1995) The scope and limitations of emergency mental health services in the community. In M. Phelan, G. Strathdee and G. Thornicroft (eds), *Emergency Mental Health Services in the Community*. Cambridge, Cambridge University Press.

Kendrick, T., Sibbald, B., Burns, T. & Freeling, P. (1991) Role of general practitioners in care of long-term mentally ill patients. *British Medical Journal*, **302**, 508–510.

Kiev, A. (1965) Psychiatric morbidity amongst West Indian immigrants in urban general practice. *British Journal of Psychiatry*, **111**, 51–56.

King, M., Coker, E., Leavey, G., Hoare, A. & Johnson-Sabine, E. (1994) Incidence of psychotic illness in London, comparison of ethnic groups. *British Medical Journal*, **304**, 1115–1119.

King, M. & Nazareth, I. (1996) Community care of patients with schizophrenia: the role of the primary health care team. *British Journal of General Practice*, **46**, 231–237.

Kingdon, D. & Jenkins, R. (1996) Adult mental health policy. In G. Thornicroft & G. Strathdee (eds), *Commissioning Mental Health Services*. London, HMSO.

King's Fund Commission (1992) *London Health Care 2010*. London, King's Fund.

Kisley, S.R., Gater, R. & Goldberg, D.P. (1995) Results from the Manchester Centre. In B. Unstun & N. Sartorius (eds), *Mental Illness in General Health Care*. Chichester, John Wiley.

Kleinman, A. (1980) *Patients and their healers in the context of culture*. Berkeley, CA: University of California Press.

Kleinman, A. (1988) *Rethinking psychiatry*. New York, Free Press.

Knapp, M.R.J., Chisholm, D. & Astin, J. (1995) *Community health and hospital consequences of residential provision for people with mental health problems: is there a London differential?* Final Report to the King's Fund, London.

Knapp, M.R.J., Chisholm, D., Astin, J., Lelliott, P. & Audini, B. (1997) The cost consequences of changing the hospital–community balance. *Psychological Medicine* (in press).

Krause, I.B. et al. (1991) Sinking heart: a Punjabi communication of distress. *Social Science and Medicine*, **2**, 563–575.

Kumar, A. (1991) *The ethnic minorities mental health development project of Tameside and Glossop association of mind. An evaluation report, Feb 1990 to Dec 1991*. Tameside and Glossop MIND

Kurtz, Z., Thornes, R. & Wolkind, S. (1994) *Services for the Mental Health of Children and Young People in England – A National Review*. Maudsley Hospital and South Thames (West) Regional Health Authority.

Kurtz, Z., Thornes, R. & Wolkind, S. (1996) *Services for the Mental Health of Children and Young People in England, Assessment of Needs and Unmet Need*. Report for the Department of Health (in press).

Lago, C. & Thompson, J. (1996) *Race, culture and counselling*. Buckingham, Open University Press.

La Grenade, J. & Bhugra, D. (1996) Community organisations expectations of mental health statutory services: a pilot study. Manuscript submitted.

Leach, J. (1979) Providing for the destitute. In J. Wing & R. Olsen (eds), *Community Care of the Mentally Disabled*. Oxford, Oxford University Press.

Leff, J. (1993) All the homeless people: where do they all come from? *British Medical Journal*, **306**, 669–670.

Leff, J. (1988) *Psychiatry Around the Globe, A transcultural view*. Gaskell Series. Royal College of Psychiatrists.

Leff, J. (1996) What Lessons Can We Learn from the TAPS Project? An Overview of Past Research and Future Direction. Presentation at the TAPS 11th Annual Conference, London 18th July 1996.

Lelliott, P., Sims, A. & Wing, J. (1993) Who pays for community care? The same old question. *British Medical Journal*, **307**, 991–994.

Lelliott, P. & Wing, J. (1994) National audit of new long-stay psychiatric patients. 2. Impact on services. *British Journal of Psychiatry*, **165**, 160–169.

Lelliott, P., Audini, B. & Darroch, B. (1995) Resolving London's bed crisis, there might be a way, is there the will? *Psychiatric Bulletin*, **19**, 273–275.

Lelliott, P., Audini, B., Knapp, M. & Chisholm, D. (1996) The Mental Health Residential Care Study, Classification of facilities and description of residents. *British Journal of Psychiatry*, **169**, 139–147.

Lewis, S. (1995). A search for meaning: Making sense of Depression, *Journal of Mental Health*, **4**, 369–382.

Lewis, G. & Booth, M. (1992) Regional differences in mental health in Great Britain. *Journal of Epidemiology and Community Health*, **46**, 608–611.

Li et al. (1994) The collection of general practice data for psychiatric service contracts. *Journal of Public Health Medicine*, **16**(1), 87–92.

Light, D. & Bailey, V. (1992) *A Needs Based Purchasing Plan for Child Mental Health Services*. North West Thames Regional Health Authority. Obtainable from Hounslow Department of Child and Adolescent Psychiatry, London TW3 3EL.

Light, D. & Bailey, V. (1993) Pound Foolish. *Health Service Journal*, 11 February, pp 16–17.

Lindesay, J., Briggs, K., Lawes, M., Macdonald, A. & Herzberg, J. (1991) The domus philosophy. A comparative evaluation of a new approach to residential care for the demented elderly. *International Journal of Geriatric Psychiatry*, **6**, 727–736.

Littlewood, R. & Cross, S. (1980) Ethnic minorities and psychiatric services. *Sociology of health and illness*, **2**(2), 194–201.

Littlewood, R. & Lipsedge, M. (1989) *Aliens and Alienists. Ethnic minorities and psychiatry.* London, Unwin Hyman.

Littlewood, R. (1990) From categories to contexts: a decade of the 'New cross cultural psychiatry'. *British Journal of Psychiatry*, **156**, 308–327.

Livingston, G. & Blanchard, M. (1996) Planning community mental health services for older women. In K. Abel, M. Buszewicz, S. Davison, S. Johnson, & E. Staples (eds), *Planning Community Mental Health Services for Women.* London, Routledge.

London Research Centre (1995/6) *Homelessness in London.* Bulletin 8. London, London Research Centre.

Lloyd, P. & Moodley, P. (1992) Psychotropic medication and ethnicity: an inpatient survey. *Social Psychiatry & Psychiatric Epidemiology*, **27**(2), 95–101.

Lloyd, K. & St Louis, L. (1996) Common mental disorders among Africans and Caribbeans. In *Ethnicity: an agenda for mental health.* London, Gaskell (in press).

Lloyd, K. et al. (1996) The development of the short explanatory model interview and its use among primary care attenders. Paper submitted.

McArdle, P., O'Brien, C. & Kolvin, I. (1995) Hyperactivity, prevalence and relationship with conduct disorders. *Journal of Child Psychology and Psychiatry*, **36**, 279–304.

McCarthy, B. & Craisatti, J. (1989) Ethnic differences in response to adversity. *Social Psychiatry & Psychiatric Epidemiology*, **24**, 196–201.

McCreadie, R.G., Leese, M., Tilak-Singh, D., Loftus, L., MacEwan, T. & Thornicroft, G. Nithsdale, Nunhead and Norwood, Similarities and differences in prevalence of schizophrenia and utilization of services in rural and urban areas. Accepted by *British Journal of Psychiatry* (in press).

McCreadie, R.G. (1982) The Nithsdale Schizophrenia Survey. I. Psychiatric and Social Handicaps. *British Journal of Psychiatry*, **140**, 582–586.

MacDonald, A., Goddard, C. & Poynton, A. (1994) Impact of 'open access' to specialist services, the case of community psychogeriatrics. *International Journal of Geriatric Psychiatry*, **9**, 709–714.

McGovern, D. & Cope, R. (1987) First psychiatric admission rates of first and second generation Afro-Caribbeans. *Social Psychiatry*, **22**, 139–149.

MacGregor, S., Ettore, B., Coomber, R., Crosier, A. & Lodge, H. (1990) *The Central Funding Initiative and the development of drug services in England.* University of London, Birkbeck College.

McGuffin, P., Farmer, A. & Harvey, I. (1991) A polydiagnostic application of operational criteria in studies of psychotic illness. Development and reliabiltiy of the OPCRIT system. *Archives of General Psychiatry*, **48**, 764–770.

McKeigue, P. & Karmi, G. (1993) Alcohol consumption and alcohol related problems in Afro-Caribbeans and South Asians in the United Kingdom. *Alcohol and Alcoholism*, **28**, 1–10.

Maden, A. (1996) Forensic Psychiatry. In *Ethnicity: An Agenda For Mental Health.* London, Gaskell (in press).

Maden, A., Taylor, C., Brooke, D. & Gunn, J. (1995a) *Mental Disorder in Remand Prisoners.* A report commissioned by the Directorate of Prison Health Care. Home Office (unpublished). Cited in Special Hospitals Service Authority. Service Strategies for Secure Care, 1995.

Maden, A. et al. (1995b) The ethnic origin of women serving a prison sentence. *British Journal of Criminology*, **32**, 218–221.

Maden, A., Curle, C., Meux, C., Burrow, S. & Gunn, J. (1996) *Treatment and Security Needs of Special Hospital Patients*. Whurr Publishers.

Mann, A.H. (1995) Future directions for the specialty of old age psychiatry, some suggestions for debate. *International Journal of Geriatric Psychiatry*, **10**, 87–92.

Marks, J.N., Goldberg, D.P., Hillier, V.F. (1979) Determinants of the ability of general practitioners to detect psychiatric illness. *Psychological Medicine*, **9**, 337–353.

Marshall, M. (1989) Collected and neglected: are Oxford hostels filling up with disabled psychiatric patients. *British Medical Journal*, **299**, 706–709.

Marshall, J. (1996) Homeless women. In D. Bhugra (ed.), *Homelessness and Mental Health*. Cambridge, Cambridge University Press.

Marshall, J. & Reed, J. (1992) Psychiatric morbidity in homeless women. *British Journal of Psychiatry*, **160**, 761–768.

Maudsley Hospital (1996) *Audit of the Care Programme Approach, half-yearly report*. London, Bethlem Royal and Maudsley NHS Trust.

Medical Foundation for the Care of Victims of torture (1994) *A Betrayal of Hope and Trust. Detention in UK survivors of torture*, 96–98 Grafton Rd, London NW5.

Meltzer, H., Gill, B., Petticrew, M. & Hinds, K. (1995) *The prevalence of psychiatric morbidity among adults living in private households*. OPCS Surveys of Psychiatric Morbidity in Great Britain. London, HMSO.

Menezes, P., Johnson, S., Thornicroft, G., Marshall, J., Prosser, D., Bebbington, P. & Kuipers, E. (1996) Drug and alcohol problems among individuals with severe mental illnesses in South London. *British Journal of Psychiatry*, **168**, 612–619.

Mental Health Foundation (1994) *Creating Community Care*. London, Mental Health Foundation.

Mental Health Foundation (1995a) *Mental Health in Black and Minority Ethnic people. Time for Action. The report of a seminar on Race and Mental Health. 'Towards a strategy'*. London, Mental Health Foundation.

Mental Health Foundation (1995b) *Mental Health in Black and Minority Ethnic people. The fundamental facts. The report of a seminar on Race and Mental Health. 'Towards a strategy'*. London, Mental Health Foundation.

Merson, S., Tyrer, P., Onyett, F. et al. (1992) Early intervention in psychiatric emergencies, A controlled clinical trial. *Lancet*, **339**, 1311–1314.

Midgley, S., Burns, T. & Garland, C (1996) What do general practitioners and community mental health teams talk about? Descriptive analysis of liason meetings in general practice. *British Journal of General Practice*, **46**, 69–71.

Mills, M. (1996) Shanti: an intercultural psychotherapy centre for women. In K. Abel, M. Buszewicz, S. Davison, S. Johnson & E. Staples (eds), *Women's Mental Health Services*. London, Routledge.

Mills, C. & Ota, H. (1989) Homeless women with minor children in the Detroit metropolitan area. *Social Work*, **34**, 485–489.

MILMIS Project Group (1995) Monitoring inner London mental illness services. *Psychiatric Bulletin*, **19**, 276–280.

MIND (1983) *Common Concern*. London, MIND Publications.

Ministry of Health (1962) *A hospital plan for England and Wales*. CMND 1604. London, HMSO.

Mitchell A.R.K. (1985) Psychiatrists in primary care settings. *British Journal of Psychiatry,* **147**, 371–379.

Moodley, P. & Thornicroft, G. (1988) Ethnic group and the compulsory admission of psychiatric patients. *Medicine, Science and the Law*, **28**, 324–328.

Moodley, P. & Perkins, R. (1991) Routes to psychiatric inpatient care in an inner London Borough. *Social Psychiatry & Psychiatric Epidemiology*, **26**, 47–51.

Moore, R. (1996) Lessons from the Mental Health Task Force London Project. In G. Thornicroft & G. Strathdee (eds), *Commissioning Mental Health Services*. London, HMSO.

Morris, I. (1991) Residential care. In D.H. Bennett & H.L. Freeman (eds), *Community Psychiatry*. Edinburgh, Churchill Livingstone.

Morse, G., Caslyn, R. & Burger, G. (1991) A comparison of taxonomic systems for classifying homelessness. *International Journal of Social Psychiatry*, **37**, 90–98.

Muijen, M., Marks, I.M., Connolly, J. & Audini, B. (1992a) Homebased and standard hospital care for patients with severe mental illness: A randomised controlled trial. *British Medical Journal*, **304**, 749–754.

Muijen, M., Marks, I.M., Connolly, J., Audini, B. & McNamee, G. (1992b) The Daily Living Programme, preliminary comparison of community versus hospital-based treatment for the seriously mentally ill facing emergency admission. *British Journal of Psychiatry,* **160**, 379–384.

Murdoch, P.S. & Montgomery, E.A. (1992) Revised guidelines of collaboration between physicians in geriatric medicine and psychiatrists of old age. *Psychiatric Bulletin*, **16**, 583–584.

Murphy, E. & Banerjee, S. (1993) The organisation of old-age psychiatry services. *Reviews in Clinical Gerontology*, **3,** 367–378.

NACRO (1990) *Black people, mental health and the courts: an exploratory study into the psychiatric remand process as it affects black defendants at magistrates' courts.* London, National Association for the Care and Resettlement of Offenders.

NACRO (1989) *Race and criminal justice*. London, National Association for the Care and Resettlement of Offenders.

NAHAT (1996) *Good practice and quality indicators in primary health care*. NHS Ethnic Health Unit in conjunction with Kensington and Westminster Health Authority NHS Ethnic Health Unit.

National Children's Bureau (1995) *Exclusion from School*. Highlight No. 136.

National Audit Office (1994) *Health Service day hospitals for elderly people in England*. Report by the Comptroller and Auditor. London, HMSO.

National Schizophrenia Fellowship (1995) *One in Ten*. A Report by the National Schizophrenia Fellowship into Suicide and Unnatural Deaths Involving People with Schizophrenia.

Netten, A. & Dennett, J. (1996) *Unit Costs of Health and Social Care*. Personal Social Services Research Unit, University of Kent at Canterbury.

Nguyen-Van-Tam, J. et al. (1996a) Health care experiences of Vietnamese families in Nottingham. *Health Trends*, **27**(4), 106–110.

Nguyen-Van-Tam, J. & Madeley, R. (1996b) Vietnamese people in study may have had language difficulties. *British Medical Journal*, **313**, 48.

NHS Executive (1994a) *Guidance on the discharge of mentally disordered people and their continuing care in the community.* (HSG(94)27). London, HMSO.

NHS Executive (1994b) *Introduction of supervision registers for mentally ill people from 1 April 1994.* (HSG(94)5). London, HMSO.

NHS Executive (1996a) Review of the purchasing of mental health services by Health Authorities in England.

NHS Executive (1996b) *Mental Health Services in London.* London Health Briefing Paper 1.

NHS Executive (1996c) *An Audit Pack for the Care Programme Approach.* Leeds, NHS Executive.

NHS Task Force (1994) *Black Mental Health: a dialogue for change.* NHS Management Executive, Mental Health Task Force.

NHS Trust Federation (1996) *Inner City Mental Health: A report by the NHS Trust Federation's Mental Health and Learning Disability Standing Committee.* NHS Trusts Federation.

Nilbert, D., Cooper, S. & Crossmaker, M. (1989) Assaults against residents of a psychiatric institution, Residents history of abuse. *Journal of Interpersonal Violence*, **4**, 342–349.

Norris, V. (1959) *Mental Illness in London.* Maudsley Monographs No. 6. London, Chapman & Hall.

North Thames Regional Health Authority (1995) *North Thames Regionwide Directory.* North Thames Regional Health Authority.

NW Thames Regional Health Authority (1994) *Partners in care. Developing health voluntary sector commissioning.* Office for public management. NW Thames Regional Health Authority.

Office of Population Censuses and Surveys (1993) *Mid-year population estimates. Government statistical service.* London, HMSO.

Office for Public Management (1996) *Responding to diversity: A study of commissioning issues and good practice in purchasing ethnic minority health.* Available from Full Public Management.

Onyett, S.R., Pillinger, T. & Muijen, M. (1995) *Making community mental health teams work.* London, Sainsbury Centre for Mental Health.

Onyett, S., Standen, R. & Peck, E. (in press) The Challenge of Community Mental Health Team Management. *Health and Social Care in the Community.*

O'Brien, J. (1987) A guide to life style planning: Using the activities catalogue to integrate services and natural support systems. In B. Wilcox & G. Bellamy (eds), *The activities catalogue, An alternative curriculum for youth and adults with severe disabilities.* Baltimore, Brooks.

Orrell, M. & Johnson, S. (1992) Three psychiatric day centres in a London Borough. *Psychiatric Bulletin*, **16**, 540–542.

Owen, D. (1996) Size, structure and growth of the ethnic minority populations. In *Ethnicity in the 1991 Census. Vol 1. The demographic characteristics of the ethnic minority populations. OPCS.* London, HMSO.

Parsons, C. et al. (1994) *Excluding Primary School Children.* Family Policy Studies Centre.

Parsons, C. (1995) *Final Report to the Department of Education. National Survey for LEAs Policies and Procedures for the Identification of and Provision for Children who are out of School by Reason of Exclusion or otherwise.* Canterbury and Christchurch College.

Patel, V. et al. (1995) Concepts of mental illness in medical pluralism in Harare. *Psychological Medicine*, **25**, 485–493.

Peach, C. (1996) Introduction. In C. Peach (ed.), *Ethnicity in the 1991 Census. Vol 2: The ethnic minority populations of Great Britain. ONS*. London, HMSO.

Peacock, S. & Smith, P. (1995) *The resource allocation consequences of the new NHS Needs Formula*. York, University of York.

Peck, E. (1994). Community Mental Health Teams: Challenges to the New Orthodoxy. *Journal of Mental Health*, **3**(2), 151–156.

Pelosi, A., McGinnis, E., Elliot, C. & Douglas, A. (1995) Second opinions: a right or a concession? *British Medical Journal*, **311**, 670–672.

Perera et al. (1991) Ethnic aspects: a comparison of three matched groups. *British Journal of Psychiatry*, **159** (Suppl. 13), 40–42.

Pharoah, C. (1992) Primary health care: how well are users served? In *Recent Research in services for black and minority ethnic elderly people*. London, Institute of Gerontology, King's College.

Pilgrim, S. et al. (1993) *The Bristol Black and Ethnic Minorities Health Survey Report*. Department of Sociology and Epidemiology, University of Bristol.

Platt, S., Marti, C. & Hun, S. (1990) The mental health of women with children living in deprived areas of Great Britain: the role of living conditions, poverty and unemployment. In D. Goldberg & D. Tantam (eds), *The Public Health Impact of Mental Disorders*. London, Hogrefe and Huber.

Platt, S., Micciolo, R. & Tansella, M. (1992) Suicide and unemployment in Italy: Description, analysis and interpretation of recent trends. *Social Science and Medicine*, **34**, 1191–1201.

Pleace, N. & Quilgars, D. (1996) *Health and Homelessness in London*. University of York, Centre for Housing Policy.

Pope, C. & Mays, N. Opening the black box: an encounter in the corridors of health services research. *British Medical Journal*, **306**, 315–319.

Powell, The Rt Hon J. Enoch (1961) Official Opening of Conference. In *Emerging Patterns for the Mental Health Services and the Public. Proceedings of a conference held at Church House, Westminster, 9–10 March 1961*. London.

Powell, R.B., Hollander, D. & Tobiansky, R.I. (1995) Crisis in Admission Beds, A Four Year Survey of the Bed State of Greater London's Acute Psychiatric Units. *British Journal of Psychiatry*, **167**, 765–769.

Priest, R.G. (1991) A new initiative on depression. *British Journal of General Practice*, **41**, 487.

Prins, H. (1993) *'Big, black and dangerous'*. Report of the Committee of Inquiry into the death in Broadmoor Hospital of Orville Blackwood and a review of the deaths of two other Afro-Caribbean patients.

Pritchard, C. (1992) Is there a link between suicide in young men and unemployment? A comparison of the UK with other European Community countries. *British Journal of Psychiatry*, **160**, 750–756.

Prosser, D., Johnson, S., Kuipers, E., Szmukler, G., Bebbington, P. & Thornicroft, G. (1996) Mental health, 'burnout' and job satisfaction amongst hospital and community based mental health staff. *British Journal of Psychiatry*, **169**, 334–337.

Raleigh, V. et al. (1990) Suicides amongst immigrants from the Indian sub-continent. *British Journal of Psychiatry*, **156**, 46–50.

Ramsay, R., Gorst-Unsworth, C. & Turner, S. (1993) Psychiatric morbidity in survivors of organised state violence including torture: a retrospective series. *British Journal of Psychiatry*, **162**, 55–59.

Randall, G. (1992) *Counted out: an investigation into the extent of single homelessness*. London, CRISIS.

Raftery, J. (1992) Mental health services in transition. *British Journal of Psychiatry*, **161**, 589–593.

Rea Price, J. & Pugh, G. (1995) *Championing Children*. Manchester City Council.

Refugee Arrivals Project (1994) *Refugee Arrivals Project Annual Report*. Room 2005, 2nd floor, Queen's Building, Heathrow Airport, Hounslow, Middlesex.

Revolving Doors Agency (1994) *The management of people with mental health problems by the Paddington Police*. London, Revolving Doors.

Revolving Doors Agency (1995a) *The use of section 136 of the Mental Health Act in three inner London police divisions*. Report to the Home Office. London

Revolving Doors Agency (1995b) *People with mental health problems in contact with the criminal justice system*. Report on a service mapping project in Camden and Islington. Part One.

Richman, N. (1993) Children in situations of political violence. *Journal of Child Psychololgy and Psychiatry*, **34**(8), 1286–1302.

Richman, N. (1985) Disorders in pre-school children. In M. Rutter & L. Hersov (eds), *Child and Adolescent Psychiatry, Modern Approaches*. Oxford, Blackwell Scientific Publications.

Ritchie, J. & Spenser, E. (1994) Qualitative data analysis for applied policy research. In A. Bryman & R.G. Burgess (eds), *Analysing Qualitative Data*. London, Routledge.

Ritchie, J.H., Dick, D. & Lingham, R. (1994) *The Report of the Inquiry into the Care and Treatment of Christopher Clunis*. London, HMSO.

Robertson, G. et al. (1994) A follow-up of remanded mentally ill offenders given hospital orders. *Medicine, Science and the Law*, **34**, 61–66.

Robertson, G., Pearson, R. & Gibb, R. (1995) The mentally disordered offender and the police. Home Office Research and Statistics Department. Research Findings No. 21.

Robertson, G. et al. (1996) The entry of mentally disordered people to the criminal justice system. *British Journal of Psychiatry*, **169**, 172–180.

Robins, D. (1992) Nafsiyat: a psychotherapy centre for ethnic minorities. In *Community Care: Department of Health funded research*. London, HMSO.

Rogers, A., Pilgrim, D. & Lacey, R. (1993) *Experiencing Psychiatry*. London, Macmillan.

Rose, S., Peabody, C. & Stratigeas, B. (1991) Undetected abuse among intensive case management clients. *Hospital and Community Psychiatry*, **42**, 499–503.

Royal College of Physicians (1994) *Homelessness and ill health*. London, Royal College of Physicians.

Royal College of Physicians and Royal College of Psychiatrists (1995) *The Psychological Care of Medical Patients: Recognition of Need and Service Provision*. London, Royal College of Physicians and the Royal College of Psychiatrists.

Royal College of Psychiatrists (1978) The role, responsibilities and work of the child and adolescent psychiatrist. *Bulletin of the Royal College of Psychiatrists*, July, p. 1.

Royal College of Psychiatrists (1986) Working Party Report. The role, responsibilities and work of the child and adolescent psychiatrist. *Bulletin of the Royal College of Psychiatrists*, **10**, 202–206.

Royal College of Psychiatrists (1987) Guidelines for regional advisors on consultant posts in the psychiatry of old age. *Bulletin of the Royal College of Psychiatry*, **11**, 240–242.

Royal College of Psychiatrists (1992) *Mental Health of the Nation: the Contribution of Psychiatry.* Council Report CR16. The Royal College of Psychiatrists.

Royal College of Psychiatrists (1996) *Report of the working party to review psychiatric practice and training in a multi-ethnic society* (in press).

Rutter, M. & Smith, B. (1995) *Psychosocial Disorders in Young People: time trends and their causes.* Chichester, John Wiley.

Rutter, M.T., Tizard, J. & Whitmore, K. (1970) *Education, Health and Behaviour.* London, Longman.

Rutter, M.T., Cox, A., Tupling, C., Berger, M. & Yule, W. (1975) Attainment and adjustment in two geographical areas, 1. The prevalence of psychiatric disorder. *British Journal of Psychiary*, **126**, 493–509.

Sashidharan, S. (1994) *The need for community based alternatives to institutional psychiatry.* SHARE newsletter. Issue 7: 3.

Scheuer, M., Black, M., Victor, C. et al. (1991) *Homelessness and the utilisation of acute hospital services in London.* London, King's Fund.

Schneider, J. (1996) Costing specialist work schemes. In A. Netten and J. Dennett (eds), *Unit Costs of Health and Social Care.* Personal Social Services Research Unit, University of Kent at Canterbury.

Scott J. (1993) Homelessness and mental illness. *British Journal of Psychiatry*, **162**, 314–324.

Scrimshaw, S.C. & Gleason, G.R. (1992) *RAP: rapid assessment procedures. Qualitative methodologies for planning and evaluation of health related programmes.* Boston, INFDC.

Secretaries of State for Health, Wales and Scotland (1989) *Caring for People.* London, HMSO.

SELHA (1993) Tackling Drugs Together: Towards a Strategy for Drug and Alcohol Misuse Services.

Shah, A. (1992) The burden of psychiatric disorder in primary care. *International Review of Pyschiatry*, **4**, 243–250.

Shapiro, S., Skinner, E. & Kramer, M. et al. (1985) Measuring need for mental health services in a general population. *Medical Care*, **23**, 1033–1043.

Sheehan, J. et al. (1995) Social deprivation, ethnicity and violent incidents on acute psychiatric wards. *Psychiatric Bulletin*, **19**(10), 597.

Shepherd, G. (1991) Day treatment and care. In H.L. Freeman & D.H. Bennett (eds), *Community Psychiatry: The Principles.* Edinburgh, Churchill Livingstone.

Shepherd, G., Muijen, N., Dean, R. & Cooney, M. (1995) *Inside Residential Care: The realities of hospital versus community settings.* London, The Sainsbury Centre for Mental Health.

Shepherd, G., Beadsmore, A., Moore, C., Hardy, P. & Muijen, M. (in press) The shortage of acute psychiatric beds – what are the options? *British Medical Journal.*

Shepherd, M., Cooper, B., Brown, A.C., Kalton, G. (1966) *Psychiatric illness in general practice.* Oxford, Oxford University Press.

Sheppard, D. (1996) *Learning the Lessons. Mental Health Inquiry Reports Published in England and Wales Between 1969–1994 and their Recommendations for Improving Practice.* Second edition. London, The Zito Trust.

Sheridan, M., Henrion, R., Robinson, L. & Baxter, V. (1990) Precipitants of violence in a psychiatric in-patient setting. *Hospital and Community Psychiatry*, **41**, 776–780.

Smaje, C. (1995) *Health, Race and Ethnicity. Making sense of the evidence.* London, King's Fund.

Smaje, C. (1996) The ethnic patterning of health. Directions of theory and research. *Sociology of Health and Illness*, **18**, 139–166.

Smith, H. (1996) A framework for the development of crisis services: Identifying the functions of emergency psychiatric care. *CMHSD Mental Health Review*, Issue 1, March 1996.

Smith, P., Sheldon, T.A. & Martin, S. (1996) An index of need for psychiatric services based on in-patient utilisation. *British Journal of Psychiatry*, **169**, 308–316.

Social Services Inspectorate and Ofsted (1995) *Education of Children who are Looked after by Local Authorities.* DOH Health Publication Unit or Ofsted, Kingsway.

Soni-Raleigh, V. & Balarajan, R. (1992) Suicide and self-burning among Indians and West Indians in England and Wales. *British Journal of Psychiatry*, **161**, 365–368.

South Thames Regional Health Authority (1995) *South Thames Region: A Pocket Guide.* South Thames Regional Health Authority.

South Thames Regional Health Authority (1996) *A strategy for the provision of NHS care for mentally disordered offenders.* London, South Thames Regional Office.

Special Hospitals Service Authority (1995) *Service Strategies for Secure Care.*

Standing Conference on Public Health (1994) *Housing, homelessness and public health.* London, Nuffield Provincial Hospitals Trust.

Stefan, M. & Catalan, J. (1995) Psychiatric patients and HIV infection, a new population at risk? *British Journal of Psychiatry*, **167**, 721–727.

Stein, L.I. & Test, M.A. (1980) An alternative to mental hospital treatment. I. Conceptual model, treatment program, and clinical evaluation. *Archives of General Psychiatry*, **37**, 392–397.

Strathdee, G. (1993) *The Nunhead service: A community mental health service with a focus in primary care.* PRiSM Occasional Paper 13, Institute of Psychiatry, London.

Strathdee, S. & Thornicroft, G. (1992) Community Sectors for Needs-Led Mental Health Services. In G. Thornicroft, C. Brewin & J.K. Wing (eds), *Measuring Mental Health Needs.* London, Royal College of Psychiatrists, Gaskell.

Styles, W. McN. (1991) Training experience of doctors certified for general practice in 1985–1990. *British Journal of General Practice,* **41**, 488–491.

Summerfield, D. (1995) Addressing Human Response to war and atrocity. Major challenges in research and practices and the limitations of western psychiatric models. In R.J. Kleber, C.R. Figley & B.P. Gersons (eds), *Beyond Trauma: cultural and societal dynamics.* New York, Plenum Press.

Stuart, O. (1996) Yes we mean black disabled people too. In W. Ahmad & K. Atkin (eds), *Race and Community Care.* Buckingham, Open University Press.

Tang, M. & Cuninhame, C. (1994) *Focus groups, access to primary health care and the Deptford Vietnamese projec*t. Save the Children Fund, UK and European Programmes Department, London Division.

Task Force to Review Services for Drug Misusers (1996) *Report of an Independent Review of Drug Treatment Services in England*. London, Department of Health.

Taylor, P.J. (1985) Motives for offending among violent and psychotic men. *British Journal of Psychiatry*, **147**, 491–498.

Taylor, P.J. (1986) Psychiatric disorder in London's life sentenced offenders. *British Journal of Criminology*, **26**(1), 63–78.

Taylor, P.J. (1996) Mentally Disordered Offenders. In E. Paykel & R. Jenkins (eds), *Prevention in Psychiatry*. London, Gaskell.

Thomas, A. & Niner, P. (1989) *Living in temporary accommodation*. London, HMSO.

Thomas. C.S., Stone, K., Osborn, M., Thomas, P.F. & Fisher, M. (1993) Psychiatric morbidity and compulsory admission among UK born Europeans, Afro-Caribbeans and Asians in central Manchester. *British Journal of Psychiatry*, **163**, 91–99.

Thompson, D. (1990) Psychiatric morbidity in the homeless. In B. Pitt, & R. Priest (eds), *Mental Health and Homelessness*. London, Royal College of Psychiatrists.

Thornicroft, G. (1991) Social deprivation and rates of treated mental disorder, developing statistical models to predict psychiatric service utilisation. *British Journal of Psychiatry*, **158**, 475–484.

Thornicroft, G, Margolius, O. & Jones, D. (1992) The TAPS Project 6, New long-stay psychiatric patients and social deprivation. *British Journal of Psychiatry*, **161**, 621–624.

Timms, P. & Fry, A. (1989) Homelessness and mental illness. *Health Trends*, **21**, 70–71.

Timms, P. (1996) Homelessness and mental illness: a brief history. In D. Bhugra (ed.), *Homelessness and Mental Health*. Cambridge, Cambridge University Press.

Tooth, G.C. & Brooke, E.M. (1961) Trends in mental hospital population and their effect on future planning. *Lancet*, **i**, 710–713.

Torrey, W., Becker, D. & Drake, R. (1995) Rehabilitative day treatment versus supported employment, consumer, family and staff reactions to a program change. *Psychosocial Rehabilitation Journal*, **18**, No 3.

Travers, T. & Minors, M. (1995) (eds) *London 95*. London, London Research Centre.

Tumim, S. (1990) *Report of a review by Her Majesty's Chief Inspector of Prisons*. London, HMSO.

Turton, P. & Tylee, A. (1995). Evaluation in setting up a large-scale educational programme – principles and problems. *Education for General Practice*, **6**, 226–229.

Trostle, J. (1988) Medical compliance as an ideology. *Social Science and Medicine*, **27**(12), 1299–1308.

TUC (1995a) *Black and Betrayed: a report on black workers experience of unemployment and low pay in 1994–95*. Trades Union Congress.

TUC (1995b) *Race and Social security: a report on access and discrimination in the benefits system*. Trades Union Congress. October.

Turner et al. (1992) Mentally disordered persons found in public places. Diagnostic and social aspects of police referrals (section 136). *Psychological Medicine*, **22**, 765–774.

Turner-Crowson, J. (1992) Long term strategies for system change. The US community support problem (CSP), *Journal of Mental Health*, **1**, 90–92.

Turner-Crowson, J. (1993) *Reshaping mental health services, Implications for Britain of the US experience. Research report no. 16*. London, King's Fund.

Turton, P. & Tylee, A. (1995) Evaluation in setting up a large-scale educational programme – principles and problems. *Education for General Practice*, **6**, 226–229.

Tyrer et al. (1994) The effect of personality on clinical outcome, social networks and adjustment: a controlled trial of psychiatric emergencies. *Psychological Medicine*, **24**, 731–740.

Tyrer, P., Morgan, J., van Horn, E., Jaryakody, M., Evans, K., Brummell, R., White, T., Baldwin, D., Harrison-Read, P. & Johnson, T. (1995) A randomised controlled study of close monitoring of vulnerable psychiatric patients. *The Lancet*, **345**, 756–759.

Ustun, B., Goldberg, D., Cooper, J., Simon, G.E. & Sartorius, N. (1995) New classification for mental disorders with management guidelines for use in primary care: ICD10–PHC Chapter five. *British Journal of General Practice*, **45**, 211–215.

Vanstraelen, M. & Cottrell, D. (1994) Child and adolescent mental health services: purchasers' knowledge and plans. *British Medical Journal*, **309**, 259–261.

van Os, J. et al. (1996) The incidence of mania: time trends in relation to gender and ethnicity. *Social Psychiatry and Psychiatric Epidemiology*, **31**, 129–136.

Vincent, C. & Lewith, G. (1995) Placebo controls for acupuncture studies. *Journal of the Royal Society*, **88**, 199–202.

Victor, C., Connelly, J., Roderick, P. & Cohen, C. (1989) Use of hospital services by homeless families in an inner London health district. *British Medical Journal*, **229**, 725–727.

Victor, C. (1992) Health status of temporarily housed populations and residents of North West Thames region. *British Medical Journal*, **305**, 387–391.

von Abendorff R., Challis, D. & Netten, A. (1994) Staff activity patterns in a community mental health team for older people. *International Journal of Geriatric Psychiatry*, **9**, 897–906.

Wallace, S., Crown, J., Cox, A. & Berger, M. (1996) Health Care Needs Assessment. *Child and Adolescent Mental Health* (in press).

Wang, Y. & Xiang, K. (1995) Chinese and Vietnamese people. In C. Harding (ed.), *Not just black and white: an information pack about mental health services for people from Black communities*. London, Good Practices in Mental Health.

Warner, R., Gater, R., Jackson, M.G. & Goldberg, D.P. (1993) Effects of a community mental health service on the practice and attitudes of general practitioners. *British Journal of General Practice*, **43**, 507–511.

Warr, P., Jackson, P. & Banks, M.H. (1988) Unemployment and mental health, some British studies. *Journal of Social Issues*, **44**, 47–68.

Watters, C. (1996) Representation and realities: black people, community care and mental illness. In W. Ahmad & K. Atkin (eds), *Race and Community Care*. Buckingham, Open University Press.

Wattis, J.P. (1994) The pattern of psychogeriatric services. In J.R.M. Copeland, M.T. Abou-Saleh & D.G. Blazer (eds), *The Principles and Practice of Geriatric Psychiatry*. Chichester, John Wiley.

Webb-Johnson, A. (1991) *A cry for change. An Asian perspective on developing quality mental health care*. London, Confederation of Indian Organisations.

Webb-Johnson, A. (1993) *Building on strengths. Enquiry into health activity in the Asian Voluntary sector*. London, Confederation of Indian Organisations.

Weller, M., Tobiansky, R., Hollander, D. & Ibrahimi, S. (1989) Psychiatry and destitution at Christmas. 1985–1988. *Lancet*, **ii**, 1509–1511.

Wessley, S. (1991) Schizophrenia and Afro-Caribbeans: a case control study. *British Journal of Psychiatry*, **159**, 795–801.

Westermeyer, J. (1991) Working with an interpreter in psychiatric assessments. *Journal of Nervous & Mental Disease*, **178**, 745.

Wilson, M. (1993) *Britain's Black Communities. NHS Management Executive*. London, Mental Health Task Force & King's Fund Centre.

Wilson, M. & MacCarthy, B. (1994) GP consultation as a factor in the low rate of mental health service use by Asians. *Psychological Medicine*, **24**, 113–119.

Wilson, M. (1995) *Alternatives in Black mental health. The Sanctuary model*. London, King's Fund Centre.

Wing, J.K. (1992) *Epidemiologically-based needs assessment; Review of research on psychiatric disorders*. London, Department of Health.

Wing, J.K. (1994) Health Care Needs Assessment. In A. Stevens, & J. Raftery (eds), *Health Care Needs Assessment*. Oxford, Radcliffe Medical Press.

Wing, J.K., Curtis, R.H. & Beevor, A.S. (1996) *HoNOS: Health of the Nation Outcome Scales. Report on Research and Development, July 1993–December 1995*. London, Royal College of Psychiatrists' Research Unit.

Wolkind, S.N. & Rutter, M. (1985) Socio-cultural factors. In M. Rutter & L. Hersov (eds), *Child and Adolescent Psychiatry: Modern Approaches*. Oxford, Blackwell Scientific Publications.

Woodley Team Report (1995) *Report of the Independent Review Panel to East London and the City Health Authority and Newham Council*.

Wright, J.D. (1987) The National Health Care for the Homeless Program. In R. Bingham, R. Green & S.B. White (eds), *The homeless in contemporary society*. Newbury Park, CA, Sage.

Wright, J.D. (1989) *Address Unknown: Homeless in America*. New York, Aldine de Gruyter.

Yee, L. (1996) *Improving support for black carers. A source book of information, ideas and service initiatives*. London, King's Fund.